# Place and Practice in Canadian Nursing History

*Edited by Jayne Elliott, Meryn Stuart,
and Cynthia Toman*

# Place and Practice in Canadian Nursing History

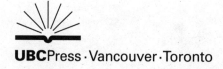

**UBC**Press · Vancouver · Toronto

17 16 15 14 13 12 11 10 09 08     5 4 3 2 1

Printed in Canada on ancient-forest-free paper (100% post-consumer recycled)
that is processed chlorine- and acid-free, with vegetable-based inks.

---

**Library and Archives Canada Cataloguing in Publication**

   Place and practice in Canadian nursing history / edited by Jayne Elliott, Meryn
Stuart, and Cynthia Toman.

Includes bibliographical references and index.
ISBN 978-0-7748-1557-4 (bound)
ISBN 978-0-7748-1558-1 (pbk.)
ISBN 978-0-7748-1559-8 (e-book)

   1. Nursing – Canada – History. 2. Nurses – Canada – History. I. Elliott, Jayne,
1949- II. Stuart, Meryn Elisabeth III. Toman, Cynthia, 1948-

RT6.A1P59 2008               610.73'0971               C2008-903380-9

---

Canadä

UBC Press gratefully acknowledges the financial support for our publishing
program of the Government of Canada through the Book Publishing Industry
Development Program (BPIDP), and of the Canada Council for the Arts, and
the British Columbia Arts Council.

This book has been published with the help of a grant from the Canadian Federation
for the Humanities and Social Sciences, through the Aid to Scholarly Publications
Programme, using funds provided by the Social Sciences and Humanities Research
Council of Canada.

Printed and bound in Canada by Friesens
Set in Stone by Artegraphica Design Co. Ltd.
Copy editor: Stacy Belden
Proofreader: Stephanie VanderMeulen
Indexer: Noeline Bridge

UBC Press
The University of British Columbia
2029 West Mall
Vancouver, BC V6T 1Z2
604-822-5959 / Fax: 604-822-6083
www.ubcpress.ca

# Contents

# Illustrations

**Figure**

**Table**

# Acknowledgments

This book builds on the connections and enthusiastic debates generated by the first Hannah Conference on Canadian Nursing History, which was held in Ottawa in June 2005. Thank you to Associated Medical Services Inc. (AMS) for its generous financial support of the conference. We also acknowledge the support of the School of Nursing at the University of Ottawa which was, at that time, under the direction of Sylvie Lauzon, as well as that of the Faculty of Health Sciences. Conference organizer Linda Soulière's work in making the Hannah Conference such a memorable occasion through her expertise and attention to detail is also appreciated.

AMS was established in 1936 by Dr. Jason Hannah as a pioneer prepaid not-for-profit health care organization in Ontario. With the advent of medicare, AMS became a charitable organization supporting innovations in academic medicine and health services, specifically the history of medicine and health care, as well as innovations in health professional education and bioethics. In conjunction with the 2005 conference, and in partnership with the University of Ottawa, AMS sponsored the establishment of the Nursing History Research Unit (AMS NHRU) at the School of Nursing at the University of Ottawa. The Unit has a mandate to foster the production and dissemination of new knowledge in Canadian nursing history through education, research, and public outreach. This collection is the first publication produced under its auspices. We are grateful for the generous counsel and encouragement of former AMS CEO Dr. Bill Seidelman, and of Dr. Mary Ellen Jeans, current CEO and president. With this level of support, AMS has taken the lead in funding this field of inquiry in Canada.

Nursing history is a small albeit growing area of study in Canada, and many scholars, especially those employed in schools of nursing, conduct their research and writing in relative isolation. We are therefore particularly indebted to the contributors for the effort they put into preparing their chapters. This book could not have taken shape without their dedication and hard work, and we hope that the exchange of ideas, from which both editors and authors have benefited, will make the field of nursing history stronger in the end.

Each of us has relied on the help and advice of archivists and museum staff across the country, and we would particularly like to express our gratitude to those who aided our search for photographs for the book. We also appreciate the constructive comments from the anonymous peer reviewers, suggestions that we have tried to keep in mind as we revised our chapters. Käthe Roth ably translated Johanne Daigle's paper.

Copy editor Stacy Belden helped sharpen and clarify our writing and smoothed out the rough edges. Jean Wilson and Ann Macklem, our expert editors at UBC Press, have been congenial and thoughtful guides in the process of shepherding the manuscript through the final stages of production.

# Introduction

*Jayne Elliott, Cynthia Toman, and Meryn Stuart*

In June 2005, historians working in the field of Canadian nursing history gathered together in Ottawa for the purpose of exploring the dual themes of identities and diversities. The Hannah Conference on Canadian Nursing History was one of two meetings that bracketed the opening of both the first national exhibit on the history of nursing mounted at the Canadian Museum of Civilization, and the Associated Medical Services Nursing History Research Unit at the University of Ottawa.[1] Encompassing roughly a one-hundred-year period from the late 1800s to the 1970s, the work of the invited presenters looked at Canadian nurses, broadly defined, who were engaged in healing work in medical institutions, the military, and out in the community over a wide geographical area both within Canada and abroad. Despite the wide range of material covered, enthusiastic discussions began to highlight common threads and fruitful directions for further research. At the same time, historians and nurse educators attending the conference, along with history and nursing students, engaged in a productive public debate over the role and meaning of nursing history within nursing programs.

One of the issues for nursing history that continues to have relevance for current health care debates concerns the category of "nurse": who is a nurse, what constitutes nursing work, and to what degree (if any) is "nurse" a universal category of identity.[2] Various professionalization movements throughout North America exacerbated these debates during the early twentieth century. Nurse leaders, following a successful campaign by physicians to gain control over their practice, sought to establish dominance over nursing practice through the standardization of educational curricula and legal authority to credential graduates of recognized hospital-based training programs. In the process, the public came to perceive nurses and hospitals as being inextricably linked through training programs and, following the Second World War, increasingly through employment opportunities. Hospital-based training and work environments aimed to standardize nurses, nursing knowledge, and nursing care, creating the illusion of a universal nurse category while devaluing the vast diversity of persons who did nursing work as well as the many formal and informal settings in which nursing took place.

Historians of nursing now call for a closer examination of nurses and nursing as well as of the meaning of nursing for those who have practised it, suggesting a need to nuance our analyses and qualify *which nurses* and *which settings* as well as in *which time frames*. American nurse historian Patricia D'Antonio, for example, noted that nursing "took on different meanings for different nurses at different times"[3] and that historians need to consider alternative perspectives, practitioners, meanings, and stories to produce "a more inclusive history of health care that privileges new meanings about nursing's work and worth."[4] Scholars working in nursing history, like those in other fields, now use increasingly complex analytical concepts and perspectives within their research. We are only now just beginning to understand how issues of gender, race, ethnicity, class, and religion have served to structure the occupation in ways that include some while excluding many others.[5] Celia Davies has suggested it is time to "explore the way that inequalities of race, class, and gender work out, sometimes unintentionally, as health care personnel and health care systems travel across an international stage" – through analytical frameworks of imperialism, colonialism, post-colonialism, and globalization as well as nurses' relations to the state.[6] Sioban Nelson critically appraised the field for a need to connect nursing history with broader historical scholarship, shifts in historiographical thinking, and efforts to situate nursing history in relation to mainstream histories.[7]

This collection seeks to disrupt and decentre assumptions about the relationship of nurses to hospitals and to the medical profession, which are found both in public perceptions and in much of the writing in nursing history. Focusing on alternate settings and places, it highlights a variety of persons who provide nursing care while performing different roles that come under the rubric of nursing work. We seek to complement the valuable text *On All Frontiers: Four Centuries of Canadian Nursing*, the first general survey on Canadian nursing history in more than half a century, which was published to coincide with the opening of the Canadian Museum of Civilization's exhibit.[8] Our authors have expanded and deepened many of the themes raised in this text, adding to the wide-ranging research on nursing and its practitioners that had been previously highlighted in the two special editions of the *Canadian Bulletin of Medical History*, produced in 1994 and 2004, respectively.[9] We anticipate that the broad scope of research presented in this text will suggest new pathways of investigation that will mirror the varied nature of current nursing practice and the diversity of its practitioners. We intend that the articles will help fill a gap for those who have lamented the dearth of historical sources[10] relating to their questions on nursing history. Our ultimate hope is to encourage a deeper understanding of the historical roots of issues that continue to challenge nurses and others in the health care system in the present.

## "Place" in Nursing History

The idea of "place" provides an important heuristic device in organizing and situating the articles in this collection.[11] None of our contributors locates her investigations entirely in the hospital-based workplace, which, at least since the mid-twentieth century, has provided the highest number of paid positions for nurses. Only one of the chapters is partially situated within the context of hospitals and hospital training schools. In this chapter, Anne-Marie Arseneault studies the transition to secular university nursing education in a New Brunswick francophone community. The rest of the authors centre their exploration of nurses and their work primarily outside the walls of urban medical institutions. A shift in location or place of nursing work has frequently served to reshape nurses' roles as well as their personal and social lives. As nurses moved further away from traditional settings such as hospitals, many leveraged more flexibility to challenge conventional expectations and meanings associated with nursing work.

Both Cynthia Toman and Meryn Stuart focus on Canadian military nurses from the First World War who worked in military hospital settings. These facilities bore some resemblance to the traditional civilian hospitals of the time and thereby reinforced gendered expectations for nurses and women who served in this male domain of war, but their distance from Canada and the conditions under which the nurses worked also served to disrupt expectations. Yearning for adventure and a place in history, fired with patriotism, and determined to take care of enlisted boyfriends and brothers, these military nurses coveted the limited number of overseas postings. While travel and sightseeing in off-duty hours did indeed make military service a grand adventure for many, nursing brutally mangled soldiers under canvas, in extreme conditions of weather, dirt, insect infestations, or even under fire, severely tested nurses' mettle. Toman centres her discussion on nurses who were sent to several areas in the Mediterranean, where they nursed mostly Allied, but not Canadian, soldiers in a "foreign" part of the world. Using diaries, letters, published materials, and archival documents, she argues that Canadian nurses experienced multiple shifting identities of gender, race, and class. As uniformed representatives of the British Empire, they simultaneously identified themselves as "imperials" with all of the privileges of officer status and whiteness and as "colonials" who were relegated to second-class status in relation to British-trained nurses. As members of the military, they aspired simultaneously to "soldier on" without complaint, as men were expected to do, while preserving their femininity and reputation as good women.

Stuart takes advantage of the prolific letter writing of First World War nursing sister Helen Fowlds to focus on the social life of military nurses. Fowlds' letters (and even her diaries) concentrated much more on social activities and relationships with fellow officers, both male and female, than they did on the often distressing conditions of wartime nursing with which she and her colleagues were confronted. While these letters served on one level to reassure Fowlds' family back home that she was safe, Stuart argues that news and gossip about shopping, clothes, and parties also constructed her as feminine and heterosexual. Stuart points to the tensions within the male-dominated military that encouraged these identities as the "normal" behaviour of women nurses but that also worked to constrain and contain the nurses' sexuality.

Place was also an active agent in constructing nurses' identities and nursing work, particularly as most nurses trained in large urban hospitals and inculcated white, upwardly aspiring, middle-class perspectives from their training into their practice as graduate nurses.[12] Shifting time and place to late-nineteenth and early-twentieth-century western Canada, for example, Kristin Burnett raises questions about just whom we identify as a nurse. In her exploration of the relationships that developed between Aboriginal and white settler women, Burnett examines the small areas of contact that opened up between these two groups of women during the beginning stages of settlement, at the same time that official policy was working toward the assimilation, or even the suppression, of Native life. She sheds light on the desperate need for the healing and midwifery practices of indigenous women within the white settlement communities. Aboriginal women, she notes, often possessed a thorough knowledge of local plants and herbs, an expertise on which many white families relied especially for help in childbirth and in fighting the potentially fatal illnesses contracted by their children. Yet, acknowledgment of these skills is largely missing from the official documents of the period as well as from the traditional accounts of anthropologists and others. In their speeches and writings aimed at a public audience, missionaries also tended to ignore or deny the aid that they had received, obscuring the significant role played by indigenous women that ensured the very survival of white settler families. On a broader scale, failing to consider the healing work carried out by all of those outside the boundaries of formal nurse training not only leaves a gap in Canadian nursing history but also negates their contribution to the building of the Canadian nation.

Myra Rutherdale studies nurses who worked with First Nations and Inuit peoples in the Canadian North, reminding us of the importance of paying attention to the diverse identities that nurses may assume or project, often unconsciously, even when practising in similar sets of circumstances. She identifies three prototypes of nurses who chose this environment, categorizing them as cleansers, cautious caregivers, or optimistic adventurers. Cleansers, she suggests, were the most interventionist in the lives of community residents. Often wives of missionaries, they zealously drew connections between cleanliness and godliness and equated both with good citizenship. Cautious caregivers approached their work in their communities with prudence, willing to observe and learn, and they often doubted the wisdom of applying southern solutions to medical problems in the North and the role of white nurses in implementing those practices. Optimistic adventurers went north primarily for adventure. Independent by nature, they embraced what they saw as the challenges of environment and geography and were impatient with those who complained about the perceived lack of southern amenities. Although they were sometimes critical of their patients, they more readily accepted the community practices that were already in place.

Marion McKay examines the development of visiting nurse associations in the urban centre of Winnipeg in the early twentieth century. While gender and class are important factors in this article, McKay adds to this mix the significance of both region/place and religion in shaping the response of those concerned with the need for social reform. In many areas of the country, middle-class women were the first to organize these services, which were later taken over by a male-dominated government bureaucracy. Winnipeg was no exception. Newly created by the city's commercial and political classes as the "gateway" to the West, Winnipeg was also the headquarters of evangelical Protestantism. At the same time, it was coping with the highest immigration rate of any Canadian city during this period, and both women and men of the white Anglo-Canadian elite viewed the growing numbers of Eastern European residents "with a mixture of loathing and compassion."[13] The Margaret Scott Nursing Mission, which began at the turn of the last century under the direction of lay city missionary Margaret Scott, and the Victorian Order of Nurses, which did not take root in the city until 1907, were visible manifestations of the desire to address this perceived problem by sending nurses out into immigrant communities.

Linda Quiney and Johanne Daigle (with Nicole Rousseau) contribute to the growing body of historical research on outpost and outport nursing in rural and remote Canadian communities.[14] Quiney focuses on nurses employed during the early years of the outpost program operated by the Manitoba Division of the Canadian Red Cross Society. As part of the national organization's peacetime program, which was launched immediately following the First World War, the division established a small number of nursing stations for returning war veterans and immigrants being settled on often marginal land in remote areas of the province. The presence of "suitable" (white, middle-class, and female) nurses was intended not only to address the basic health care needs of this population but also, in a similar way to McKay's study, to connect with the nation-building agenda of "Canadianizing" immigrants. Daigle and Rousseau study nurses working with the Medical Service to Settlers in Québec, which was one of the few outpost nursing programs in Canada initiated and directed by government officials. Searching for a solution to alleviate the effects of the Depression and partnering with militant nationalist clergy who wanted to protect and regenerate the French Canadian "race," the state looked to the North as the ideal physical and ideological space for preservation and renewal. Colonization projects settled large numbers of poor French Canadian families in northern and isolated sections of the province. Unable to attract physicians to work in these settlements, the government hired nurses to attend to the medical needs of the settlers and, in particular, to provide maternity care for women. Even after the colonization project ended, the government continued to supply nurses to remote communities into the 1960s. The authors interviewed a large number of former nurses involved with the project, using analytical concepts of "contact zones" and isolation to understand the nurses' different perceptions of the people and their work in these communities.

Isolation, non-traditional settings, and shifting identities were a part of the immigrant nurse's experience as well. Jayne Elliott bases her study on a decade of letters that Louise de Kiriline, who arrived in Canada in 1927, wrote regularly to her mother back home in Sweden. Although de Kiriline worked for most of this time as an outpost nurse with the Ontario Division of the Canadian Red Cross Society and was then employed as the first charge nurse of the Dionne quintuplets, she clearly considered nursing as only one aspect of her identity. De Kiriline claimed other social identities: she was a recent immigrant, a self-supporting single woman, and, perhaps most importantly, an attentive daughter to her distant mother. Elliott investigates the ways in which de Kiriline constructed her multiple simultaneous identities, arguing that the particular shape taken by her perspectives on race, gender, and class functioned as "markers of familiarity" to her mother. As editors of other immigrant collections of letters have suggested, de Kiriline's wish to remain the daughter her mother knew helped to maintain the close relationship between the two as she adapted to a new life on her own in a northern Canadian environment.[15]

Francophone nurse education outside of Québec, as examined by Anne-Marie Arseneault in her study of changes in nurse training for students in northern New Brunswick during the 1960s, highlights the significance of both place and religion in shaping, in this instance, the "appropriate" education for nurses. Suggesting that religious orders and secular government competed for control over university education for New Brunswick nurses, Arseneault discusses the confluence of ideas, individuals, and groups that came together to establish the first university nursing program for franco-phone students at the newly formed Université de Moncton in 1965, a form of education already in place for anglophone nursing students at the University of New Brunswick. These developments, which took place within the context of sweeping social changes introduced by Premier Louis J. Robichaud and his government during the 1960s, were meant to discourage the marked regionalism between the northern and southern areas of the province and to provide equal access to public services for all New Brunswick residents. The opening of the *École des sciences infirmières* in Moncton in the southern part of the province, however, led directly to the closure of the baccalaureate nursing program under the Religious Hospitallers of Saint Joseph at their Collège Maillet, which had long been situated in the north of the province. The Hospitallers were a group of religious women who had a long history of involvement in health care in the North through their hospitals and nursing schools. Their presence had added much to the local economy of the region, but their struggle to maintain the programs in nursing education ultimately proved futile and was only one manifestation of the demise of the significant role played by religious congregations throughout the province in francophone higher education in general.

Overall, this collection of articles attempts to decentre the strong connection between nursing and hospital work that persists within the writing of nursing history and within the public perception of nurses and their workplaces. The studies suggest that place needs to be considered as a significant variable, in conjunction with gender, race, class, war, and religion, in shaping nursing identities and nurses' work. Paying attention to place reveals considerable diversity in the ideas, concepts, and meanings associated with nursing work, providing a framework through which to interrogate the meanings that nurses ascribed to their own practice as well as the meanings that historians, among others, attribute to nurses' work.

# 1

## "A Loyal Body of Empire Citizens": Military Nurses and Identity at Lemnos and Salonika, 1915-17

*Cynthia Toman*

Trained civilian nurses enlisted with the Canadian Army Medical Corps (CAMC) during the First World War as part of a general rush from the dominions to show support for Mother England. Granted officer status and the military rank of nursing sister (NS), they shared a strong desire, along with many other soldiers, to be part of "history in the making" through participation in what was supposed to be "the last great war."[1] Canadian nursing sisters were generally eager to serve in forward medical and surgical units during the war, anticipating postings to the western front. They argued that such an assignment was "real" war nursing. Safer postings in England and Canada, where an increasing number of convalescent and rehabilitation soldiers needed nursing care, were far less desirable, according to Matron-in-Chief Margaret Macdonald, who noted the reticence among civilian nurses to enlist for these positions.[2]

However, most nursing sisters never imagined that several hundred of them would spend nearly two years in the Mediterranean theatre as members of one of the five CAMC units posted in support of the British forces at Lemnos, Salonika, and Cairo during the Gallipoli campaign, although there were no Canadian fighting troops involved in this military theatre of war. NS Mabel Clint described the posting announcement as causing a good deal "of consternation, as we had thought of the war in terms of the western front, though the campaigns in the near east had made us realize the vast scale of operations, and some international problems involved. The majority had rather expected that we should be attached to the Canadian Corps."[3] It was considered inappropriate, even scandalous, during this period to have women close to an active theatre of war, but the level of carnage made medical and nursing care a necessity. As NS May Bastedo wrote to her family, "You didn't think when I went abroad that I would have a Mediterranean trip, did you? ... 50 miles from Galilpoli [sic], too close to guns for me, thank you."[4] Their postings lasted between six months and two years (from mid-1915 to mid-1917), depending on the particular medical unit and on the nurses' state of health, which often deteriorated in these settings reputed to be the worst conditions of the war for soldiers – both men and women.

Military nurses are conspicuously marginalized in the historical scholarship on women and war, partially because the association of nurses with war and killing runs counter to conventional accounts of nurses as idealized women who epitomize both femininity and pacifism. The failure to distinguish between volunteer and trained nurses, as though their experiences were identical, is an important limitation within the scholarship.[5] When trained nurses are the subjects of inquiry, historians typically treat them as a single, homogeneous group comprising a chapter or two within larger studies. Gail Braybon noted in particular the very narrow range of sources used by those who do study women and war, contending that "women's wartime history was, and often still is, overlaid with myth. They have their own stereotypical roles to fill. There is scope for them to be seen as victims, villains or heroines, depending upon the viewpoint of the writer."[6]

Recent scholars have pointed to the importance of context-specific studies as sites of evidence to explore these often contradictory and ambivalent behaviours.[7] Braybon, too, called for historical research to specifically examine small cohorts, individual lives, and/or the events of a few days or weeks that can then be situated into the larger context of lives before and after the war, eschewing grand narratives and macro history in favour of "looking closely" at the small parts of the jigsaw while taking care to fit them together.[8] No historians have studied the Canadian nursing sisters within context-specific situations from the perspective of diverse intersecting identities or as subjects within military-medical contexts.

This chapter explores the contingent and often contradictory workings of identity from the perspective of the First World War Canadian military nurses who were stationed primarily at Lemnos and Salonika, where they were perceived, and perceived themselves, as both "imperials" and "colonials." As NS Clint wrote when embarking for the Mediterranean, "It seemed now that we should lose our identity, and be side-tracked [from the western front in France, which was considered the main focus of war activity]."[9] What did it mean for these nursing sisters to be simultaneously British and colonials, officers and soldiers, women and nurses in these settings? Would they prove to be worthy representatives of the Empire? How would they measure up against two dominant colonialist discourses that portrayed Canadians as hardy, adventurous, accustomed to primitive conditions, and efficient at "making do" but which also positioned them as being inferior in comparison to proper British-trained nurses?[10]

On the one hand, the Canadian nursing sisters represented British power and superiority as military officers of an Allied force and as members of the

British Empire. On the other hand, they were members of the territorial forces – that is, they were "colonials" from the dominions and they increasingly resented colonialist discourses. NS Mildred Forbes, for example, was quite critical of the presence of Canadian medical units in the Mediterranean when there were no Canadian troops stationed there. She maintained that the British were using dominion nurses as test cases for the harsh conditions. At the same time, she staunchly determined that Canadian nurses would not be found lacking or inferior to British-trained nurses. As Forbes wrote, "I suppose by sending the Canadian and Australian nurses to Lemnos first ... [the British] could see how they stood it before venturing to send theirs over. But we will show them of [sic] the stuff we are made of."[11]

The Mediterranean postings were portals to the Orient or "Near East," where the nursing sisters encountered what they perceived to be "strange" exotic races, languages, and cultural practices as well as competing discourses regarding imperial, colonial, and national identity. The near Orient, bordering on the Mediterranean Sea, was within easy reach and had been a favourite place for Europeans to travel to and write about since the early nineteenth century. Yet it had become associated with backwardness, degeneracy, inequality, and, in particular, with ideas about the "biological bases of racial inequality."[12] Scholar Edward Said described the western European perspective of the "Orient" as a "semi-mythical construct" that privileged whiteness along with the institutions, vocabulary, scholarship, imagery, doctrines, colonial bureaucracies, and colonial styles associated with whiteness.[13] Furthermore, for members of the Empire, "to reside in the Orient is to live the privileged life, not of an ordinary citizen, but of a representative European whose empire (French or British) *contains* the Orient in its military, economic, and above all, cultural arms."[14]

In this article, Empire carries dual meaning. It refers specifically to the British Empire of the early twentieth century as well as to an extensive colonial network of goods, economies, and politics. Prevailing discourse on the British Empire portrayed an "idealized notion of the national character as comprised of the 'manly' qualities necessary for military triumph and successful colonization: independence, fortitude, courage, daring, resourcefulness, and paternalistic duty."[15] As Catherine Hall and others have pointed out, "Empire was about the political, military, economic, and cultural exploitation and domination of the British over subject peoples." It included a range of practices and discourses affecting both the metropole and the colonial periphery, including the "justification of conquest and domination."[16] Anne McClintock argued for a gendered perspective on empire – the idea that men and women experienced imperialism differently and that various categories of difference were brought into being "*in and through* relation to each other – if in contradictory and conflictual ways." She contended that "the rationed privileges of race all too often put white women in positions of decided – if borrowed – power, not only over colonized women but also over colonized men. As such, white women were not the hapless onlookers of empire but were ambiguously complicit both as colonizers and colonized, privileged and restricted, acted upon and acting."[17] Katie Pickles also referred to the need "to gender national, imperial, and colonial spaces" and suggested that women participated in distinctly gendered forms of female imperialism associated with nurturing and caring activities.[18]

The First World War is portrayed typically as a defining moment for Canadian identity formation. Carl Berger was one of the earliest historians to explore the emergence of a Canadian national identity within the context of the early 1900s, arguing that the country deliberately chose to maintain and build stronger ties with Britain during this war in order to demonstrate that Canada deserved more power within the dominion structure. At the same time, politicians wanted to show that the country was ready for independence from England.[19] More recently, a growing body of literature has broadened the conceptualization of national identity from definitions contingent on geography toward conceptualizations of national identity as "imagined communities and spaces" that people perceive as bonding themselves to one another.[20] The nursing sisters, for example, consistently sought opportunities to care for "our boys," referring to the Canadian soldiers, while increasingly calling themselves Canadian rather than British although there was no official Canadian citizenship until 1947. And far from geographical Canadian territory, they sought to recreate Canadian-style living conditions, traditions, and celebrations. As Barbara Lorenzkowski and Steven High have recently pointed out, "if the vast body of recent scholarship on nationalism shares a unifying concern, it is with the fluidity, complexity, and shifting boundaries of national belonging, the role of gender and race in shaping narratives of empire and nation, and, indeed, the tendency to regard the nation itself as a 'text.'"[21]

As others have shown, transnational spaces, such as those the nursing sisters encountered in the Mediterranean, were significant in the construction of national identity. Historian Cecilia Morgan, in her study of English-Canadian travellers to Britain during the pre-war period, examined how the concepts of nation and empire were both staged and performed during the late Victorian and Edwardian periods. Morgan argued that "many tourists arrived with preconceived notions of themselves as 'Canadians' and as members of the British Empire," which subsequently "complicated their reactions to the staging of empire that they encountered."[22] Canadian military nurses found themselves in somewhat similar positions at Lemnos and Salonika, embedded as they were within the military hierarchy and highly visible as uniformed representatives of white British military might, and yet they were considered second class because they were nurses from the dominions. It was in resisting such a preconception that they began to share an emerging self-awareness of Canadian difference.

Nursing sisters' accounts frequently illuminate the interplay of empire, race, and gender through portrayals of hardship and danger on the one hand and portrayals of opportunity, marvels, and curiosities on the other.[23] These women left a relatively small body of first-hand accounts, which include several memoirs, diaries, a few sets of letters, collections of photographs, autograph books, and a small body of oral histories. One can also glimpse their presence and find references to their activities by reading traditional archival documents and records, medical unit histories, and an official history of the CAMC "against the grain." Nurses' accounts were constructed by individuals who appeared to be very aware of their unique situation as women privileged by occupational status to participate in an otherwise all-male domain of war. Their accounts vary considerably in both quantity and content, partially due to individual characteristics and to their intended audiences. NS Clint, for example, had previous publication experience related to her involvement with the Imperial Order Daughters of the Empire.[24] Some nurses wrote themselves into personal histories through their diaries and memoirs, punctuating everyday activities with visits from royalty or excursions to local tourist attractions. Clint, Katharine Wilson-Simmie, and Maude Wilkinson waited until the 1930s and 1970s, respectively, to publish their accounts, requiring readers to take the passage of time and post-war reconstructions of collective social memory into account, among other problematic aspects of these personal accounts.[25]

For the most part, nursing sisters maintained a proper official silence regarding the contentious or controversial aspects of their war experiences, as good soldiers were supposed to do. They were subject to military regulations that included the censorship of personal mail, although they creatively avoided censorship sometimes by sending letters back to England with friends who posted them outside of the military system. They also self-censored their accounts, as NS Helen Fowlds illustrated through her adherence to the soldier's unwritten code in writing to her family: "Already its [sic] getting to be a case of *in* the army or *not* and those who are, don't discuss their troubles with those who aren't."[26] As Meryn Stuart points out in her chapter in this volume, for example, NS Fowlds was a prolific letter and diary writer, especially during her time at Lemnos and Salonika where she explicitly warned her family not to divulge the contents of her letters and not to publish them in the newspapers for public viewing: "We have been cautioned repeatedly against allowing any of our letters to be published and we are to make all our friends understand that thoroughly. Some of the letters from the first caused a great deal of comment in military circles. One Nova Scotia nurse wrote of admitting a soldier covered with vermin. He said 'Sister – keep away. I'm covered with vermin,' and she said, 'Brother, I honour every louse on your body.' Did you ever hear any thing more disgusting? That was copied into dozens of eastern papers and was very severely criticized so warn anyone I might be likely to write to – in case I forget."[27] Given these various constraints, the small but significant collection of surviving sources are nonetheless remarkable and useful for study.

## "Soldiering" for the Empire

Nurses from the white dominions were particularly favoured as recruits to the British nursing services, even during the pre-war period. A survey of the British nursing supply at the beginning of the war, published as the *Report of an Advisory Committee Appointed by the Army Council to Enquire into the Supply of Nurses,* clearly gave preference to nurses from the dominions and warned nursing services to "abstain from recruiting in the United States or foreign countries."[28] When the British War Office issued a call for dominion nurses to supplement the British units as war became imminent, 314 Canadian civilian nurses joined the Queen Alexandra Imperial Nursing Service (QAIMNS) prior to the mobilization of nursing sisters for the CAMC.[29]

Many nursing sisters held strong pro-British stances. NS Clint, who was part of the first Canadian contingent, described the 1914 arrival in England with this jingoistic passage in her memoir: "Back from this western continent came a loyal body of Empire citizens, eager to aid in defence of the old home. Into the famous Devon seaport, which no enemy had ever penetrated, sailed a very different 'Armada,' to add a significant episode to the long and memorable pageant it had witnessed down the centuries. Most of the First Contingent were born in 'these Islands,' and as they crowded to the rigging, whatever emotions they felt were those of familiar sights, home reminders, and unchanging affection the beauty of England inspires."[30] British citizenship was one of the basic requirements for enlisting with the CAMC. The majority of Canadian nursing sisters already had strong British roots as either first- or second-generation Canadians. According to the demographic analysis of 1,133 attestation records, at least 13 percent of the nursing sisters were born in Britain, Scotland, Ireland, or Wales. They also shared in a prevailing British post-industrial revolution discourse regarding a moral obligation to "save" and "civilize" the rest of the world. Their specific imperial mandate was to "save the world" through the care of sick and wounded soldiers, and they believed that they could limit war's devastation by doing so. Nothing in their prior experiences, however, had prepared them for the conditions at Lemnos and Salonika.

The Mediterranean expedition began as a naval campaign in March 1915 to divert German actions against Russia by opening a second front. It ended in a "reverse," according to most accounts. Combined British, Australian, and French troops landed on the Gallipoli peninsula of Turkey, sustaining heavy losses and making very little military progress against Turkey and Bulgaria, who were aligned with Germany. By January 1916, the Allied forces had to evacuate the peninsula. Canadian nursing sisters cared for thousands of these soldiers from the ill-fated Gallipoli campaign, primarily at two field hospitals on the island of Lemnos and two in Salonika in Greece, under some of the worst conditions of the war. Between 1915 and 1917, the five CAMC units supported Allied troops, although there were no Canadian combat units involved in the area. It was a relatively brief but horrendous period for the units on Lemnos, but the units in Salonika remained there for almost two years.

Lemnos was bleak and barren, a sandy, rocky wasteland with few trees, where there was no comfortable season for tented hospitals. It was extremely hot in the summer, flooded and muddy during the rainy season, and freezing cold with snow during the winter. At least one medical unit was situated over a previous camp's sanitation dump, and water had to be transported from Alexandria or distilled onboard supply ships in the harbour. The lack of water and sanitary conditions caused as many or more deaths as battle wounds.[31] Both men and women soldiers experienced the bleakness of Lemnos, but, according to NS Clint, at least one soldier declared the island as "no place for Sisters" (read: women). Clint further claimed that they were the first cohort of nurses to arrive there to care for more than 97,000 sick and wounded soldiers, although the Gallipoli campaign had been going on for seven months already when they arrived.[32] When Canadian hospital units withdrew from Lemnos, one moved to Salonika to join the other units already there in support of British troops fighting in Albania and Serbia (1915-17).

NS Fowlds collected her colleagues' stereotypical expectations about Lemnos en route to the island in an autograph album that she titled "It has been said." In this album, NS Cecily Galt wrote, for example: "No nurses or white women at all – only Greeks ... We will all be very black both from the sun and not having any water to wash with. A very dirty place." NS Frances Upton, in a more soldierly tradition, wrote: "I have heard that we are going to Lemnos, and also that whoever suggested sending white women there, should be shot. However, it's up to Canada."[33] In her memoir, NS Clint described life and work on Lemnos after the nurses had been there for several weeks as follows: "Chief characteristic: Flies! Small flies, big flies, flies of all colours, historic flies, up-to-date flies, 7,350 types ... It's a long way home." One could not "eat or drink without swallowing flies, the tables swarmed with them; every patient's dressing removed required another to stand by fanning vigorously as a cloud of pests prepared to settle. Pus and maggots abounded and wounds would not heal."[34]

Hunger was an immediate and persistent problem for men and women alike on Lemnos. Matron Eleanor Charleson of No. 1 Canadian Stationary

Hospital (CSH) reported upon arrival that there was "nothing to eat except malted milk tablets" for two days until the British navy finally arrived with food and water. Throughout their stay, nurses wrote consistently about how hungry they were.[35] NS Katherine Wilson painted a particularly bleak picture at No. 3 CSH, where "Matron Jaggard sat at the head of the table; she made no excuse for the lack of table linen, or china dishes that make a table attractive. She simply asked us to remember the men in the trenches, and that we were all part of the army, all working for a victory that would come ... She finished with the quotation 'Ours not to question why, ours but to do or die.' Looking down at the pale gray bread and wax margarine, I wondered, 'How soon?'"[36] Entries from nurses' military personnel files support these personal accounts, qualifying their discharges from the CAMC for reasons such as "debility," weight loss, anemia, or being "medically unfit due to the conditions of service."[37]

In comparison to Lemnos, conditions at Salonika were slightly different, partially because these medical units arrived later in the season and with better systems of provisioning. Forty-six-year-old NS May Bastedo, for example, arrived at Salonika with No. 4 Canadian General Hospital from Toronto (CGH) during November 1915.[38] She described the unit's setting as located five miles from the town of Salonika, overlooking the main harbour, with Mount Olympus visible about forty miles away. No. 5 CGH from Vancouver was expected to join them, and did eventually, although they were diverted for some weeks to Cairo and then bombed on arrival to the harbour. Bastedo's tented hospital had been in existence for only two weeks. Both patients and staff lived in tents with two coal-oil stoves per tent and straw mats for flooring. According to her letters home, it rained all day, creating dreadful mud everywhere and necessitating the use of rubber boots, raincoats, and hats. Like Lemnos, however, "the water supply is the problem as it has to be brought so far, then it is boiled and chlorinated and even the soup tastes of it."[39] Bastedo was in charge of the isolation tents, where illnesses combined with December snow and freezing rain to increase the misery: "I have the Isolation tents, six and my own tent in a field. I have two orderlies and now the special one. We have been here nearly three weeks and the hospital has been fine. We have had a good many patients in & were a regular clearing station for a while ... A good many men came in with frozen feet as well as influenza, colds and rheumatism ... My duty tent is in the centre and I have to walk back and forth to the others. They are all infectious diseases."[40] In addition to cases of frostbite, the medical units had to deal with typhoid, malnutrition, black water fever, malaria, and other assorted fevers of undiagnosed varieties.[41]

A few Canadian nurses served briefly at Malta and Cairo. The island of Malta was primarily a transfer point for patients evacuated from the Gallipoli peninsula to Lemnos, Salonika, or back to England. It was also a respite

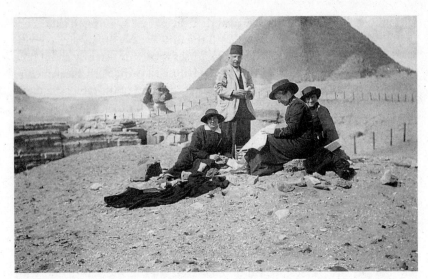

Lunch at the pyramids with Nursing Sisters Johnston, Mildred Forbes, and Laura
Holland. Exploiting all opportunities for travel, many nursing sisters wrote about
and photographed their settings as an exotic world of adventure. They described
themselves primarily in terms of whiteness, femininity, cleanliness, and British-ness,
in contrast to Blackness, masculinity, dirtiness, and Greek-ness. Some of their diaries,
letters, and photographs resemble travelogues in which they naturalized their own
presence and authority while representing contexts "new" to them through
pejorative images.
*Courtesy of Trent University Archives, 69-001, Helen Marryat Fonds*

posting for medical and nursing staff who might need an extended recovery
period from their own illnesses or from the harsh conditions encountered
at the other sites. NS Luella Lees noted, for example, that Malta was an easy
and pleasant assignment.[42] No. 5 CSH, which converted into No. 7 CGH
during its brief eight-month stay in Cairo, was redirected to Europe and the
western front. On occasion, hospital units in transit or individual nurses in
need of rest spent short periods of time in Cairo, while the authorities determined where to send them next. Cairo offered multiple tourist attractions
to be enjoyed during off-duty furloughs, especially by the nurses who staffed
a British hospital located within sight of the pyramids at Giza and Sakkara.
NS Elsie Collis, for example, was one of six nurses with No. 5 CSH at Heli-
opolis during December 1915, where she described in her diary the "magic"
of the pyramids during several moonlight expeditions.[43]

Performing the expected behaviours of good soldiers (which nursing sisters
readily called themselves) was an important aspect of proving oneself a
worthy member of the Empire. It included enduring all manner of wartime

conditions, exhibiting a willingness to die for the Empire, and adhering to the soldier's code of silence – all without complaint. Canadian military nurses were determined to forge an exemplary professional and military reputation, in spite of the conditions and risks. After all, as NS Wilson wrote, this was "real soldiering."[44] They had enlisted with the anticipation of some hardships and a lack of conveniences associated with civilian hospitals and private duty work. Yet they had also expected to work in relative safety under the protection of the Geneva Conventions, and it is doubtful that they seriously considered their work dangerous.[45] Although they did experience occasional shelling and infrequent bombing from Zeppelins, the main Mediterranean threats were poor nutrition, exposure to diseases, and unsanitary conditions. Even Matron-in-Chief Margaret Macdonald, who played down the apparent failure to adequately provision nurses at Lemnos and Salonika, acknowledged the rugged, inhospitable conditions as being "quite unsuited to the presence of women. The nursing sisters were surely tried, yet, of such soldierly material were they constituted, that complaint was rare."[46]

During September 1915, for example, it was the unsanitary conditions and lack of water that took its toll, as medical officers, nursing sisters, and orderlies succumbed to dysentery one by one. NS Clint wrote that "everyone was temporarily or permanently poisoned at Lemnos," and at one point "only three out of thirty-five nurses were on duty at No. 1."[47] Matron Jessie Jaggard and NS M. Frances Munro of No. 3 CSH died as a result of the severe dysentery. Eulogizing their burials on Lemnos, Matron Jean Cameron-Smith wrote in her report: "What nobler death could any have than theirs? Serving their King and Country, in a time of stress and strain, such as the world has never seen, and yielding up their own lives in this greatest of all services – the service of humanity – they have not died but have entered into immortality. Their story will be told in the pages of Canada's history and *read* by the children of generations to come."[48]

According to NS Clint, special preparations were made in the anticipation of the death of more nurses, wherein a "trench to hold six was dug in the Officers' lines. A laconic notice-board bore the legend: 'For Sisters only' ... But whether or not the hilarity with which the premature preparation was received cured our invalids I know not, but no more [nurses'] deaths occurred in the Canadian hospitals ... a corner that is forever Canada."[49] NS Fowlds found the funerals chilling reminders of their obligations as soldiers, recording in her diary: "Such a desolate place for a woman to be buried and everything so different from what it would have been at home ... all jarred terribly on one's nerves. It was so absolutely matter of fact, and military, strictly active service."[50]

These "unsuitable" working conditions were also threats to nurses' femininity and womanliness, which would potentially harden them through their exposure to such unheard-of filth and disorder. NS Myra Goodene asked

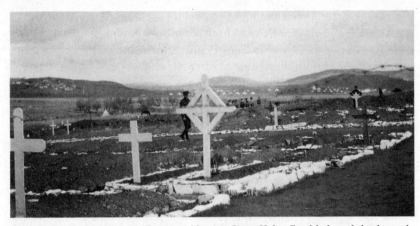

Graves of Canadian sisters at Lemnos. Nursing Sister Helen Fowlds found the funerals chilling reminders of their obligations as soldiers, recording in her diary: "Such a desolate place for a woman to be buried and everything so different from what it would have been at home ... all jarred terribly on one's nerves. It was so absolutely matter of fact, and military, strictly active service."
*Courtesy of Trent University Archives, 69-001, Diary #1, 15 September 1915, Helen Marryat Fonds*

one of the medical officers, for example, "if he saw much change in us, having known us when we first came. He thinks we all look older and a bit seedy. Certainly the lye here has told on us, whether we like to admit it or not. Our skin is roughened, our hair is getting grayer and worst of all our teeth are in a sad state. The iron in the water seems to be the cause – when disturbed the water is brickish in colour, settling in time. Have not had a hot bath for 6 months."[51]

However, retreat from the conditions was not acceptable, at least to those nurses who left accounts. NS Fowlds was particularly scathing and sarcastic about the efforts of her matron at No. 1 CSH to have their unit returned to England due to the hardships. Fowlds had served under Matron Eleanor Charleson, nicknamed Birdie, for a long time, and her diaries are full of grievances and complaints against the matron who apparently also had problems with her feet. The ultimate insult was the threat that Matron Charleson posed to the nurses' personal and professional reputations, as Fowlds described in the following passage:

Our Matron of course – you know by reputation – for I think I've written you about her. She is an extraordinary creature [,] a very poor talker but quite a plausible writer. She is fed up and it's evident she wants to go home. Well she is trying to work it that the entire unit – Sisters at least will be recalled and of course the reason given will be that we couldn't get along at all out here – She could have stood it but that the Sisters were discontented etc. We are doing our best to "fix her feet" as none of us is anxious to leave. This is our really first chance of making good. We are needed out here and we have a splendid unit. In France we were of no account. To be *recalled* from here would be awful and we are all prepared to resign if necessary though of course we won't ever come to that. But to have the Matron [unclear] us with everyone we will not stand.[52]

Fowlds described another situation at Lemnos during November 1915 when the nurses, who were ordered off night duty due to the bitter winter conditions, resisted the order. The matron "was furious at her domain being invaded – called a meeting of the Sisters. Wrote a verbose sickly sentimental letter to Williams [the officer commanding] about our utter lack of thought for our health when the soldiers 'our brave lads' needed care. The meeting was as per usual, simply to back her up. Everything she wanted to say always goes in as coming unanimously from the Sisters ... The hardship of night duty under existing weather conditions were thought too great."[53] Like Fowlds, other nurses resented any implications that they might desert their duties because of the difficult conditions, choosing to represent themselves as loyal, self-abnegating, and sacrificial. NS Forbes expressed her resignation to the situation as follows: "I only hope we will all get home intact! But it is no use worrying – we must all 'play the game' ... I hear malaria is apt to be prevalent later on – it is a nasty thing to get but cannot beat dysentery – which we had to fight before."[54] Forbes was eventually placed on the "casualty list" for a series of boils that she developed, typically caused by staphylococcal infections, first on her arm and then on her eye. At least two of the boils required surgery to drain the infection, followed by hot fomentations to heal them. At this point, she admitted that she was "getting sick of roughing it."[55] NS Upton contracted malaria and required several lengthy convalescent leaves that delayed her full return to civilian work until 1921. Other nurses decided that they had had enough of war, however, and used either their length of service or debility and illness incurred in the Mediterranean theatre as an excuse for requesting an early return to England as invalids suffering from the "conditions of service." Less conspicuously, still other nurses simply resigned their commissions "in order to marry," a socially acceptable end to harsh wartime service.

Eventually, according to NS Clint, "news leaked to Canada of our sorry plight ... The Canadian Government was communicated with, and a cable to London authorities had a quick reaction on Lemnos. The A.D.M.S. [assistant director of medical services] was instructed to inspect the hospital and redress disabilities. He happened to be one of those old-style officials ... who fully believed Colonials were still pioneers and 'accustomed to roughing it,' as he said."[56] There is good evidence from both NS Fowlds' diary and the correspondence of NS Forbes to Canadian senator Cairine Wilson in Ottawa that "leaks" to the Canadian government originated at least partially with the nurses themselves, some of whom had political connections in Canada through family members.[57]

It is difficult to know just how deliberate the leaks were, but, regardless of the intent, the complaints and leaks violated the soldier's code of silence and put into question, in effect, a nurse's behaviour as a good soldier. The leaks fuelled debates within Canada regarding the country's participation in what many citizens considered a "foreign war" or "England's war." They also fuelled emerging power struggles within the military organization that involved the surgeon general, a minister of Parliament, and high-level military authorities, resulting in a controversial investigation of the CAMC as a whole.[58] Ultimately, all Canadian units were withdrawn from Lemnos in January 1916, and the last Canadian nurses left Salonika by August 1917.[59]

### Identity and Empire

Historian Adele Perry has pointed out that while the construction of white women as a symbol of empire might have constricted the parameters of their experience, it also "accord[ed] them levels of power and authority usually denied women on the grounds of sex." In racialized contexts, where there were few white women, they generally benefited from deferential treatment regardless of their social positions "back home."[60] Historian Dea Birkett, in her study of nurses in colonial West Africa, also found that "for many women, the sense of importance instilled by imperial duty, combined with the promise of adventure, was strong enough to draw them away from more comfortable positions in Britain."[61] As members of the Allied military forces, Canadian nursing sisters were inextricably linked to the British Empire's long history of dominance and privilege, which constructed "Others" as inferior, backward, degenerate, and unequal, based on perceived racial and class differences. Empire and race intersected with their work and off-work activities, disrupting their self-perceptions of identity, professional roles, and competencies.

Nursing sisters were doubly privileged as white women and officers, in spite of the harsh conditions at Lemnos and Salonika. Their privileges included occasional opportunities to be tourists as well as to benefit from the surveillance and protection of military men with whom they served. They were supposed to "know one's position," however, and behave according to the socially constructed expectations of uniformed representatives of the Empire. In particular, they were to maintain "proper" class and race relationships in relation to the local inhabitants. NS Clint perceived the Canadian nurses, rightly or wrongly, to be "the first white women, other than the natives, and they were not very white, to set foot on this classic ground."[62] Illustrating the extent to which gender, race, and empire intertwined in discourses regarding the maintenance of "proper" relations in these settings, she wrote: "It was noticeable that men and women from other parts of the Empire did not know how to treat the natives with that indescribable mixture of *benignant aloofness* ... learned by Great Britain in centuries of administration of other Races and Religions. The natives understand it perfectly, and it is not really a barrier. Limitations are mutually recognized, and not overstepped."[63] Clint took her superior status and British-ness as both natural and given. She clearly differentiated herself from the other (read: non-white) parts of the Empire at the same time, claiming membership in the dominant "we" and assuming a mutual acceptance by local peoples.

Exploiting all opportunities for travel, many nursing sisters wrote about and photographed their settings as an exotic world of adventure. They described themselves primarily in terms of whiteness, femininity, cleanliness, and British-ness in contrast to Blackness, masculinity, dirtiness, and Greekness. Some of their diaries, letters, and photographs resemble travelogues in which they naturalize their own presence and authority while representing contexts "new" to them through pejorative images.[64] There are, for example, many descriptions of devious "dusky" Turkish and Egyptian men. NS Mabel Lucas called Malta an "international place" where they "wouldn't dare walk alone."[65] She characterized one group of people as infantile and another group as devious: "The Soudanese are a much finer type of humanity than the Egyptians: great, ebony, good-natured, biddable children, always grinning, willing, and loyal ... But my impression of the Egyptians on the other hand was of a mysterious, furtive, evasive scheming people, always ready to double-cross their benefactors, the British."[66] An anonymous nurse in Salonika portrayed French, Greek, and Serbian patients as subservient, passive, and childlike rather than dangerous: "They were always most courteous, agreeable, docile patients, and always absurdly grateful and devoted."[67]

Racial and cultural differences are most frequently described in unflattering ways. The nursing sisters' accounts typically portrayed local peoples and conditions as unkempt, unruly, or divergent from European standards of neatness, cleanliness, and order.[68] NS Fowlds described Salonika: "The streets are very narrow and paved [with] cobbles, and absolutely filthy. They say it is not safe in the city after dark, and I can easily believe it, for such a rough looking lot of people I never saw before. English, French, Greek, and a few Serbian soldiers, hordes of refugees and villanous [sic] looking Turks and Greeks ... The place was full of spies."[69] NS Wilson recounted her experience in Alexandria, Egypt: "In front of some shops sat old men, smoking large pipes resting in bowls of water on the ground. From these extended the long curved pipe stem decorated with many coloured tassels. But ugh! Such filth, flies, and odours. It might all look very well on canvas, but at close range it was far from beautiful. I shuddered and thanked my lucky stars we had two strong Canadian padres as guards."[70]

Although inextricably linked to the Empire, the nursing sisters perceived themselves as being variously positioned within it. As historians Barbara Lorenzkowski and Steven High pointed out, "although Anglo-Canadians prided themselves on their 'senior' position in the imperial family, the 'British world' was far more ambiguous about the status of Canadian 'colonials.'"[71] Many Canadian nursing sisters shared NS Clint's strong sense of identification with the Empire, at least initially. They expected British nurses to welcome them warmly and treat them as professional equals. Not long after their arrival in England, however, the British nurses made it clear that they were the senior and superior nursing service. NS Clint bristled vigorously that both public and professional discourse "just assumed" that Canadians "would not be worth much professionally."[72] Canadian nurses especially resented being referred to as "colonials," a derogatory designation that positioned them as inferior in relation to the British-trained QAIMNS. The designation reflected systemic inequalities wherein imperials subordinated colonials, relegating them to less desirable settings and work and expecting deference accordingly. Historian Jan Bassett, for example, referred to the Australian nursing sisters as "pawns in an imperial game" in Salonika and India. She argued that colonial nurses were deliberately assigned to the dirtiest settings (the "backwaters of war") and that British authorities considered them as being good only for the nursing care of Greeks, Turks, and Bulgarians.[73]

Major sources of tension between QAIMNS and Canadian nurses concerned issues of officer's rank, pay, and privileges that the CAMC nurses had and the QAIMNS nurses did not. As this jealousy over rank grew, the QAIMNS nurses were guilty of treating their dominion colleagues very poorly. One medical officer described the Canadian nurses in Malta as having had a "rotten time" with "hardly enough to eat," being made to "sleep in the same quarters as the servants," and enduring "nasty remarks about them wearing a uniform with lieutenant's stars and receiving lieutenant's pay." It is doubtful that Canadian nurses were entirely innocent parties to these controversies. They were always proud to be officers, ready to claim the privileges and capitalize on whatever opportunities the status might afford them. When sturdier and more protective facilities were built in Salonika in 1917 for incoming British nursing sisters, the Canadian medical units made haste to occupy them and assert "squatters' rights" to the more comfortable amenities.

Officer rank inverted expected relationships, where colonial or dominion nurses were to show deference to the QAIMNS nurses, which exacerbated imperial-colonial tensions. Both NS Clint and Fowlds often referred to the British as "they" and to the Canadian contingent as "we." Fowlds, for example, wrote: "You say we embarrass the British. Well maybe – ... They were prepared to find us crude and in every sense of the word 'common Canadians' and when we don't look and act the part they are sore over their disappointment. A Canadian ... was saying yesterday that an English doctor ... was jeering at the 'Two star freaks' – meaning Canadian Sisters – said he prayed that if he were sick he'd never fall into our clutches.[74] Fowlds also resented British nursing sisters who refused to give up their privileged position during the evacuation of Lemnos. She felt that the Canadian nurses should have received priority for evacuation based on the "sacrifices" they had endured, writing that "#27 Gen. [a British hospital unit] has been kicking up a row & insisted on going, and suggested – the nerve! – that *we* stay. They who have never seen active service, came straight from England, have only been here a month or so and who have 600 patients. We sent our 7 patients over there & they refused to take them saying they were to send their patients to us. They certainly have played a dirty game."[75]

Still other contentious issues concerned the differences between the British and Canadian uniforms, which were closely linked to perceptions of femininity. Even prior to her postings at Lemnos and Salonika, NS Fowlds reported that "the English nurses are openly jealous of our uniform and every day we notice little changes they are making in order to look like us – and imitation in this case is certainly flattery. They all say 'Your uniform is so becoming and ours makes us look like maids' ... No English women can criticize Canadian feet – our girls are much better shod. They all wear heavy tan boots while the English affect strap slippers with French heels – and usually run over at the ankles."[76] Here again, Canadian nursing sisters were probably not as innocent as they portrayed themselves to be. They were exceptionally proud of their official wardrobe, referring often to its flattering design, soft fabric, and smart looks.

At the same time that these tensions were growing between the QAIMNS and CAMC nurses, a sense of national belonging was also developing, which both unified the Canadian nursing sisters and differentiated them from the British nurses. Canadian nurses who had served temporarily at British hospital units and adopted British mannerisms generated antagonism upon their return to the Canadian units. According to NS Fowlds, "Some of the girls who have been in Imperial Hospitals all winter used to make us wild, they were so darned English – the name Canadian was almost distasteful to them. They talked English ... and they ran down everything Canadian. Now of course they are full of pride to belong to the country – Isn't it sickening? I wonder they scruple to take Canadian money."[77]

The tensions went further than appearance and mannerisms, extending to the domain of nursing practice skills – in the same way that graduates of different training schools typically competed with one another to assert that their way of doing things was better than any other. One newspaper account, for example, published the "Impressions of a Canadian Nurse: On the English Methods Caring for the Sick and Wounded." It criticized the number of nurses available for patients, the different techniques of doing dressings, and the amount of training. For example, the author wrote: "We notice, for instance, that your fully-trained [three years] nurses does [sic] not appear to have had an experience as varied as our own nurses, and take certain subjects as 'extras,' which are taken by ours in the ordinary course."[78] NS Fowlds went so far as to summarize the differences in this way: "It's a case of oil and water and we're better kept apart. Our ways are not their ways."[79]

Context-specific studies, such as those of the experiences of Canadian military nurses on Lemnos and in Salonika, allow us to examine the complexity of national identity as well as the significance of time and place in shaping the contradictory and ambivalent behaviours related to identity formation. Nursing sisters' occupational status positioned them uniquely as white women serving with the Canadian army in exotic settings of the Mediterranean and as officers who shared associated military privileges usually reserved for men. Both positions assured them of protection by the British army. Furthermore, they were simultaneously "imperials" and "colonials" in relation to the British Empire, which served to unsettle pre-war discourses regarding citizenship and national identity. Through their work of salvaging war's waste, First World War nursing sisters were engaged in the process of nation building. In addition to saving Canadian soldiers' lives, they re-created an imagined Canadian community through everyday social activities and relationships within the CAMC, while differentiating themselves from both the British and the non-whites they encountered. Identity among these military nurses was fluid and shifting, contingent on what was at stake and how such claims might be parlayed into opportunities, either professionally or personally.

## 2

# Social Sisters: A Feminist Analysis of the Discourses of Canadian Military Nurse Helen Fowlds, 1915-18
*Meryn Stuart*

"Feminist ideology" is another word for trying to understand in the life of a woman, the life of the mind, which is ... not coldly cerebral but impassioned.
– Carolyn Heilbrun, *Writing a Woman's Life*

This chapter examines the experiences of Helen Fowlds, a Canadian nursing sister who worked in France and the Mediterranean during the First World War. Using her copious letters home to her mother, as well as her diaries for 1915-17, I analyze the ways in which she constructed and expressed ideas of femininity and sexuality in her military social life. Historian Joan Scott warned against seeing experience as "incontestable" and as the unassailable evidence of the truth of a life. I do not treat Fowlds' words as *transparent* of her actual thoughts or actions. Rather, I confront questions of the *constructed nature of experience* and how subjects (such as female nurses) constituted themselves in the context of war.[1]

The Great War was Canada's first military engagement to employ significant numbers of nurses, and both military officials and nursing leaders strove to provide a "proper" space for women within a male-dominated sphere. Nurse training that emphasized skill and discipline, uniforms linked to the imagery of religious habits, and rules and regulations that governed both the on- and off-duty hours of nurses all worked together to promote an idealized portrait of nurses as protected and dutiful daughters of the military. Like many of the women who eagerly signed up for the front lines, however, Fowlds had never experienced the excitement of travel to unknown places nor had she ever before considered herself free in a man's world. In reading through her letters, we can see how she constructed herself as a young, modern "new woman" of the 1910s and 1920s who was coming of age through these wartime experiences and looking for self-fulfillment and sexual equality within the context of the war.[2] She was unafraid to express, even

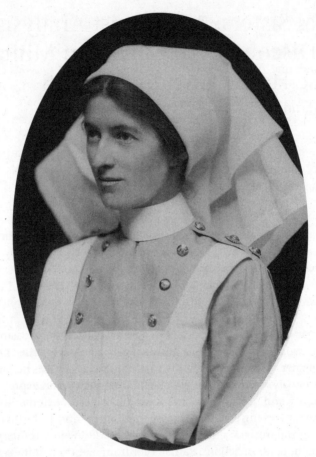

Helen Lauder Fowlds as a young nurse. Linked to the imagery of religious habits and promoting the images of authority and femininity, nursing military uniforms idealized nurses as protected and dutiful daughters of the military.
*Courtesy of Trent University Archives, 69-001, Helen Marryat Fonds*

to her mother, her pleasure in the numerous social activities in which she took part that involved men as well as women, and her letters and diaries also reveal the ways in which she often disregarded prescribed regulations concerning appropriate nursing behaviour.

Helen Lauder Fowlds was born in 1889 in Hastings, Ontario, the only daughter of a middle-class, but not wealthy, family. She entered the Grace Hospital training school for nurses in Toronto and graduated at age twenty-five just before the outbreak of the Great War.[3] She immediately enlisted with the Canadian Army Medical Corps (CAMC) and by December 1914 was in Québec receiving military training. In February 1915, Fowlds sailed on the SS *Zeeland* with nurses and soldiers and, after arriving in England, wrote to her mother every few days while she waited to go to France. She finally sailed for France for "active service" near Boulogne on 18 March 1915, telling her mother that "we are all in good spirits and not a bit nervous."[4] In April 1915, just after arriving at the front, Fowlds wrote: "I wouldn't go home for a million dollars. To have missed this!! I can't even think about it."[5]

In her discussion of Maritime women and their diaries and letters to each other, Canadian historian Margaret Conrad noted that so much of women's history is carried on in the private sphere that "failure to consult their personal documents could seriously warp the portrayal of women's history."[6] Since letters like those of Fowlds have rarely come into the public domain, however, we have had little opportunity to learn about the social lives of First World War military nurses. Torpedoed supply ships, officially censored letters, fear of letters being published in newspapers at home, and self-censoring all limited letter writing (and the receiving of letters) for nurses as well as soldiers in the field.[7] As the only extant letters of a CAMC nursing sister who regularly discussed her social life and sexuality, Helen Fowlds' ninety-four letters to her mother and her three irregularly written diaries afford a unique opportunity to analyze the construction of sexuality and femininity. Other nurses' first-person published accounts based on diaries do not discuss sexuality, although Nursing Sister (NS) Maude Wilkinson alluded to male "friends" in her memoirs.[8]

Yet, as feminist historian Karen Duder made clear, in order to see conformity *as well as* resistance to patriarchal norms in women's first-person accounts, we need to pay attention to the "not said" and the "not seen" as "conceptual tools" for feminist analysis.[9] What has not been "said" in secondary sources on military nurses is the portrayal of their relationships with men, specifically male officers in the case of Canadian nurses. The amount of space that Fowlds devoted to these relationships in her letters and diaries betrayed her intense social interest in men in a way that her mother and grandmother would likely never have expressed.[10] This chapter thus subverts the saintly image of the nurse as an asexual, dutiful "daughter" of the military. This one nurse, at least, was constructing herself as (hetero)sexual and felt free to write about it.

## Women, Nurses, and War

After war was declared in August 1914, over 3,000 nurses, known by title as nursing sisters and by rank as officers, quickly volunteered. Approximately 2,000 nurses and matrons went overseas with the CAMC before the war was over.[11] As historian Susan Mann (and others) have argued, these women wanted to do their duty to help heal the men and to show their patriotism and commitment to winning the war.[12] Families also expected nurses to watch over the health of their beloved enlisted brothers and cousins and to fly the flag for the Empire and for Canada.

However, female nurses were not combatants, and, therefore, the silence in official war histories about their experiences and work is profound. According to Mann, the nurses themselves may have wanted "oblivion" and so failed to reply to pleas for post-war recollections.[13] Canadian military historian Tim Cook, in his 2006 analysis of the official histories of the world wars, only briefly mentioned nurses and their lack of an official history. Although he included Sir Andrew Macphail's 1925 official history of the all-male medical service in the First World War,[14] Cook concentrated on the histories of male soldiers in combat. As he wrote, "military history is, ultimately, about examining the terrifying, brutal and exhilarating experience of battle."[15] Nurses were not perceived as soldiers in "battle," and Canada seemingly forgot its military nurses except in relation to their place in the CAMC under the authority of physicians.

Women's historians, however, have published work dedicated to First World War military nurses. Jan Bassett and Mary Sarnecky have each produced comprehensive commissioned histories of First World War nurses in Australia and the United States, respectively.[16] Popular histories of Canadian military nurses exist,[17] although some of the work on Canadian military nursing care is on women with the Voluntary Aid Detachment who were not trained nurses. Linda Quiney, for example, has written an excellent history of the Canadian Voluntary Aid Detachment corps.[18] With the noted exception of one published master's thesis, the edited war diaries of NS Clare Gass and the first biography of Matron-in-Chief Margaret Macdonald represent the only published monographs by a Canadian academic historian.[19] These two books are particularly valuable because they present little-known aspects of nurses' day-to-day lives and work and demonstrate the decisions made on behalf of nurses by their military nursing superiors.

Of the published histories on military nurses that exist, few historians have used sexuality as an analytic concept in relation to nurses and war.[20] In her biography on Macdonald, Susan Mann not only discussed Macdonald's social experiences and her single marital status but also explored her habit of tacitly encouraging heterosexual relationships and marriage for "her" nurses.[21] Historian Katie Holmes used several nurses' letters and diaries to study First World War Australian military nurses and the way in which they constructed their sexuality. Australian nurses were "honorary" officers with rank by 1916, so the opportunity for relations with enlisted men was "severely restricted," although Holmes stated that nurses were not "averse to some insubordination."[22] She found that nurses assumed various roles: as mothers for the wounded or shell-shocked soldiers, as sisters for recovering patients to assist them in restoring their masculinity, and as lovers or potential lovers to soldiers who were not their patients.

**The Diaries and Letters of Helen Fowlds**

As previously mentioned, wartime conditions make it impossible to determine if all of the letters that Fowlds wrote reached their destination. On her death in 1965, she bequeathed all of the letters and diaries her mother had saved to Trent University Archives, where they now form part of a virtual exhibition on her wartime experiences. Fifty-three letters survive from 1915. Many of these were written after she was sent with her hospital unit (No. 1 Canadian Stationary Hospital [CSH]) to the Dardenelles campaign in August. At this time, she was posted to Lemnos, which was considered to be the most disastrous nurses' posting of the war because of the alleged military ineptness and the blatant disregard for nurses' and soldiers' living conditions.[23]

Fowlds was still in the Mediterranean (at Lemnos, Cairo, and Salonika) in 1916. The letters she wrote decreased dramatically in number to twenty-one, in part because she was ill with a chronic respiratory infection from April to September. She returned to England as an invalid in September 1916 by ship, via the island of Malta, and wrote from there and later from England. It is unclear if all of her letters were received in Canada or, perhaps, if she wrote only infrequently until the end of 1916. Certainly, she reported receiving letters from her family that were months old and complained of the bad mail service to Lemnos and Salonika. Just eleven letters exist from 1917, and the most major event she described was receiving the Royal Red Cross at Buckingham Palace in February. Eleven letters also remain from 1918. Perhaps additional letters from this year were simply lost, but she may also have been exhausted and saddened by the death of her brother Don on the front lines. In a rare letter to her father, she declared that on opening the communiqué announcing his death "it seemed as if the world was ended."[24]

Historian Katie Holmes has argued that letters and diaries could help nurses cope with the chaos of war and "articulate and recreate their lives" through them. She explained that writing letters home maintained a link between the past and present, while diaries, which were not censored, recorded the things that the nurses could not put into their letters (such as descriptions of their lovers) and "chart[ed] change."[25] Letter writing was an expected ladylike activity for middle-class girls and women who had reached the level of high school literacy. Especially in her early days overseas, most of Fowlds' letters were cheerful, social, and chatty. Gossip and news about friendships made and lost with colleagues filled the pages, and she tried to include news about her brothers and friends from home who were at the front. Fowlds eagerly anticipated news from her family, and if letters were too slow in coming from her mother or aunts, she grew anxious and urged her relatives to continue to write. Writing letters in this way helped to spare her family, and particularly her mother, any concern. "I hope you are not worrying about me," she wrote from France, "we are as safe and safer than at home, for we are protected in every way. We are busy but as I have said before it really isn't as hard on one as the work in a big base at home."[26] Even when living conditions appeared daunting, she appeared to recover quickly in her letters. On her arrival in Salonika, she wrote to her mother: "I should have written before, but when I first come to a place I can't think of anything except what I shouldn't write about." A few lines later, however, she went on to say lightly that there were five women in her tent and they had "heaps of fun."[27]

Although often written sporadically, Fowlds' three diaries span the years 1915 to 1918, the third being kept into the 1930s. As Conrad observed, "diaries are women talking to themselves."[28] In contrast to her letters, Fowlds' private thoughts expressed in her diaries seem at times more serious. The diaries often contain "bad" news instead of encouraging, uplifting news, and in them she mentioned more difficult issues such as her sorrow at attending nurses' funerals, battles gone wrong, and her own persistent health problems. Nonetheless, descriptions of her social encounters and those of her tent mates also abound in her diaries, though they include more specific details, such as the names of nursing colleagues' male "lovers," than are included in her letters. Most intriguing are the pages neatly sliced out of her diaries – did Fowlds herself censor material before depositing them for public consumption?[29]

## Nurse Training and Gendered Ideology

According to both the Canadian army officials and Canadian nursing leaders, trained female civilian nurses made ideal military nurses, based on a shared gendered ideology about their expected work and behaviour. The discipline of the hospital training school and the way in which patient care was organized from the end of the nineteenth century into the mid-twentieth century enabled the trained nurse to fit seamlessly into the "military machine" of war because she had already acquired both the requisite skills and attitudes. Indeed, as American historian Susan Reverby pointed out, "the domestic order created by a good wife, the altruistic caring expressed by a good mother, and the self-discipline of a good soldier were to be combined in the training of a good nurse."[30]

Graduates of the large, urban schools (where it was believed that students could receive a broader experience) benfited from the four basic threads of training school and became the most sought-after nurses for enlistment into the military. First, nursing superintendents were to select the "right" sort of character for training, choosing women they believed were physically, intellectually, and psychologically superior as well as sexually chaste and unmarried. Ideal characteristics included good manners, pious attitudes, feminine appearance, and executive skills so that they could supervise servants and patients alike. Daughters of the middle classes were preferable since it was believed that they learned the necessary behaviours at home.

Second, supervisors socialized their female students within a regime of strict discipline and trained them to be loyal to their superiors and obedient, polite, reliable, and efficient in caring for patients. Hospital training schools wanted to produce the "good" nurse, who was a woman displaying the right feminine altruistic attitude as well as automatically meeting the needs of the hospital first. As ideal front-line care providers, these women arguably influenced the entire success of the hospital endeavour in the early twentieth century.

Third, nurses were to be taught self-abnegation and strict obedience in their relationships with physicians, to always follow orders, and to meet the doctors' needs on the wards. A widely used textbook in 1885 put it this way: "To the doctor, the first duty is that of obedience – absolute fidelity to his orders, even if the necessity of the prescribed measures is not apparent to you. You have no responsibility beyond that of faithfully carrying out the directions received. [In hospital] military discipline should prevail, and implicit, unquestioning obedience should be the first law for the nurse, as for the soldier."[31]

Finally, the good student nurse was also careful to keep romantic encounters separate from working relationships with doctors and male patients. Nurses were exposed to the ideology of the "dangers of impurity and the rewards of a pure life" in their own churches and schools as they grew up in the 1880s and 1890s. Heterosexual relationships were not forbidden, but it was expected that young women would be chaperoned and not meet young men on their own. Appropriate "ladylike" attitudes, including feminine dress, were a clear benchmark of success in training schools across the country in the early twentieth century.[32]

## Military Context: Rules and Regulations

The inculcation of obedient caregiving and femininity associated with hospital training schools allowed nurses to fit well into the sexual division of labour on the wards of military hospitals.[33] In general, superiors expected nurses to manage wards as they would a middle-class home and to take responsibility for all domestic issues such as cleaning and beautifying, ordering food supplies, looking after their "boys" (the patients), and supervising "servants" (the orderlies and scrubbers). In addition to performing actual nursing care and organizing the wards, they planted gardens outside their huts and sewed curtains and sleeping bags. The army also expected them to boost the morale of discouraged patients by writing letters home for them and decorating the wards for holidays and parties.[34] It relied upon nurses to buy food treats to tempt the sickest patients, to distribute Red Cross supplies such as pajamas, socks, and cigarettes, and to "interest themselves in the home circumstances of men being invalided as permanently unfit," reporting such men to the matron.[35] The army also wished nurses to serve tea to medical officers and visiting dignitaries.

In her directive *Instructions for Members of Canadian Army Medical Corps Nursing Service (When Mobilized)*, Matron-in-Chief Macdonald set out a series of forty-two instructions outlining the duties of the matrons under her and regulating the lives of the nursing sisters. Most of the rules related to the provision of nursing care, but the verbs used included "should," "will," and "must," leaving no doubt that these were commands. Discipline and good order on the wards were each matron's responsibility. She was to report "neglect of duty or impropriety of conduct," whether on the part of the sisters, patients, or visitors, to the commanding officer. She was required to submit "confidential reports" on all nurses under her command, detailing each one's "capability" but also their "tact, zeal, judgment, and personal conduct."[36]

Nursing sisters were warned to "comply" with any orders from the matron and the medical officers. Signifying the desire of superiors that nurses should be considered "ladies" at all times, they were instructed to be "careful to exercise due courtesy and dignity in all relations with officers, NCOs [non-commissioned officers], men, and patients."[37] Echoing the 1885 nursing textbook, the final instruction commanded them to "bear in mind that unquestioning obedience and loyalty to [their] superior officers are an obligation."[38]

The instructions set out how nurses would act under "the immediate supervision" of their superiors, whether they were on the wards or on off-duty time. Matrons had complete control over their nurses' off-duty time since the hospital was staffed twenty-four hours per day and the nurses slept and ate in female-segregated tents or huts close to the hospital wards. The matron-in-chief, who oversaw how these instructions applied to the nurses, was directly responsible for all of the nurses' "recreation" – the word recreation being a trope for the maintenance of both professional and sexual propriety. The rules forbade nurses from visiting the wards when they were not on-duty and from accepting "presents of any kind from any patient, or friend of any patient, whether during his illness or after his death, recovery or departure." Nurses were to "retire to their rooms by 10:30" at night and have all lights out by 11:00 "unless special permission was given."[39] Although not explicitly addressed, attending church services, vacationing, and socializing with other nurses while off-duty appear to have been acceptable activities. Unspoken assumptions of the instructions, however, were meant to keep nurses from becoming involved in compromising situations: unsuitable entertainment, excessive partying, and, in particular, contact with men that was considered too close.

## Threads of Discourse: Femininity, Sexuality, and Resistance to Rules

As a young middle-class woman and a graduate of a respected Toronto-based hospital, Fowlds represented the ideal type of nurse desired by the military. The manner in which she constructed herself through her letters and diaries demonstrates that in many ways she conformed to the notions of femininity expected of her social position and training. Nonetheless, the letters and diaries reveal some resistance to prescriptive military rules, especially in Fowlds' social life, and she was critical of her superiors, illustrating that she often failed to meet the imagined expectations of the military and nursing leaders. Fowlds' letters reassured her mother that at the same time that she was exploring her role as a newly independent professional woman, she was also living a "normal" life for a young and sociable middle-class woman of her age. The following discussion will examine the ways in which her writing about shopping habits, clothing, both civilian and military, and active social life helped to construct Fowlds' femininity and sexuality, albeit in a particular middle-class manner: modest, stylish (but not garish), and respectable.

Many of Fowlds' letters were concerned with organizing the sending and receiving of goods. Fowlds asked for everything from stockings to letter paper and camera film to be sent to her from Canada.[40] From France, she wrote that "stockings are an outrageous price over here and a few pairs of tan cashmere every month or two would be mighty welcome ... One pair a month would be heaps. That is all I need – I think."[41] On another occasion, she wrote: "And before I forget, did I leave behind me a pair of black pumps with velvet buckles ... Send them along if you find them."[42] From Lemnos, she asked: "If you can send me a couple of rolls of film every little while in with clothing or something of the sort I'd love to have them as it is very difficult to get them in [,] being contraband. Declare the other things in the parcel and take a chance."[43] Her mother, in turn, sent food, especially cakes and coffee, to accompany the letters, and some of these items Fowlds sent on to her brothers Eric or Don, who, as soldiers, were never far from her mind. Fowlds also bought gifts that she sent back to her family, items such as Turkish brass or Belgian lace that were undoubtedly exotic and prized souvenirs in a North American, middle-class home.

Erika Rappaport, in her research on letters sent between colonists and their relatives back home, argued that money and goods circulating between parents and children created and sustained middle-class identities, families, and economies throughout Britain and its Empire.[44] While the kinds of goods that circulated between Fowlds and her relatives may not have been critical to maintaining the Fowlds' family economy in quite the same way, the amount of time and energy devoted in Fowlds' letters to the sending, receiving, and redistributing of items tended to fix Fowlds' identity within her family. Despite her status as an independent woman working for wages far from home, she remained a good, dutiful, middle-class daughter, still leaning on her parents for support, caring for her brothers overseas with her, and thinking of them all even as she experienced new and exciting adventures on her own.

### Shopping and Feminine Clothes

NS Fowlds loved to shop. Indeed, in reading her letters of 1915 and 1916, one would think that little nursing work was done! Fowlds and her friends, especially NS Myra Goodene, seemed to take every free opportunity in France, Egypt, Greece, and England to shop for clothes, especially feminine silk underwear, pajamas, and other goods, and to have shampoos and manicures: "Miss Goodene, Boultbee and I spent our afternoon in Boulogne, and certainly had a time. We had a bath at the [Crislot], bought a wonderful cake, and inspected most of the stores. The lingerie shops are a great temptation and I must lay in a stock while I am over here."[45] After a trip to Cairo, she wrote that she "got half a dozen prs. of Silk Knickers made – 4 of pongee Aunt Hattie sent me and one pink and one blue pair. We found the silk best as it took up little space and was easily laundered. I also got a cheap pair of Chinese silk pyjamas – I like them better than night-gowns."[46]

The nurses also bought and sold civilian clothes among themselves when they were leaving a posting: "I sold that linen hold all trimmed with pink ribbon (which I never used) for $3.00!!! to a girl who is crazy about pink. I also sold two white linen shirt-waists I had at the 'Children's' for a dollar each to a girl who hadn't anything to ride in. Altogether I took in £9. It may sound like a daylight robbery but when a girl about my size and build went home without offering to sell a thing, I was furious. The girls all said it was the best sale they'd ever been at. I had a knitted jacket all made except to put a border on and Brock took that."[47]

Nurses had purchasing power and good salaries for single women of the time. Their shopping echoed the consumer culture of early twentieth-century society, when women's "material needs, wants and desires" began to take precedence over other pastimes.[48] With the increased development of department stores in the middle of the nineteenth century in England and the United States, women's public and private spaces merged through the pleasures of "looking" for goods and clothes. Stores became what sociologist Rudi Laermans called "female leisure centers," transforming "active buying into passive shopping."[49] Erika Rappaport analyzed "a new era of shopping" in London with the opening of Selfridges department store on Oxford Street in 1909. According to her, Selfridges' "scale and intensity" transformed the nature of shopping and also of bourgeois femininity.[50] By the middle of the war, shopping for pleasure in the urban centres of England, Europe, and the Middle East attracted Fowlds and her friends, along with other women of their class and income. By the end of the war, she had clearly bought into the trappings of an affluent middle class, spending her savings on furs and a stylish hat and illustrating a continued consciousness of being feminine and well dressed. She wrote, "At last I have got my furs. I saved all winter and got a set of black fox when I was in London. They cost $125, and are quite good value. I am delighted to have them as furs always make you look clothed. I got a very pretty hat too, made from a model."[51]

Despite Fowlds' many purchases on her shopping trips, she and her fellow nurses could wear civilian clothes only when they were on leave, playing tennis, or riding in England. All of their time elsewhere, especially in France, was spent in military uniform. Matron-in-Chief Macdonald was a "stickler for proper dress," insisting at all times on professional, military, and regulation attire and refusing to permit embellishments such as jewellery, even when off duty.[52] Like most nursing sisters, Fowlds was clearly proud of her distinctive uniform, which consisted of both "full" dress and "working" dress. The latter consisted of a blue linen uniform with gilt CAMC buttons, collars and cuffs, rank badges of two stars on both shoulders, a tan leather belt with a heavy CAMC clasp, white apron, and one yard of muslin for the veil.[53] She struggled to keep her uniforms looking new. "It cost a small fortune to have my uniforms dipped," she wrote her mother. "They were all so faded. Some of the girls are appearing in gorgeous new ones of heavy silk or linen."[54]

Veils were especially important to the nurses, perhaps because American nursing sisters did not have them and commented on the fact. Keeping veils clean and white must have been difficult, particularly under the trying conditions in Lemnos. When she became desperate, Fowlds asked her mother for veils and sometimes the material to make them: "How I have blessed you for those two veils which arrived in good condition today. My stock is very low. If you could send me about two or even three a month it would be heavenly especially while we're out here. There is a very fine material almost like bolting cloth that makes up beautifully and stays fresh ever so much longer than the others. The ones we made out of that piece of lawn were no good at all – too small and too heavy."[55]

Several scholars have studied the symbolic nature of the military nurse's uniform. As Kathryn McPherson pointed out, artists and sculptors have represented military nurses in almost proto-feminine roles as nurturer, morale builder, caretaker of the sick, ideal servant, and companion to men. Several paintings in the Canadian War Museum, for example, as well as the better-known marble frieze in the Hall of Fame in the Parliament buildings in Ottawa, which Canadian nurses helped erect after the First World War, feature the large female figure of "humanity" as a generic symbol of female caregiving.[56]

Nurses' billowing white muslin veils, white aprons, and soft, bright blue cotton uniforms had roots in the habits of religious sisters, and thus they also represented religious symbolism. In the well-known three-panelled painting of nurses in No. 3 CSM at Doullens, France, nurses care for patients and assist physicians with a statue of Mary in bright blue robes standing high on the wall above the hospital ward.[57] Military nurses' uniforms also functioned as symbols of authority and femininity. Literary critic Sharon Ouditt argued that uniforms of British military nursing volunteers offered the "illusion of a coherent identity" and "helped to subdue expressions of individuality that might border on the sexual."[58] Nonetheless, white veils were feminine, even mysterious and seductive, and projected a certain image of heterosexuality, particularly through their relationship to those of a Christian bride in white.

## The Construction of (Hetero) Sexuality

According to historian Carroll Smith-Rosenberg, the critical issue for the generation of "New Women" born in the 1880s and 1890s was sexuality, which was linked with identity and freedom.[59] As a woman of this generation, Helen Fowlds was herself exploring the kind of freedom seldom available to women before her time, and she was unafraid to write home about it. The nurses often had fun together, and they were not above gently mocking people who in other times might have commanded their respect. "You'll think by my letters we are having far too much fun for 'active service,'" she wrote to her parents from France. "Our greatest enjoyment is in the evening parties – just as it is with nurses the world over I think. We all get together in some one's [sic] tent and have something to eat and MacCullough mimics everyone in the place. The padre at No. 8 British is a remarkably handsome man, young and very much in love. He brings divine love and human love into all his sermons till it is a regular by-word. He does a great deal of moving around and hitches up his surplice a lot too – and Mac can imitate him exactly."[60]

Many of her letters were filled with her interest in men and the opportunities for meeting them. On board the ship to Lemnos, Fowlds enumerated the ratio of men to women: "We all rejoiced at the thought of two more days on board – for it has been a most delightful trip. There are 85 Can. Sisters, about 60 M.O.'s [medical officers] – 24 English sisters and 7 R.A.M.C. men besides the ships officers – and we have all enjoyed every minute."[61] Once on Lemnos, she wrote her parents that "our afternoon teas are functions. To-day we had a lieut. and two of the dearest middies from the Glory and officers from most of the thousand odd English regiments around here, and Sundays there isn't standing room ... We have a ripping lot of girls in

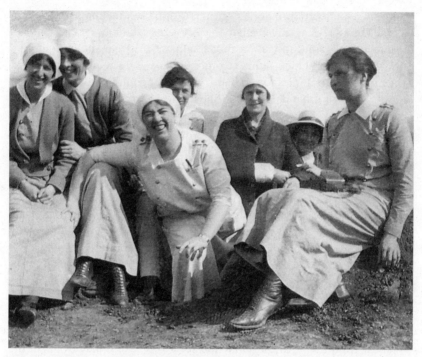

Helen Fowlds (on left) sharing leisure time with colleagues. Living in cramped and difficult quarters and sharing the work and life experiences of nursing overseas often brought military nurses close together. Photos such as this one would also reassure parents back home that their daughters were enjoying "normal" activities of young womanhood despite their proximity to the dangerous and masculine theatre of war. *Courtesy of Trent University Archives, 69-001, Helen Marryat Fonds*

this unit and the men certainly like to come here."[62] She was delighted to be "meeting men here who come from every corner of the world ... [We try to make it] pleasant for the boys from all the regiments stationed near here and ask them up for tea and make them feel they have a place to come to. Tea is our salvation – every day we have actually dozens of men." Suggesting that perhaps she had been less than adept at relationships with men before she left home, she continued her letter by "thanking God every minute for being one of the lot sent out here. Women are very much in the minority here and we have had to develop whatever conversational powers we possessed. I know it's done me worlds of good."[63]

Some of Fowlds' letters mention dances and parties with the men, and her matron seems to have promoted certain heterosexual activities between nurses and fellow officers. Contrary to what was allowed for the English nurses, Matron-in-Chief Margaret Macdonald approved of nurses dancing with fellow male officers, "because nurses who were surrounded with an

atmosphere of depression needed the recreation both mentally and physically."[64] The nurses arranged many such events (suitably chaperoned) in
hospital units around special occasions such as Christmas and Halloween.[65]
They were not forbidden to marry officers, but if a nurse married while in
the military, official rules forced her to resign her commission even though
her new officer-husband did not. While Fowlds' letters likely comforted her
family that she was not in immediate personal danger, they may also have
reassured them that she was engaging in activities considered "normal" for
a healthy young woman.

Nonetheless, comparing Fowlds' letters to her diaries suggests that there
were limits to what she could write to her mother. Before leaving for Lemnos,
she admitted in her diary that that she could not help staring at "such
*splendid big men*" as the Canadians: "I was far too busy watching their faces
as they went by to pay attention to shopping. I met Reg Runnels, looking
*so big and brown and manly.*[66] In one diary entry, she outlined the layout of
the "tea room," a description that did not make it into her letters perhaps
since it took on overtones of a somewhat sexualized space: "The tea room
looks so homelike & pretty. Blew sent up a sick carpenter from her ward who
made two huge davenports which are padded with biscuits – half mattresses
and covered with brown blankets – with heaps of bright cushions they are
the most comfortable and ornamental seats you could imagine."[67] In the
same entry, as well as in others, Fowlds noted the names of her nurse friends,
the names of the men they especially liked, and the indications of affairs,
which, again, were not mentioned in letters to her mother.[68] She commented
once that "[NS] Scoble up to her old tricks – entertained [Capt] Carmichael.
[Nurse] Blew having heavy affairs with Dixon, Tom Young and Col Davis
and Alfred" and wrote later that same week that "Micky has a heavy affair
on with Pierce."[69]

Although all matrons were responsible for the "recreation" of the nurses
under their command, it is unclear to what extent they had control over
the nurses' social life and conduct, especially in Lemnos and on board ships.
What is clearer is the fact that some nurses had very little respect for some
of their superiors. Fowlds wrote that "Charleson [whom they called Birdie]
is unspeakably awful as a Matron. She acts like a common servant and if
there is anything that should be left unsaid she always says it."[70] Fowlds
continued to disparage her in her diaries, explaining that once the nurses
had a "supper party" and NS Mae and "Blew" made fun of Birdie by imitat-
ing her return from a trip to Cairo.[71] When Birdie was "mentioned in French's
[sic] dispatches [sic] – Christmas list," Fowlds wrote that she was "running
around to everyone asking 'Have you nothing to say to me this morning?'
etc. No one would congratulate her, except her usual henchmen. In the la-
trine this morning she said to [NS] Clint, 'Did you know I'd been mentioned
in dispatches?' Clint said 'What for?'"[72]

The disdain of Fowlds and the other nurses for superior officers suggests some resistance to being governed by military regulations or instructions, but it also reveals the fact that nurses could "break the rules." As she explained, "We aren't fond of our matron but we might have got worse ... She knows nothing about what goes on in her unit and thank God ... we have a lot of girls who have a good time but know the limit. You could stay out all night every night in the week for all she'd know. I think we have as little scandal as any unit there is, but no thanks to her."[73]

Historian Peter Bailey argued that there was an understanding of sexuality (or parasexuality as he named it) during this period that was linked to consumption and the practices of bars and barmaids in urban centres. Parasexuality was sexuality that was "deployed but contained, carefully channeled rather than fully discharged."[74] I am not comparing nurses to barmaids but, rather, using Bailey's view that nurses were part of the "new women" of the early twentieth century who were athwart the public/private divide in a sexualized commercial culture.

## Conclusion

As NS Helen Fowlds reveals through her letters, she was a modern young woman who expressed her femininity and sexuality through a love of shopping and an active social life with men, despite the restrictions of military life. We cannot generalize Fowlds' experience as it compares to other military nurses, but in terms of the contemporary mass consumer culture, she may not have been unusual even in the context of war. Modern women were beginning to believe "in the possibilities of personal transformation" through changes brought about by urban living, mass production, and speed of travel.[75] New opportunities for work and education in an increasingly secular society meant that middle-class white women such as Helen Fowlds might have experimented with their lives even as they constructed it.

# 3
# The Healing Work of Aboriginal Women in Indigenous and Newcomer Communities
*Kristin Burnett*

Examining the curative services that Aboriginal people, especially women, made available to European Canadians offers an opportunity to explore the complex sets of relationships that existed between indigenous people and newcomers during the late nineteenth and early twentieth centuries in western Canada. Beginning with the fur trade and extending well into the period of settlement, non-Aboriginal people sought out the healing and caregiving expertise of Aboriginal women. Historians have largely ignored the therapeutic labour of Aboriginal women, and the health care services that indigenous women provided, particularly in obstetrics, have remained invisible. The healing and caregiving work that Aboriginal women performed created an informal network of health care in western Canada and formed an important conduit of cross-cultural relations during the early period of settlement. Even after the arrival of white doctors and nurses, these informal networks of health care continued, for a period, to operate alongside Western biomedical institutions.

Before 1890, western Canada was sparsely settled and organized, and institutional Western health care was not available to most western Canadians. As a result, European Canadians sought out practical alternatives to Western medical care and treatment. Some settlers used home remedies, other settlers turned to family members and neighbours, and still others relied on local Aboriginal groups.[1] Even after 1890 when municipalities began to build hospitals and the number of doctors and nurses in western Canada grew, acquiring the services of a graduate nurse or doctor remained prohibitive due to cost and distance. Thus, during the late nineteenth and early twentieth centuries, indigenous women played essential roles within their own and newcomer communities as midwives, healers, and repositories of medicinal plant knowledge. Indeed, Aboriginal women's work around healing and caregiving constituted a kind of contact zone during this early period of settlement.[2] However, the frequency and nature of this contact that revolved around health and healing was not static, and it changed in response to historical circumstances associated with white settlement and nation building.[3] Nevertheless, the decline of indigenous women's curative work was not uniform, and in some areas of western Canada, the healing labour of Aboriginal women persisted.

Tracing the patterns of indigenous women's healing work allows nursing and medical historians an opportunity to address the invisibility of indigenous women's therapeutic expertise and knowledge. Indeed, by including such labour as part of the repertoire of skilled and unskilled curative labour that women performed, this study offers a broader definition of what constitutes women's healing and caregiving work. In addition, investigating the curative roles of Aboriginal women presents the opportunity not only to acknowledge the existence of a vibrant indigenous therapeutic culture but also to consider health as a potential and particularly gendered site of contact.

Locating indigenous Plains women and their work within the historical record is extremely difficult. Aboriginal women's roles were often less public and spectacular than more masculine activities, such as the buffalo hunt, and therefore contemporary observers were less likely to document it. For instance, amateur ethnographer and naturalist George Bird Grinnell provided a brief description in 1892 of the plants eaten by the Blackfoot but devoted an entire chapter to hunting.[4] The lack of interest paid to indigenous women's activities also extended to their healing abilities. Ethnographers often overlooked the mundane and more concrete curative skills in Plains culture in favour of the public and spectacular healing ceremonies that were usually performed by men. This is particularly true in regard to those therapeutic skills surrounding the rituals of childbirth.

Contemporary scholars have perpetuated this oversight by paying very little attention to women's reproductive and healing activities in Plains communities. Feminist scholars have offered several reasons for this omission. Historian Patricia Jasen argued that derogatory representations produced about Aboriginal women by European fur traders and explorers in eighteenth- and nineteenth-century texts have led to a distortion of birth culture in indigenous society.[5] During this period, European explorers characterized Aboriginal women as possessing animal-like natures, implying that Aboriginal women gave birth painlessly. Since many European Americans believed such racialized and gendered images, the study of obstetrics among indigenous people appeared to be unnecessary.[6]

Historian Maureen Lux proposed perhaps the most compelling explanation. She contended that scholars investigating the colonial project in North America have focused almost exclusively on disease and death in indigenous communities. Academics have inadvertently perpetuated the myth of the "vanishing Indian" by emphasizing ill health, death rates, poor living conditions, and social disintegration in indigenous communities at the expense

of cultural persistence, resistance, and change. Such a focus in colonial scholarship has masked the survival of certain cultural practices such as obstetrics
among Plains people.[7] Recent works by sociologists and anthropologists have
attempted to redress such misconceptions and to acknowledge an extensive
tradition of midwifery in Aboriginal communities. These works, however,
deal only with northern Aboriginal people in the present.[8] This study seeks
to outline the midwifery services that indigenous women made available to
White settlers and, in doing so, insert the healing work and obstetrical expertise of Plains women into the history of western settlement.

### The Changing Landscape of Western Canada

The late nineteenth century was a period of rapid social and economic
change for indigenous Plains people. The negotiation of treaties and the
establishment of reserves in the 1870s, the consolidation of the Indian Act
in 1876, and the decline of the buffalo fundamentally altered the lives of
Aboriginal peoples in western Canada.[9] Following the Northwest Rebellion
in 1885, the federal government instituted a pass system and used the North
West Mounted Police (NWMP) to restrict and monitor the movements of
Aboriginal people. This pass system required Aboriginal people to obtain
permission from the Indian agent or farm instructor whenever they wanted
to leave the reserve for whatever reason.[10] Such measures served to isolate
Aboriginal people on reserves and eroded their ability to practise subsistence
strategies and participate in local economies.

With the creation of reserves in the 1870s, the federal government began
its formal assault on the social and cultural activities of indigenous people.
In the late 1880s and early 1890s, the federal government formed a partnership with Protestant and Roman Catholic organizations to make Western
education and basic medical services available to Aboriginal people on
western reserves. Both the educational and medical services possessed a
strong religious component and were intended to replace existing social
structures. In an effort to undermine the fabric of indigenous communities,
the federal government amended the Indian Act in 1885 and in 1895 began
to criminalize community-based ceremonies such as the potlatch and sundance.[11] Building schools, providing Western medical services, and passing
restrictive legislation reflected the federal government's agenda to assimilate
Aboriginal people into a settler society based on European-North American
culture and values. However, such efforts by the federal state and missionary
organizations did not produce the desired results, and Aboriginal people did
not assimilate but, instead, continued to rely on those cultural practices that
were a vital part of day-to-day life.

Although the 1870s had witnessed growing numbers of farm families
migrating west from eastern Canada and north from the United States, by
the 1880s few European-Canadian women occupied the territories west of

Manitoba. The Dominion Survey in 1872, which was intended to settle the western landscape, left white settlers cut off and isolated from one another. The district of Alberta in 1885, for example, had an Aboriginal population of 9,500 in contrast to only 4,900 non-Aboriginals.[12] These demographic disparities ensured that European-Canadian settlers, particularly women, needed the healing and caregiving aid of indigenous women. Even after 1890 when the settlement of western Canada increased dramatically, and European-Canadians began to outnumber Aboriginal people, encounters that dealt with health continued, and the obstetrical work of indigenous women played a central role in the settlement of western Canada. In spite of the federal state's best efforts, easily identifiable and drawn boundaries did not exist between settlers and indigenous people, and the midwifery services that indigenous women made available to female settlers best illustrate the complicated social and spatial terrain of western Canada.[13]

## Aboriginal Women's Healing and Caregiving Work

The vital help and caregiving work that Aboriginal women performed for fur traders, missionaries, the NWMP, and early settlers (often recent immigrants to Canada) remained an important part of the informal health care networks that operated across western Canada before and after Confederation. Two types of healing encounters occurred between indigenous people and newcomers. The first revolved around the provision of medicinal plant knowledge, practical medical aid such as the treatment of cuts and the mending of bones, and general nursing care by indigenous women. The second healing encounter took place almost entirely between Aboriginal and European-Canadian women and was premised upon a shared experience of childbirth.

Some of the earliest records providing descriptions of indigenous and newcomer relations are those left behind by fur traders. Fur trade journals, correspondence, and company records reveal that newcomers did require medical treatment by western North-American Aboriginal people. For example, the chief factor at Fort Pelly, located at the northeastern elbow of the Assiniboine River, used the services of a local Aboriginal woman to treat his employees. An entry in the fort's daily log dated 14 February 1863 indicates that an "old native woman was paid six yards of printed cotton for doctoring Thomas Favell."[14] The daily log does not reveal whether the woman lived at the fort or how the chief factor acquired her services. What it does suggest is that non-Aboriginal people recognized that indigenous women possessed a certain degree of useful medical knowledge and were willing to pay for their skills.

In much the same way, missionaries, who arrived well before any significant white settlement, also availed themselves of the curative knowledge of the Plains people. The following three examples illustrate how important indigenous healers were to male missionaries and their wives during a period when no other medical help or assistance was available. The earliest example, noted in a local community history, involved Robert T. Rundle, the first Methodist missionary to arrive at Fort Edmonton in 1840. Rundle fell from his horse and broke his arm in 1847 while visiting the Blackfoot and relied on Blackfoot healers to set his arm and care for him.[15] Thirty years later, the wife of John Maclean, the Methodist missionary at the Blood reserve during the 1880s, developed an infection in her finger from a cut. Before he left to travel his circuit, Maclean advised Annie to see the local Aboriginal healer, commenting that the problem would be cleared up in less than a week if she did. Unfortunately for Annie, she failed to heed Maclean's advice and was forced to have her finger removed at the knuckle.[16] Charlotte Selina Bompas, wife of the well-known Anglican bishop of Athabasca William C. Bompas, faced a difficult situation in the 1870s when she became very sick. Alone and unable to care for herself or her daughter, Bompas was nursed back to health by Madeline, a Cree woman with whom Bompas had been trading for food. Bompas even went so far as to refer to Madeline as her "little wife."[17]

The fact that missionaries used the healing knowledge of indigenous people highlights just how much the experience of living in the mission field differed from the very public statements that missionaries made about indigenous people and culture. As agents of social change, missionaries had a vested interest both in promoting their work and justifying its utility.[18] Historian Myra Rutherdale's insightful analysis of the encounter between Bompas and Madeline suggests that while "intimate relations were not part of the dominant colonial discourse ... the context of living in the mission field allow[ed] for a challenge to the preconceived notions held by missionaries."[19] Missionaries were dedicated to reshaping indigenous culture. That missionaries used the curative and caregiving capabilities of Aboriginal people was at odds with the negative representations missionaries produced about Aboriginal culture and medicine. If we read only the celebratory and public accounts, we might think that Bompas' experience was unique. Indeed, it was not, and it is at the disjuncture between discourse and practice that we find such contradictory stories.

Official histories describing the settlement experience for European-Canadian settlers in western Canada rarely acknowledge the presence of indigenous women. The continued mobility and importance of indigenous Plains people sits awkwardly on top of narratives of empire building. By the late 1870s, Aboriginal people in the West were supposed to be confined to reserves, and their economic and environmental knowledge was meant to be no longer a factor in an economy based on farming and ranching. The labour of indigenous people, however, did not fade into irrelevance, and indigenous women continued to provide timely aid and care during medical emergencies. In the 1880s, an unnamed woman from the Moosomin district in present-day Saskatchewan wrote: "The Indian woman took in the situation at a glance. She pushed aside the terrified Mother and picked up the ailing child. By signs she indicated hot water from the kettle on the stove. Into it she put a pinch of herbs from the pouch slung around her waist. She cooled the brew and forced some of it between the blue lips of the infant. Soon the gasping subsided, and sweat broke to cool the fevered skin. The baby relaxed into a peaceful, natural sleep, cradled in the arms of the crooning Indian woman. That mother to her dying day remained grateful."[20]

Similarly, the wife of François Adam fell ill during haying time at the east end of Crooked Lake in the summer of 1892. Adam's farmhand immediately fetched Father Bellivaire, the local Roman Catholic priest, who arrived shortly accompanied by two indigenous women and their children. After setting up their tents, the women proceeded to steep various twigs and roots for several hours before giving the mixture to Mrs. Adam, who drank it and immediately felt better.[21] Although Adam may not have known which Aboriginal women in the area were willing to offer their curative skills, he was aware that the neighbourhood priest did. Such networks were a common part of life in the Prairies.

Settlers were familiar with the botanical knowledge of Aboriginal women. European Canadians frequently recalled that their districts had one or two Aboriginal women who served as both doctors and caregivers. Some of them remembered Mrs. Longmore, wife of Johnny Saskatchewan, a Native woman who "knew all the places where she could gather the leaves, the berries, the barks, and the roots which formed her materia medica, and to her knowledge of their efficacy, and skill in their use, many a woman in those days attributed her safe return from the valley of the shadow."[22] Memoirs of early settlers and local community histories reveal that indigenous communities shared a wealth of knowledge with newcomers about the resources of western Canada. Historians make similar arguments regarding the early period of the fur trade and the important roles that indigenous women played at the fur trade forts and for the mobile voyageurs, but they have not written much about the agriculturalists and ranchers who settled the Prairies less then one hundred years later. As Effie Storer, an early resident of the Battleford District, wrote, "Down through the ages [Native women] have gathered various roots in their season, and buds from different trees and shrubs which they kept or prepared for medicinal use amongst the tribe. And indeed at times helped the early settlers in their need. Many of the elder women proved quite adept at diagnosis and in prescribing the correct herb-tea, the taste of which was long remembered by the patient as in most it proved efficacious. Lint from the cotton wood tree and the hairy fuzz of the anemone seed pod were frequently called into requisition."[23]

A local history of southern Alberta notes that the Blackfoot used a "ball shaped fungus, similar to a mushroom, which ... when tied over a wound would stop bleeding and was used as an anaesthetic."[24] The white community was familiar even with treatments dealing with more personal and, at the time, illegal issues such as birth control and abortion. Scholar Elaine Silverman conducted interviews with women who had lived in Alberta from 1880 to 1930. Describing how indigenous women dealt with birth control, one women stated: "I guess the priests didn't approve, but the women figures [sic] that's the Indian way, not the white man's way. They sewed a black bag from the bladder of a bear. They'd dry it, then mix it with some liquid, and then they'd lose the baby. There must be some medicine in that. They figure that's okay. It's from the land they figure it didn't do any harm. Well the priest didn't know about it. Nobody told him about it."[25] In some cases, the healing expertise of Aboriginal women was used in conjunction with Western medicine. For instance, the local doctor was unable to help pioneer Charles Bray's sister-in-law, who was suffering from dysentery. A Blackfoot woman cured her with white prairie flowers steeped in tea.[26] Mrs. Reid from Battleford, Saskatchewan, found it was fortunate that there were indigenous women who "possessed remarkable knowledge of the simples to be found in the various parts of the West."[27]

## Obstetrics

Obstetrical knowledge and skills of indigenous women played an important role in the establishment and maintenance of a contact zone premised upon health and healing. Given the nature of settlement in the West, many European-Canadian women were without the assistance of doctors, nurses, or female family members during childbirth. As a result, Aboriginal women were often a timely and welcome presence during labour because they possessed skills that enabled white women to survive childbirth, eased their pain during labour, and provided advice following the birth. The wives of fur traders, missionaries, government employees, and settlers all made use of Aboriginal women as midwives.

One of the first accounts of a European-Canadian woman requiring the services of an indigenous midwife occurred during the fur trade. The story of Marie-Ann is included in the collection of stories about "trail blazing" women written by Alberta's popular historian Grant MacEwan. Following her marriage to Jean-Baptiste Lagimodière, a French Canadian voyageur, Marie-Ann decided to accompany her husband on his trip to present-day Manitoba in 1807. The "brave and mighty" Marie-Ann gave birth to their first child the following year at Pembina in the Northwest Territories. Jean-Baptiste had prepared for the birth by making arrangements with a local Cree woman, the wife of an Aboriginal trapper, to remain near his cabin so that she could assist his wife during labour. During the labour, the woman used herbal tea to ease Marie-Ann's pain and, following the birth, introduced Marie-Ann to the practicality of a moss bag.[28] The woman's labour and the

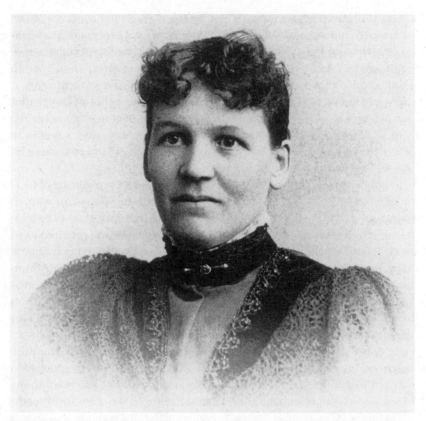

Eliza McDougall, wife of Methodist missionary John McDougall, and her sister-in-law Annie, relied heavily on the midwifery skills of Mary Cecil, a Cree woman who attended them both. Neither of the McDougall women acknowledged this help, however, in their many public presentations to church groups.
*Courtesy of Glenbow Archives, NA 1677-6*

assistance of the indigenous midwife does not figure prominently in the tale nor is the midwife recognized as being responsible for safely bringing the "first legitimate white baby" in western Canada into the world.

Much like the missionaries' use of indigenous healers, their use of obstetrics also reveals experiences in the mission field that did not conform to or become part of the dominant narrative of the missionary encounter. Eliza Boyd McDougall, the wife of the Methodist missionary John McDougall, and her sister-in-law, Annie McDougall, were both attended by Mary Cecil, a Cree woman who worked as midwife, nurse, and servant.[29] Annie McDougall remembered Mary Cecil affectionately. Although she had initially feared her, "she had soon become very fond of her because of her kindness and faithfulness. For twenty-eight years I had not better servant or friend, and the children loved her as well as any white woman."[30]

Likewise, European-Canadian women who married employees of the Department of Indian Affairs also relied on the services of experienced indigenous midwives to assist them during labour. In an unpublished collection of reminiscences, F.C. Cornish, the Indian agent for the Sarcee from 1887 to 1890, recalled that his eldest son had been born while he was employed at the Sarcee reserve. As Cornish wrote, "in those days it was not an easy matter making provision for such an event. The nearest doctor was in Calgary. Nurses were unattainable."[31] Fortunately, Mrs. Cornish had been able to obtain the obstetrical services of the interpreter's wife, a Sarcee woman who was well known as a good midwife.[32]

In isolated and under-serviced areas, female settlers also made use of local indigenous women during childbirth. Once European-Canadian women found out that they were pregnant, they would often make plans to be with female relatives or friends close to their due date, but these plans often went awry. Following her marriage in 1864, Susan Allison lived with her husband, John, on his ranch in the Similkameen Valley, British Columbia.[33] Allison recounted giving birth to two of her children during the late 1860s and early 1870s with the help of indigenous midwives. On the first occasion, Allison had intended to travel to Hope, British Columbia, to be with her mother for the birth but was caught by surprise when the baby was born two months early. John fetched the sister of one of the Aboriginal workers from the neighbouring ranch. Suzanne, the midwife, calmed Allison by giving her whiskey to dull the pain.[34] Allison recalled that "Suzanne was good to me in her way – though I thought her rather unfeeling at the time. She thought that I ought to be as strong as an Indian woman but I was not."[35] Allison's second birth was also attended by the wife of an Aboriginal man that John knew.[36]

Thirty years later, a recent immigrant from Ontario, Annie Greer, shared a similar experience. During her first winter in Dauphin, Manitoba (1893-94), Greer lived in a log and sod hut and was by herself when she went into labour.[37] She gave birth to her first child with the assistance of the local midwife, Caroline, who was the wife of the chief on the neighbouring reserve. Caroline came prepared with a satchel full of herbs, roots, bark, and leaves. She saved the mother's life and refused payment for doing so.[38] A decade later, Mary Lawrence of northern Alberta made a similar choice when securing help to deliver her first child. Lawrence preferred the presence of an indigenous midwife over her other alternative, her father-in-law.[39]

Even when hailed, physicians in many cases were unable to reach women in time because so few doctors worked in rural districts. Physicians preferred to practise in urban areas where there was a better chance of making a decent living.[40] Most were not guaranteed a steady income and supplemented their practices with other paid employment.[41] Even doctors from the Department of Indian Affairs could not support themselves on their salaries. For example,

Dr. Lafferty worked as the medical officer for the Blackfoot for over twenty years. In addition to his work for the Department of Indian Affairs, Dr. Lafferty had a practice in Calgary, ran a ranch, was a banker, ran a dry goods store, and was periodically the mayor of Calgary.[42]

Given the shortage of physicians, many stories depict settler women who gave birth by themselves while their husbands went for the local doctor. Effie Storer used the obstetrical services of an indigenous woman while she was stationed at Whitefish Lake in the Northwest Territories (in present-day Alberta) with her husband, an officer for the NWMP. Storer recalled that her daughter Irene was born on 30 March 1894, and since the closest doctor lived in Edmonton, she was forced to rely on the services of an "old medicine woman." The following year when her husband was transferred to Battleford, Northwest Territories (in present-day Saskatchewan), her daughter Muriel was born prematurely, and, once again, an indigenous midwife was called in to oversee the labour.[43] It is telling that during a period in which the NWMP were actively involved in restricting the physical movements of Aboriginal people through the pass system, indigenous women were able to circumvent such restrictions when they attended the wives of NWMP officers.

Some doctors appreciated the expertise of indigenous midwives. Harriet Sayese, a midwife who lived near Frog Lake, wrote that while her mother never received an education, she "was a wonderful help and much was accomplished among our Native people on the reserve. When people were sick mother was called on to help, often being midwife. She even helped Dr. Miller at times, as midwife, in the old hospital he had set up in his home at Elk Point in the early 1920s."[44] Many doctors throughout the Canadian West relied on local midwives to help with births that they knew they might not be able to reach in time. Mrs. Walker was an experienced midwife and medicine women whom Dr. Isman, the physician from the village of Wolsely, frequently asked to manage those births he was unable to attend.[45] Ellen Smallboy, a Cree woman born in 1853 near James Bay, remembered that the Indian agent, who was a doctor, had taught one of the midwives on the reserve techniques that enabled her to be more adept at dealing with difficult obstetrical cases.[46]

Geography was not the only factor that constrained the access of European Canadians to physicians and hospitals. The women's branch of the United Farmers of Manitoba recorded that prior to 1920 a doctor's visit could cost anywhere from twenty-five to fifty dollars.[47] Given the boom-bust nature of the western economy, few farmers could afford to call on the services of a doctor. Additionally, those settlers who wanted to use a hospital could not do so because the cost of inpatient care remained prohibitive. Familiarity and comfort also drove the choices that European-Canadian women made about their birth attendants. Several women from southern Saskatchewan preferred the services of a skilled midwife to the unappealing medical alternatives available to them. As Maggie White and Ellen Hubbard explained, there were only three doctors available in their district: one doctor who was very nice but old and deaf, another who had been a doctor in the army and had little patience for women, and a third doctor who drank too much.[48]

In spite of the potential importance of indigenous women's aid, European Canadians were often hesitant to recognize their neighbours' help. When congregations invited the McDougall women to speak about their experiences, for example, their stories did not include the work of indigenous women. In an address that Eliza gave at the evening service at the Pincher Creek United Church on 6 June 1935, she described her experiences in terms of the deprivation that missionaries' wives experienced: "In the main the men could take care of themselves, but what of women? Without companionship of their own sex, except the squaws, sharing all the hardship and privations of frontier life, bearing their children without medical or nursing aid, these are some of the sacrifices made by the noble generation of women."[49] Indeed, in the nearly twenty addresses to church audiences that Eliza McDougall and her sister-in-law Annie delivered, none mention their intimate and important relationships with indigenous women. Nor does John McDougall's publication mention these encounters. However, in an interview with journalist Elizabeth Bailey Price in the late 1920s, Annie revealed that Mary Cecil was very important in ensuring the well-being of the McDougall women. Evidence of Indian Agent Cornish's wife using an indigenous midwife also does not appear in official departmental correspondence. Rather, the indigenous midwife emerges years later in undated archival documents written by Cornish.[50] Similarly, John Maclean's advice to his wife that she consult an indigenous healer is documented in personal correspondence, but in his speeches and published texts, Maclean represented indigenous healing practices as "medical folk-lore" and superstitious beliefs that rely on harmless objects to affect cures.[51] Maclean's writing, like other missionary texts at the time, portrayed traditional therapeutic knowledge as ineffective and hazardous.[52]

European-Canadian women and their husbands eulogized white women's roles as "harbingers of civilization" and lamented the lack of white female companionship and proper medical care. Historian Sarah Carter has commented on the historical amnesia that has written Aboriginal women out of the official histories of the West.[53] Jennifer Brown has pointed to a comparable silence in the published texts of Egerton Ryerson Young, who did not acknowledge the influential role that the Cree nanny, Little Mary, played in his son's life.[54] Andrea Smith has called the invisibility of indigenous women in the colonial imagination a "present absence."[55] It is not surprising then that evidence of Aboriginal women's midwifery and healing sits awkwardly amid the broader colonial narratives about the process of settlement and nation building. Settler women only begrudgingly acknowledged their debt to the indigenous women who helped them.

Acknowledging the labour of Aboriginal women may have been particularly awkward given the growing efforts to constrain indigenous women in their own communities and homes. As an employee of the Department of Indian Affairs, Cornish was responsible for "stamping out" indigenous cultural activities, and Mrs. Cornish was expected to teach indigenous women European-Canadian values and domestic skills. They may have felt conflicted about relying on indigenous women's healing skills. Amendments to the Indian Act in 1885 and 1895 regarding the criminalization of religious ceremonies served as mandates for officials of the Department of Indian Affairs. Prior to 1884, the Indian Act had dealt primarily with issues of property acquisition and disposal, Indian government, and education.[56] A law banning all potlatch or "giveaway" ceremonies was passed in 1885, and in 1895 section 114 prohibited the practice of the sundance and similar ceremonies. These amendments provided agents with the necessary legal tools to suppress indigenous medicine.

Indigenous women were targeted in particular ways. Negative images of Aboriginal women led many Westerners to regard the presence of indigenous women within the physical boundaries of cities and towns as a social and moral concern.[57] Stereotypes that characterized indigenous women as shameless prostitutes were particularly powerful.[58] After 1892, legislation in the Criminal Code and under the Indian Act made it easier to convict indigenous women for prostitution.[59] At the local level, incidents such as the 1884 conflict in which Aboriginal women were denied access to a ball held at Fort Macleod's NWMP barracks reflected popular mechanisms of constraining Aboriginal women's movement.[60] After 1885, an indigenous woman in Battleford, Northwest Territories, had her hair chopped off as punishment for being in town without a pass.[61] In Calgary, town residents were cautioned against buying anything from Aboriginal women or hiring them to work.[62]

In these circumstances, the fact that missionaries and Indian agents and their families welcomed Aboriginal women into their homes speaks to the tremendous need for obstetrical and health care help and highlights the uneven effects of colonial power. By the end of the nineteenth century, however, interactions between indigenous and European-Canadian women may have declined. In a study of childbirth on the Canadian Prairies, Nanci Langford examined the diaries and letters of seventy-eight female homesteaders in Saskatchewan and Alberta.[63] Only a few of these women admitted to using indigenous women as birth attendants, perhaps because the majority of Langford's evidence pertains to the decades after 1900 when European-Canadian settlements were neither as small nor as isolated as in previous decades.

## Conclusion

The stories that settlers told regarding their use and awareness of indigenous medical practices differ from nation-building discourses that have erased Aboriginal women from the narrative of settlement and have emphasized the strict social and spatial boundaries that separated indigenous people and European Canadians. In fact, such stories expose the discrepancies between the official and unofficial record. Not everyone used the healing abilities of indigenous women, but the available evidence suggests that Aboriginal women worked as midwives, nurses, and caregivers for many white settlers. Indigenous women provided essential services during periods when there was no one else. When white trained female nursing personnel became available, they gradually supplanted the role of indigenous women. Since nurses, doctors, and hospitals remained expensive and not freely available, however, this development did not take place until well into the twentieth century. This transition was also not seamless, as European Canadians continued to rely on Aboriginal women's therapeutic expertise.

The history of women's healing work, health, and colonialism has concentrated to a large degree on the work of white women, the provision of Western biomedicine to Aboriginal peoples, and the establishment of what many have considered inadequate systems of health care. Few scholars have looked at the informal systems of health care that already existed in western Canada and that were extended to newcomers during the early period of settlement. Healing, nursing care, and obstetrics constituted a contact zone predicated upon a sexual division of labour and shared experience of gender. Indeed, an examination of midwifery in western Canada offers an opportunity to investigate how two cultures came into contact and were sensitized to one another, however unequally, through obstetrics.

# 4
# Cleansers, Cautious Caregivers, and Optimistic Adventurers: A Proposed Typology of Arctic Canadian Nurses, 1945-70
*Myra Rutherdale*

In the fall of 1950, Donalda McKillop Copeland arrived at Southampton Island, about 600 miles north of Churchill, Manitoba. Copeland hailed originally from Dauphin, Manitoba, where her mother was a nurse and her father was a Presbyterian minister.[1] She was accompanied by her husband Harold Copeland, the new welfare officer and schoolteacher for the community, and their four-year-old daughter Patsy. Donalda was to serve as the nurse to the Inuit of the community, and she was also meant to share some of the teaching responsibilities with her husband. Since their new community of Coral Harbour/Salliq did not have a nursing station, she set up her work facilities at home and would, over the next five years, see patients there. She would also carry out many home visits.[2]

Copeland's family home and nursing station soon became a hub for patients and social calls. Even apart from patients dropping in, young Patsy had an active social life with many visitors. Like previous newcomers to Arctic communities, the Copelands were welcomed by the Inuit, who offered them warm hospitality. Children especially were shown reverence. Donalda Copeland found that all of the children in the community were well loved by their parents, either natural or adoptive, and therefore it seemed quite easy for the Inuit to extend that same love to Patsy: "They loved especially the white child who had come to live among them and their attitude toward her was always benevolent and protective."[3] Children were equally fascinated and curious about Patsy.

One little girl, Nana, became Patsy's best playmate and, as her mother wrote, "the pair immediately became inseparables [sic]. When it was too cold for outdoor play, I permitted them the use of our sun-porch. Gradually Nana became an accepted part of our household, sharing all our rooms and our meals. Gradually, too, without any objection from the child or from her family, I took over the regular washing and bathing of the little girl and the care of her clothing, supplementing it with pieces I made up for her myself."[4]

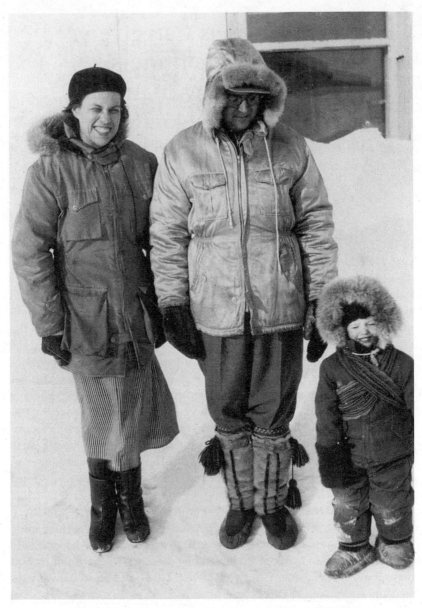

Donalda McKillop Copeland and family, Southampton Island, 1950s.
*Courtesy of Glenbow Archives, NA 3366-9*

Nana became a regular member of the Copeland household and added to
the comings and goings of the Copeland family. However, her presence also
brought out in Donalda McKillop Copeland a certain predisposition to clean,
or what I call in this chapter the characteristics of the "cleanser" type. The

hustle and bustle following the Copelands' arrival in the community can be read as a case of successful adaptation. However, the evidence also suggests that Copeland was determined to impose her habits of hygiene on others, not only providing clean Western-styled clothing for Nana but also washing and scrubbing her body.

The home base of Dorothy Knight, another nurse who settled in the Arctic, was also a busy place, and, as in Copeland's case, we can learn much about Knight from her first responses at the time of her arrival. Knight, a native of Sarnia, Ontario, arrived in the eastern Arctic community of Lake Harbour/Kimmirut, ninety miles (140 kilometres) west of Frobisher Bay/Iqaluit, in the spring of 1957. Unlike Copeland, however, Dorothy Knight found both a nursing station and a home in Lake Harbour/Kimmirut. Her nursing station and clinic was an abandoned United States army Quonset hut. It was especially appealing since it was large, but oddly it came complete with mosquito netting on the windows because it had been originally intended for Pearl Harbour, not Lake Harbour/Kimmirut.[5] Nonetheless, upon her arrival, the nurse's new home was a beehive of activity. Knight was first introduced to her interpreter, a man called Ishawakta, and a few minutes later she met Oola, Ishawakta's mother-in-law, who Knight learned was hired to help out around the house. These first few hours in her new home were recalled in her biography, yet it is striking that Knight hardly shared the same response to her surroundings as Copeland: "She saw that Oola was in the kitchen, clattering with the stove. She must think I'm such a fool, Dorothy thought, trying the radio again. It produced static as usual. I don't know how to set the stove. I don't know how to dispose of my own wastes. I don't even know yet how I can be of help to these people."[6] Dorothy's first encounter with her new neighbours filled her with doubt and anxiety. She wondered if she was up to the task of northern nursing. This sense of anxiety suggests what I will go on to describe as characteristic of the "cautious caregiver" type.

Visitors at the nursing station in Fort McPherson/Teet'lit Zhen, Northwest Territories, provoked yet another set of responses from a twenty-five-year-old nurse, Lucy Wilson, a response that differed from those of both Copeland and Knight. Wilson was born and raised in Grande Prairie, Alberta. In a letter to her parents written in the fall of 1962, she revealed the slight anxiety she felt over an impending visit from her zone supervisor, an anxiety that was caused by matters beyond nursing: "But poor Hank will have to be nonexistent for a few days as we are anticipating a visit from Miss Kelly tomorrow. Miss Kelly is the zone supervisor of nurses – our boss. So we have to remove all evidence of Hank & he'll have to stay at William's place while she's here. I don't mind her coming as I like her better then Callaghan. She isn't such an old prude."[7] As we later learn, Hank was actually Lucy Wilson's recently adopted dog, a nursing station guest who would not meet with the approval of her visiting supervisor. Wilson demonstrated here a willingness to break the rules and fly by the seat of her pants. This defiance seems to be a typical characteristic of a third type of nurse that I identify as an "optimistic adventurer."

What should we make of these three quite different responses to the comings and goings of people and animals in northern nursing stations in the post-Second World War era? In reading the letters, diaries, biographies, autobiographies, and official correspondence of northern nurses and doctors, medical professionals who worked in the Arctic and in provincial and territorial northern Aboriginal communities, I often wondered what kinds of encounters they had had with the people they cared for. What did they have in mind before they left their various communities, and how did they experience the North once they arrived? How did their day-to-day experiences change their ideas about Aboriginal lifeways, and how did they write about their work and aspirations? Most importantly, I have also been curious about how race and gender figured in their day-to-day relationships.

I have focused on Donalda McKillop Copeland, Dorothy Knight, and Lucy Wilson, each of whom, I would argue, represented one of the three different approaches taken by nurses in their work and lives in the North.[8] Nonetheless, these categories are fluid. For example, it is clear that the cautious caregiver could become, on occasion, an optimistic adventurer or even a cleanser, and there were moments when a nurse such as Wilson, the optimistic adventurer, could become a cleanser. It would be extremely unlikely, however, that the cleanser type would become an optimistic adventurer.

For Copeland and Knight, I draw upon their biographies as my main sources. Copeland collaborated closely with her editor, journalist Eugenie Louise Myles, to publish her memoirs in 1960, five years after her five-year sojourn on Southampton Island.[9] Published in 1975, Knight's biography came out fifteen years after she had left the North. For Wilson, I used primarily a collection of richly detailed letters that she wrote to her parents from 1960 to 1964. Historians face challenges in reconstructing experiences through these kinds of materials. Sources such as Wilson's letters are often considered more immediate, since they were written during the time and in the exact setting where the recorded events took place. Copeland and Knight, however, told their stories years afterward. While it is tempting to suggest that the passage of time allowed for reflection on and the shaping of their narratives, letters written by Knight immediately after her time in northern Canada reinforce the same doubts about her experiences that Knight's biographer expressed almost fifteen years later.[10] Nevertheless, we must approach biographies with caution and a realization that memory can distort what would appear to the reader to be exact details. The social context can change as well. What might have appeared to be a legitimate or socially acceptable type of work for nurses in the 1950s may have been, only twenty years later, called into question as a colonizing enterprise.

## Northern Health Services

Immediately following the Second World War, the Canadian federal government increased its efforts to provide health care in the Canadian Arctic. Until 1945, Westernized health care in the North was delivered mainly under the auspices of the Anglican and Roman Catholic churches. During the war, however, it was apparent, especially to American soldiers on patrol in the Arctic, that many Inuit suffered ill health. Their complaints, inspired partly by the increase in tuberculosis, placed pressure on the federal government to compensate for their apparent neglect. Instead of the handful of federally funded doctors who periodically travelled across the North, a new Indian and Northern Health Services (INHS) branch was established. It would employ nurses in communities of over 200 members. By 1963, the branch had a staff of 2,500 people, including nurses, doctors, dentists, and administrators.[11]

Officially, the government claimed that it wanted to provide a level of health care to allow "the Indian and Eskimo people of Canada to reach and maintain health and living standards comparable with those of other citizens."[12] In many public proclamations, the INHS referred to the government's moral obligation to northern Aboriginal people and, on occasion, noted that its budget, which amounted to $25 million in 1963, represented the "medicine chests" promised in treaties.[13] While the INHS employed the language of citizenship and morality, it also increasingly brought the North and the bodies of northerners under an administrative project directed by staff in Ottawa. No doubt, the presence of the INHS' nurses and doctors did much to alleviate the ill health that the Inuit suffered, but some scholars have criticized the program for either being colonialist in approach or not offering as much as it could have. In his work on Inuit reactions to incoming nurses, medical anthropologist John O'Neil argued that "northern medical dialogue is a discourse on colonialism, influenced heavily by the medical and nursing ideologies of control and surveillance."[14] Historian Walter Vanast was not quite as critical in his treatment of the history of medical care for the Inuit of Ungava. Instead, he believed the federal government "lacked motives for providing help and humanitarian agencies were busy elsewhere."[15] According to O'Neil and Vanast, a combination of neglect, parsimony, and colonizing discourse characterized northern health services. In general, this observation is true, but what is missing from their analysis is a close reading of the relationships that developed in northern communities between Natives and newcomers. Also missing also is an understanding of the ways in which the individual personalities of the nurses shaped the entire nurse-patient dynamic. Discerning individual differences or nursing types helps lend some complexity to the history of northern nursing, and it is to the three identifiable types that we now turn.

### Donalda McKillop Copeland: Cleanser

The cleanser type was obsessed with cleanliness, hygiene, comportment, and appearance and was probably the most interventionist in terms of wanting to remake or reconstitute Aboriginal bodies. Cleansers were zealous in their attempts to clean, and they were most concerned about children, although they would have been pleased to convert adult practices too. Aboriginal people had long known the cleanser type. Missionaries in northern Canadian communities from the late nineteenth century had often tried to introduce Westernized hygienic practices. Many historians of colonization have noted how intensively colonization was actually a bodily experience. Mary-Ellen Kelm, for example, argued that missionaries and other colonial agents recognized that in order to "capture" the minds of Aboriginals, they had to "capture" their bodies first. Bodily reform was part of this process.[16]

Nurses such as Copeland were trained in the fundamentals of the "germ theory" and were therefore highly conscious about cleanliness. The extent to which they had internalized ideas on hygiene is made clear by historian Kathryn McPherson. She argued that routine cleanliness, mixed with concepts about how germs were spread, produced in nurses an amalgamation of ideas. These ideas were well expressed by one early twentieth-century Canadian nursing student, who observed that the modern nurse was "constantly during the performance of her daily duties ... in close contact with practically all kinds of bacteria or disease germs, and not only [was] she in great danger of infection herself, but there [was] the possibility also of others becoming infected through her carrying germs of various diseases."[17] If it was difficult for Aboriginal people in northern communities to change their hygienic practices, so too was it challenging for nurses to confront their own deeply held convictions or to escape from the standards of their training. Ironically, cleansers rarely acknowledged traditional Aboriginal cleansing rituals or other traditional healing practices.

Evidence of Copeland's cleanser characteristics is found in her biography. The descriptions of her relationships with the Inuit of Coral Harbour/Salliq provide an opportunity to assess the extent to which Copeland tried to change the awareness of hygiene and germs in her community. Her closest friendship would turn out to be with Eenerook, or Tommy, as she came to call him. Tommy was one of the first people to greet her and her family upon their arrival, and Copeland quickly learned that he would be the sled driver who would convey them to their new community. Tommy, the son of a whaler, had already been exposed to other southerners. He made a genuine effort from the beginning to ensure Copeland's comfort. She recalled how he expressed his concern: "'There now. Are you fine?' he asked solicitously in English, and already I sensed that in the midst of my uncertainty and bewilderment I had found a friend."[18] Copeland was intrigued with the prospect of having so quickly made a friend and, she hoped, a cultural mediator: "Through Tommy, I was to turn the key to open partway at least the door to the closed world, the world of the mysterious Innuit [sic], or Eenook, whose chosen homeland the white men had so harshly invaded."[19] The nurse's romanticized notions of the "mysterious other" would quickly disappear. Only a few moments after she had expressed her contentment in finding a new friend, she undoubtedly began to wonder about how she could negotiate her position as a nurse and as a new companion: "To my open-mouthed astonishment, the driver Tommy stepped from his place before me and moved only a few feet away. There he freely relieved himself in the hard-packed snow. As he did so, a cloudy mist of snow arose before him. Already I was too chilled and numbed to be shocked, and too melancholy to care."[20]

This newly arrived southerner was "shocked" at Tommy's lack of shame. Neither this incident nor Copeland's shock would soon be forgotten. Later, at a community dogsled race, Tommy and Copeland made eye contact after the most respected hunter on Southampton Island went ahead and committed the same "transgression": "Near me Joe Curly relieved himself on the frozen surface, much to the embarrassment of Tommy. After that first day, Tommy had quickly become aware of the proprieties in the presence of the white woman and was never again guilty of overstepping these bounds."[21] Copeland thought that Tommy was embarrassed by Joe Curly's behaviour. Perhaps he simply felt awkward because he knew that she was passing judgment, not just on the individual involved but also on the Inuit in general. While this moment of eye contact between Copeland and Tommy exposes some of the tension that existed, it also appears that, for the most part, Tommy accepted the new nurse's anxieties about hygiene and germs. In fact, he frequently demonstrated a sense of humour about cultural and linguistic matters, although Copeland was sometimes unsure about his comprehension. When she was setting up her clinic on the back porch of her house, they had their first discussion about germs. However, as she repeated the word, she remained convinced that Tommy did not know what she was talking about. He soon revealed the truth, as she explained: "From time to time the women passed steaming mugs of tea. At first, conscious of the germ-laden surroundings in these damp unhealthy huts, I had politely but firmly refused this hospitality. To Tommy I had more than once mentioned the word 'germs,' although I doubt if he ever grew to understand its meaning. He was with me the first time I declined to have a cup of tea with my Eskimo hostesses. 'Germs?' he enquired softly, a wicked grin crinkling his bronzed face."[22]

Tommy had indeed clearly understood Copeland's germ phobia. In fact, this incident prompted her to carry her own mug so that she would not "offend the rules of hospitality" nor be forced to obsess about germs when sipping hot tea.[23] Tommy felt comfortable poking fun at Copeland about this germ anxiety, and in the end she confessed that "in the matter of germs there was no doubt but that Tommy regarded me as an absolute fanatic."[24] They were able to come to a mutual understanding, which sometimes even led to humorous jousting about the significance of germs. Despite being able to joke a bit, Copeland nonetheless remained relentless in her desire to change the Inuit's hygienic practices.

Copeland's most intensive cleansing efforts, or her self-confessed "citizenship work," was saved for the children of the community. Citizenship, hygiene, and moral reform were often intricately connected. In this case, the Inuit were being offered, through the health and welfare program, the rights of citizenship, but at the same time it was a very limited citizenship in the sense that there was a limit to the services provided.[25] Copeland's citizenship work started at the schoolhouse, where she set up a clinic to carry out bodily inspections of each child. She invited boys and girls to report to the nurse's office where she was prepared with her measuring instruments: "For each child I made the usual health record of height, weight, condition of skin, eyes, ears, and throat. After each examination, I held out a comb and they understood. Soaking my comb in cuprex, thoroughly I curried each head of straight black hair. In cases where the scalp was badly marked with lesions, I persuaded them to let me cut their hair shorter, and I treated the scalp with zinc oxide."[26] In one case, this procedure did not work out so well since the father of a young girl took deep offence at this newcomer cutting his daughter's hair. Strict taboos around haircutting did not stop Copeland from trying to clean up this young girl's matted tangles, nits, and "mass of ugly sores."[27] As she recalls, "that afternoon in my kitchen I looked up startled. There was Karsinga's father, Eetook, brandishing a gun."[28] Copeland was unapologetic and tried to explain the necessity for the haircut.

Her cleansing efforts did not stop at providing school inspections of childhood growth and hygiene. This first step instilled in her the need to go further with her reform program. She fantasized about how much could be achieved if structural changes were made to the school. One day, not long after the haircutting episode, she muttered out loud, within earshot of her husband: "'What a fine thing it would be,' I sighed, 'if only we had some sort of communal wash and bathhouse.'"[29] Harold Copeland set to work to make it possible: "In the school kitchen we provided a galvanized tub. The fire in the stove had to be kept going at all times to maintain the school temperature to a degree of working comfort. So we let it be known that after school hours anyone, man, woman, or child could come to the school to bathe or wash pieces of clothing."[30]

In comparing her efforts in hygiene to those of her husband in teaching, she claimed that his progress was as encouraging as hers was discouraging: "I toiled in the most dismal of atmospheres, the unsanitary, often filthy huts among adult minds not only distrustful and suspicious but unable to accept what was new and different. I faced too the challenge of trying to improve sanitation and health habits in the most pitiful of homes in the harshest of environments."[31] Copeland lamented her results with adults, but she felt somewhat more positive about the impact she and Harold had made on the local children. In her estimation, their hygienic work, combined with their attempts at "doling out of vitamins and cod liver oil ... [and] school lunches of soup, porridge, cocoa and milk were all building betterment."[32] Betterment, according to Copeland, could be measured by visible physical change, a healthier-looking population of children.

Like a missionary, Copeland tried to spread the gospel of hygiene, but in the end she was not entirely satisfied with her accomplishments and seemed disappointed with her results. Her determination to "cleanse" the population of their practices, to clean bodies, no doubt led to this disappointment. The nurse's expectations for change were impossible to meet. Had she attempted to see the value of Inuit culture and the practical difficulties posed by her goals she may have been able to measure her success on different terms.

## Dorothy Knight: Cautious Caregiver

Dorothy Knight was by no means as much of an interventionist as Copeland. The cautious caregiver is characterized by self-questioning, which we saw evidence of in the earlier passage in which Knight wondered whether or not she could actually help the Inuit. Knight wondered whether white women should be nursing in Inuit communities, and she would eventually come to question the entire northern medical enterprise. Her initial desire to work in northern Canada was not based on her belief that she could carry out social reform. When the government representative asked "why exactly" she wanted the job, she recalled being very blunt in her response: "'Because I'm curious!' she said. She felt a flush of guilt. Well, it was true. It wasn't some missionary zeal to improve the health of the northern people or save them from disease that had prompted her to answer the advertisement."[33] Perhaps this lack of "missionary zeal" is the most significant difference between cleansers and cautious caregivers. Not eager to change hygienic and health care practices, cautious caregivers instead tended to be interested in Native medicine, keen to record observations based on cultural differences but not in judgmental ways. Cautious caregivers were much more self-reflexive and conscious of moving forward carefully, both culturally and medically.

From the moment the ship pulled into Lake Harbour/Kimmirut, Knight threw herself into her work. A medical emergency awaited her. Marg Gardener, the Anglican missionary's wife, greeted her with the news that a young girl urgently needed her attention. Knight carefully checked the patient, taking a mental note of all symptoms, when suddenly Gardener asked: "What do you think?" "'I think ...' began Dorothy. She bit her lip, trying to hide her apprehension. What *did* she think? *Nurses don't diagnose,* she remembered Miss Beamish saying in Sarnia. For one thing, it's illegal! Five years after graduation, she could still see the coldly impersonal face of the nursing director as she pounded her awed students with the Rules. Dorothy checked the thermometer. It read 106 degrees. 'I think it's meningitis.'"[34] Knight scrambled to get the child ready to be flown to the *C.D. Howe,* the medical ship from which she had just disembarked. Given Knight's training, she was understandably nervous about diagnosing. Like all northern nurses, though, she was forced into offering a diagnosis, and she most certainly felt a real sense of accomplishment when she made the right call.

While Knight was cautious about diagnosing, she did not hesitate to engage fully in her multiple tasks. There were even moments when cautious caregiving gave way to practices that we would associate more with cleansers. At least one piece of evidence suggests that she did have cleansing tendencies, yet even in these efforts we can gain some insight into how she questioned her own instincts. Knight saw many children with common skin ailments such as impetigo and scabies. One little girl with particularly bad skin became a prime candidate for a dip in the bathtub. This bath became a community event that included Knight's interpreter, Ishawakta, along with Hilda Baird, the Hudson's Bay Company trader's wife, all ready to help out. Despite the group effort, the little girl began to scream with fear, prompting an early removal from the tub: "She sat in the living room, the sobbing girl cradled in her lap. *What am I trying to do?* she asked herself glumly. *I can't put bathtubs into every Eskimo dwelling in the Arctic.* She would take the girl back to the hospital and tell her mother to wash her with a cloth from a familiar pot. She had no idea when regular bathing would become a habit among the Inuit, but she would never subject a child to the terrors of the tub again."[35] The experience of trying to bathe a child, of actually embodying the cleanser type, left Knight unconvinced that she had the correct approach. The child's screaming was a reminder not only of the difficulty of trying to change cultural practices but also of the need to change the architectural structure of Arctic homes. This southern nurse realized that the little girl would be better off in her own home, cared for by her mother.

Knight also doubted the wisdom of evacuating tuberculosis patients to southern Canada. Tuberculosis was rampant in Arctic communities during the 1950s. The federal government responded by sending patients to southern Canadian sanatoria until they were well enough to be reintegrated. Even before she arrived at Lake Harbour/Kimmirut, Knight helped out at the clinics held on board the *C.D. Howe.* Inuit were X-rayed and checked over as the ship progressed from one community to the next. During one stop, Knight found herself thinking about that day's outcome: "She wondered bleakly how many new cases of TB would be detected that day and how many families would have to face the agony of knowing that one of their members must go south for treatment."[36] She was uncomfortable with the evacuation of tubercular patients because she could see the fear evoked by the prospect of having to board flights for the south and the toll it took on family members who stayed behind. She wondered why it was not possible for tubercular patients to be looked after in their own homes.[37]

In the context of the 1950s, however, treating people in their own communities was a radical idea. Even more radical was Knight's view that the Inuit should be trained as nurses and stationed in northern communities. She thought that it would make much more sense for community members to look after their own people, especially in light of the language barrier that she herself faced. Her biographer recorded Knight's curiosity over this matter: "She wondered why Health and Welfare had not instructed her to find a bright young Eskimo to learn some of the basics of nursing and perhaps equip him or her with a first-aid manual in syllabics. After all, the Bible had been brought to the Inuit in this way. Then she laughed. Health and Welfare had even forgotten to pass out manuals to their own northern nurses."[38]

On one northern sojourn between Frobisher Bay/Iqaluit and Lake Harbour/ Kimmirut, she met an Inuk man who was very capable in English. Out of curiosity, she found herself asking Simeonee, an employee of the Hudson's Bay Company store, "if he thought the Inuit would like to do the jobs for themselves that white men and women did in the Arctic." She was not surprised when "the Eskimo took several long drags from his cigarette and looked thoughtfully over the tundra before answering. 'Lutiapik,' he said slowly, 'how do we know until we try.'"[39] In just one year, Knight had moved from a position of wondering how she could help and if there was anything she could do in the field to an awareness that the Inuit themselves should be trained to nurse each other. By the late 1950s, the INHS branch had begun to train and hire Aboriginal people but often only as orderlies, ward maids, and interpreters. It would be some time before Aboriginal nurses began to appear in northern stations.

Knight's belief in the Inuit's ability to take care of themselves was provoked in part by the fact that, although she was one of the people sent to look after them, she was often the one who was looked after. This conundrum was especially evident as she prepared for and made several trips away from Lake Harbour/Kimmirut to the floe edge or to other communities or, at times, to just outside town for fishing expeditions. These trips forced Knight to appreciate the complexity of preparation as well as the finely tuned navigational skills possessed by the Inuit. Her interpreter Ishawakta did much of the work to transport her out to the communities where her skills as a nurse were required. On one such journey, she found herself wondering just exactly how he did it: "It was hopeless for a *kabloonah* to try to understand how the Inuit found their way around the seemingly featureless barrens. She sat on the *komatik* noting a distant mountain, a cluster of hills, a tall rock, and wondered how Ishawakta navigated by these few landmarks. There seemed little to guide him to Seemeegak's remote camp in Amadjuak country."[40] She was, however, utterly confident that not only could Ishawakta get her to where she was going but that he would also have packed all the necessary supplies for their travel.

Knight's experiences as an Arctic nurse offer a fine example of the cautious caregiver. Reluctant to rush into situations and cautious about offering a quick diagnosis, she carefully weighed her comments about the Inuit in most instances. She was skeptical from the beginning about how much her efforts would contribute to the better health of the local population, yet she was always available and keen to do her duty. She believed that there was much to be learned from Inuit culture and recommended that Inuit caregivers be trained in Western medical techniques so that they could help each other. The cautious caregiver type had little in common with the cleanser, but this is not to say that Knight did not on occasion exhibit cleansing tendencies. Yet the cleanser and cautious caregiver took substantially different approaches to northern nursing. Whereas the cleanser sincerely wanted to change behaviour, especially with respect to hygienic practices, the cautious caregiver was far more likely to understand that southern hygiene could take hold only if substantial structural changes were to take place. Like a cleanser, Knight periodically found herself growing impatient with the Inuit for giving in to what she saw as their version of fate. She wanted them to be more demanding of life, as had Copeland. However, Knight did not propose a program of reform to try to change this "characteristic."

The cautious caregiver had more in common with the "optimistic adventurer." Knight enjoyed the fishing expeditions and trips that she took to camps beyond Lake Harbour/Kimmirut, where she felt she came to know the "real" Arctic. At times, she marvelled at the vast expanse that she came to understand as the Arctic and, in so doing, exhibited some attachment to the place. The Arctic landscape undoubtedly formed an important memory of her experience of northern nursing. On one occasion, while out on a fishing trip with a few Inuit women from Lake Harbour/Kimmirut, she reflected on the meaning of life in the Arctic: "Dorothy tugged the hood of her parka around her face and stretched out on the ledge. She stared across the frozen lake. The surface glimmered under the moon. It must have been well below zero, but there was no wind, her clothes were warm, and the moss was comfortable. She slept soundly, woke when she was cold to stamp her feet or move her arms or legs. Then she slept again. She sat up when it was dawn. The stars were very large in the brightening sky. One of the dogs raised his head to look at her, then whined lazily and buried his nose in his tail. There was no movement from the peacefully sleeping Inuit. At last she felt she had met the Arctic."[41] These adventures, more than anything, seemed to satiate the curiosity that Knight felt about life in the Arctic – the curiosity that had inspired her to apply for her nursing job in the first place.

## Lucy Wilson: "Optimistic Adventurer"

Another type of nurse who emerged through my investigation of oral interviews, biographies, autobiographies, and archival collections is the "optimistic adventurer." Lucy Wilson is best described as a woman who went north with a sense of adventure. This type of nurse treated her time in the North as an opportunity to learn as much as she could about the people, environment, and landscape. She participated in opportunities provided particularly by the unique outdoor activities and learned as much as she could about local history from both the Aboriginal people and the resettlers – the newcomer white population, particularly the older trappers. Optimistic adventurers tended not to want to change the Aboriginal people. They could be critical but were less likely to reinforce stereotypes. They tended to be positive about Aboriginal culture and, in some cases, sought to learn as much as possible about Aboriginal traditional healing practices. Also, these nurses were more likely to break the rules by doing things such as sheltering dogs, and they generally did not complain about the North. They did not feel compelled to question their place as white women in Aboriginal communities. They took their tasks seriously but also enjoyed other aspects of northern living.

Most outpost nurses, almost by definition, had to have some sense of adventure. They had to be willing to travel and to attempt to fit into their new communities. Whether they were travelling to Ceylon in the late nineteenth century or to Africa in the second half of the twentieth century, nurses were often captivated by the promise of new experiences, travel, and remoteness.[42] As demonstrated by historians Christina Bates, Dianne Dodd, and Nicole Rousseau, they also had to be fiercely independent. As one of these authors noted, one Québec nurse "donned breeches, cut her own firewood and negotiated with local residents."[43] Independence was the key to the outpost nurses' success, especially in northern Canada. However, according to scholar Helen Gilbert, the northern outpost nurse is often conflated with ideas about imperialism "as she implicitly follows the footsteps of the imperial explorers through the *terra* incognita ... [and] moves into a space in the colonial imaginary always already inscribed with promises of heroism, adventure and even romance."[44] Gilbert's study of recruiting advertisements for northern nurses in *Canadian Nurse* suggested to her that most narratives about nursing in northern Canada were overwhelmingly positive and simplistic: "This nurse-meets-north narrative is typically styled as a travelogue of sorts, introduced with some kind of verbal or visual hook, lavishly illustrated, and often elegiac in tone. A strong affirmation that the northern experience was, or will be, worth all the hardships invariably provides an up-beat narrative closure."[45] Gilbert would no doubt view the optimistic adventurer category with some skepticism, thinking that those who fell into it had perhaps been duped by the rhetoric of colonization and the hegemonic tropes of nordicity – of humans versus nature. There could be truth to this perception. Some women also may have been attracted to the North because it offered independence and adventure. Appealing to these instincts might have served the government's program well. While reinforcing Gilbert's concerns about romanticizing the north, Lucy Wilson's letters also suggest the appeal of the North for someone with her predisposition and training.

Wilson started her northern nursing career as a relatively recent graduate, having completed her nurse training in 1958 at the Royal Alexandra Hospital in Edmonton, Alberta. She had had six-months' experience at the Charles Camsell Hospital in Edmonton and had also worked for eighteen months for Alaska's Native Health Services. This young nurse's first INHS posting was at Cambridge Bay/Iqaluktuutiak, in present-day Nunavut, where she stayed for one year before transferring to Fort McPherson/Teet'lit Zhen in the Northwest Territories. Wilson's day-to-day duties in the nursing stations consisted of caring for maternity cases and looking after sick children, especially babies who suffered from various infections or pneumonia. On a regular basis, she also tended to standard cuts and wounds. When patients presented at the nursing station and were diagnosed with extreme illnesses, she usually arranged, if time permitted, for them to be flown to southern Canada, often Edmonton. She treated whatever illnesses she could, however, in the North.

Wilson's optimism seems apparent from the beginning of her sojourn. She arrived prepared to traipse around in snowshoes but found it more convenient just to walk on the drifts. She was pleasantly surprised by the helpfulness of both the Aboriginal woman hired to work at the nursing station and the male caretaker: "David is the caretaker also native and is a real nice fellow too. There doesn't seem to be much he can't do. He's the handyman, carpenter, water and oil checker and anything else." She noted as well that the newcomers in the community were keen to socialize: "The station here seems to be quite a popular stopping place to everybody which results in a frequent cup of tea, coffee, or chocolate. So is all very social indeed. I think I'm really going to like it here and soon we'll be settled in & become acquainted with everyone and everything."[46]

At Cambridge Bay/Iqaluktuutiak, Lucy Wilson worked with a nursing partner and quite frequently had to fly to smaller Inuit encampments when medical emergencies presented themselves. Her first voyage was to Byron

Bay and Pelly Bay, west of Cambridge by about 150 miles, where she found the residents, as she put it, a "healthy well fed looking lot," and their homes quite comfortable: "Some were igloos, some were tents with snow built over and some were small wooden shacks. All in their own way were snug and warm – everything is really piled up and stacked in. They use seal oil for fuel and coal oil or gas lanterns for light. The Pelly Bay people are quite well off as they are able to hunt lots of seal, occasional walrus, quite a few polar bear and foxes. Also the fishing is supposed to be about the best there too."[47] She observed that the community members were independent and healthy, except for minor problems such as eye infections. She felt warmly welcomed as an outside visitor. She also described in positive terms her visits with the Gwich'in along the Peel River, particularly at Fort McPherson/Teet'lit Zhen. She was pleased that most of the families spoke English, which, from her perspective, made it much easier to chat: "It is sure different to go home visiting here. You go in and have a real good conversation about many things instead of the smiling, nodding, and grunting type conversations I used to have with the Eskimos. Yet I'm rather nostalgic for them."[48]

From Fort McPherson, Wilson travelled out to communities beyond the town limits and held clinics up and down the Peel River. In her travels, she never failed to mention how much she enjoyed herself because of the encounters with her patients. They, too, were eager to visit with the nurse on her rounds and, as Wilson noted, they "usually invite[d] us for a cup of tea and maybe a piece of lovely cooked fish. At this one camp I had a piece of fish that I think was the best I've ever tasted. I'm liking these people more as I get to know them and feel right at home with them."[49]

As much as she felt right at home with the Gwich'in and the Inuit, she also enjoyed travelling and conversing with the men of the North, including the bush pilots, the RCMP, and the old trappers. In a letter written shortly after her arrival at Cambridge Bay/Iqaluktuutiak, she discussed how she travelled sometimes as the only woman in a large party of men: "You might wonder if I didn't feel a bit uncomfortable by being the only female among 20 men – I didn't. They all said I was sure good for morale and that I should travel the Dew Line. Well I told them it did wonders for my morale too so all were happy."[50]

Wilson fit in well with the newcomer men and appreciated any opportunity to get outside the settlements to visit with Aboriginal people and spend time at the Distant Early Warning Line camps. She joked about how one of these men, the cook at one of the camps, decided that she was in need of a haircut, and, after spending some time coaxing her, he took the scissors to her head of thick hair. "Well that darn so and so nearly shaved me bald! It didn't look so bad from the front for the simple reason he didn't get at the front. From the back I looked like one of the boys," she wrote her parents.[51]

Not only was she compatible with the adventurous men, but she was also inadvertently made to look like one of them. Certainly, a good sense of humour was a useful characteristic for optimistic adventurers in their northern Canadian travels.

In her usual optimistic tone, Wilson described various fishing expeditions, flight mishaps, and community sports day events as well as other special occasions in her letters home. In great detail, she described a Halloween party at which many of the newcomers and some of the Gwich'in dressed up in their favourite costumes. One Aboriginal man particularly impressed her. He had dressed as Jack London and made a great pretence of being a Klondike gold miner. As they danced together, he told her stories about all of the old timers: "He named off more characters and called them his partners more than I can recall of gold rush fame. Makes you realize that these Indians are far from illiterate or unread." The idea that Aboriginal Canadians were illiterate came from images in mainstream magazines, newspapers, and popular discourse.[52] Optimistic adventurers, however, characteristically appreciated First Nations' culture and practices and were able to see beyond the stereotypes in an attempt to broaden their horizons. Certainly, Lucy Wilson was able to accentuate the positive even when she recognized a difference.

Wilson, however, was not so keen on newcomers who complained about being in the North. Those who could or would not adapt to their new conditions tested her tolerance. She enjoyed the optimistic adventurers around her and made it clear that she wanted to work with those who were comfortable being in the North. She described one of her nursing partners as a recent convert to things northern, writing that "she has taken to curling with as much enthusiasm as she has taken to everything else up here ... She's really dug in, feeling at ease with all situations with a well-developed northern attitude of 'why get spastic?' I couldn't stand to work with anyone who insisted on getting frantic about things or was unhappy with the North."[53] She was especially critical of those who constantly complained about missing southern amenities.

Lucy Wilson was conscious of the fact that she was optimistic by nature and that she wanted to surround herself with those who were like-minded. Her goal was to keep busy and to try to see as much of the North as she could while she was there. She was as interested in the Aboriginal population and her patients as she was in the stories and antics of the newcomers. Unlike Dorothy Knight, she did not seem to question her place or wonder why the indigenous women were not being trained as nurses themselves. Nor did she, like Donalda McKillop Copeland, try to change the hygiene and bodily practices of northern children. She seemed to accept her patients and her neighbours as they were.

## Conclusion

A critical analysis of the nursing profession leads us beyond the purported goals of health care and prevention. Certainly, the Canadian federal government saw that introducing nursing stations in northern communities would help make a positive impression on a Canadian public increasingly informed about Aboriginal ill health. And as other historians have argued for other various colonial contexts, nurses risked becoming "tools of empire." The Canadian government, too, hoped that nurses would carry out "citizenship work." Yet, while these three northern nurses worked for a bureaucracy that had its own clear aims and purposes, they also had to forge day-to-day relationships that moved them beyond matters of surveillance, scientific technique, and colonial mandates. It seems quite clear to me that Donalda McKillop Copeland, Dorothy Knight, and Lucy Wilson began their work as northern nurses with the hope that they would be able to make a difference and help their northern patients. Both northern conditions and the nurses' individual personalities, however, prompted an array of adaptive responses. What emerges from the three sets of sources discussed in this chapter is a striking difference in approach, reminding us of the variety of ways that nurses reacted to their situations. They were not all colonizers bent on reshaping Aboriginal lives. Some were. They were not all post-colonialists conscious of the hegemonic health care enterprise. Some were. And they were not all optimistic adventurers, ready to make the best of whatever circumstances they faced. Some were. By sharpening our gaze to look at individual nursing experiences in localized settings, I think we can come closer to understanding the complexities and nuances of the historical record.

**Acknowledgments**
The author is grateful to the Social Sciences and Humanities Research Council for its support of her work. She would also like to acknowledge funding from the Associated Medical Services Hannah Foundation for the History of Nursing Conference held in 2005 where this paper was originally presented. Thanks also to all of the volume editors, especially to Jayne Elliott for her patience and her fine editorial work, and to Robert Rutherdale and Jim Miller for their ongoing encouragement.

# 5

# Region, Faith, and Health: The Development of Winnipeg's Visiting Nursing Agencies, 1897-1926

*Marion McKay*

In the history of public health, the emergence of visiting and public health nursing programs has received increasing attention in the past two decades. One focus of this body of work is the role that lay women played in the formation of visiting and public health nursing programs. For example, Karen Buhler-Wilkerson has examined the role of charitable visiting nursing associations, such as the Henry Street Mission, in the development of both visiting (home care) nursing and public health nursing in the United States.[1] Both faith and civic duty, she argued, underlay middle-class women's participation in the provision of bedside nursing services in the home. In her study of the development of the Los Angeles city health department, Jennifer Koslow persuasively argued that female social reformers initiated or proposed many programs that ultimately became the cornerstones of that city's public health system.[2] In Canada, lay women also established and lobbied for the provision of nursing services in the community. In addition to the national Victorian Order of Nurses that was instituted in 1897,[3] lay women were also involved in the formation of local and provincial visiting and district nursing programs such as the Lethbridge Nursing Mission, the Alberta District Nursing Service, and the Newfoundland Outport Nursing and Industrial Association.[4]

Historians have also examined nurses' experiences as the employees of philanthropic and publicly funded community health agencies. Buhler-Wilkerson has provided thoughtful answers to the perennial question of why public health nursing never attained the autonomy and prestige that early nursing leaders hoped it would achieve. The turning point for public health nurses, she argued, occurred in the 1920s, when philanthropic visiting nursing agencies began to decline and many of their programs were taken over by public health departments. These agencies constrained, rather than enlarged, the scope of nursing practice in the community. Unlike the privately funded visiting nursing associations, where nurses and lay women collaborated in the development of nursing programs, medical officers of health within publicly funded health departments shaped nursing programs according to a medical view of the community's needs.[5] In her research on the development of public health programs in British Columbia in the 1930s, Megan Davies made a similar argument, observing that "links with ... laywomen and with the older traditions of community nursing had to be severed in order for a scientific, professional model to be firmly imposed, and for the new order to be seen as legitimate in the 'male' eyes of the public health profession."[6]

Other work has also focused on the extent to which gender constrained the autonomy and scope of practice of Canadian public health nurses. In Ontario, the Ontario Board of Health, for example, employed child welfare nurses, who often worked alone and were compelled to make independent decisions about patient care. At the same time, they performed their work under the scrutiny of male medical health officers at the Ontario Board of Health as well as physicians in private practice in many of the communities in which the nurses worked. Meryn Stuart has argued that gender shaped the ambivalent and "often conflicted" relationships between the physicians and nurses.[7]

Notwithstanding the fact that the professional autonomy of visiting and public health nurses withered during their separation from the middle-class lay women who had first nurtured their practices in the community, the legacy of female-led social reform programs is mixed.[8] On the one hand, middle-class lay women played an important role in the social reform movement of the late nineteenth and early twentieth century. As individuals, their involvement ranged from friendly visiting in the homes of the poor to membership on the boards of their communities' organized charities. Collectively, middle-class women founded their own charitable organizations, which focused particularly on the needs of women and children. Often, professionally trained female social workers or nurses were employed by these agencies, and the task of providing direct services was delegated to them. Female-led social reform programs dedicated to the rescue of abandoned and abused children, the sheltering of unwed mothers, the redemption of "fallen women," and the preservation of the health of women and children are generally acknowledged as important contributions to health and welfare services during an era when the state did not necessarily provide these programs. However, female social reformers also exerted cultural control over the immigrant and working-class populations that were the focus of their interventions.[9] As a result, some historians have characterized their work with the "less fortunate" as paternalistic, conservative, and judgmental.[10]

This chapter examines the contributions that two voluntary nursing agencies, the Margaret Scott Nursing Mission (MSNM) and the Winnipeg Branch of the Victorian Order of Nurses for Canada (VON), made to the development of visiting and public health nursing programs in Winnipeg, Manitoba, between 1897 and 1926.[11] It will argue that regional ambitions and local anxieties played key roles in the development of these two organizations. In the course of providing much-needed health care services to Winnipeg's poor and immigrant populations, visiting nurses from both agencies used health teaching and direct care as vehicles for the dissemination of health and child care practices that were congruent with the ideals of the city's Anglo-Canadian middle class. As well, both agencies co-operated and interacted with a wide circle of other governmental and non-governmental agencies that concerned themselves with the Canadianization of recently arrived immigrants.

**The Regional Context**

Prior to 1919, Winnipeg's civic pride and sense of destiny outstripped its size and glossed over its geographic isolation from central Canada. The city's business and commercial elite, drawn almost exclusively from the ranks of Canadian- or British-born Anglo-Celtic Protestants, ceaselessly promoted Winnipeg as one of Canada's foremost cities and as the nation's gateway to the West. Winnipeg was to become the progressive metropolitan capital of "a new western Ontario," "loyal to the British connection, but free of the 'fogeyism' of Ottawa."[12] However, having only recently wrested political and social control of the former Red River colony from the hands of free traders, the Métis, and the employees of the Hudson's Bay Company, Winnipeg's new elite was faced with an even more pressing threat to their ongoing dominance of civic life – the immigrant problem.

The influx of Eastern European immigrants to western Canada created significant anxiety among the region's social and political elite. Some believed that the federal government's immigration policy should entirely exclude "this class" of immigrant. "Better by far," intoned the *Winnipeg Telegram*'s editor in 1901, "to keep our land for the children, and the children's children, of Canadians, than to fill up the country with the scum of Europe."[13] Winnipeg's industrial and business leaders were apparently no less convinced that Eastern Europeans were the least suitable type of immigrants arriving in western Canada, although they also realized that the presence of a large, cheap, and unskilled labour force was essential to Winnipeg's ongoing dominance of western Canada's industrial and business sector.[14]

Winnipeg's explosive population growth was an important factor underlying the class, religious, linguistic, ethnic, and political tensions that characterized the city's civic life in the early twentieth century. In 1871, the year of its incorporation, Winnipeg boasted a population of 241 citizens. However, from then until 1921, the city's population growth exceeded the rate reported by almost all other Canadian centres, propelling it from Canada's sixty-second largest city in 1871 to its third largest in 1911, a position it maintained until at least 1921. Its most rapid growth occurred between 1901 and 1916,

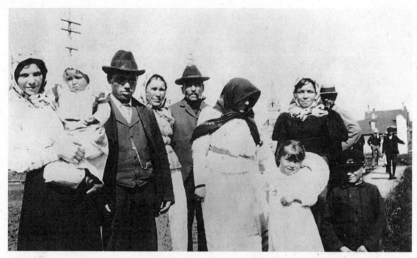

This photograph, taken in Winnipeg's North End in 1901, portrays a group of Russian immigrants. The waves of Eastern European settlers who began to arrive in Winnipeg at the end of the twentieth century threatened to transform the city's social landscape and undermine the dominance of the city's Anglo-Canadian citizens. Despite the manner in which some elite Winnipeggers represented these immigrants, the newcomers were as diverse as their Canadian- and British-born counterparts. *Courtesy of Archives of Manitoba, Immigration Collection 24, N25502*

when the population increased from 42,000 to 163,000. Eastern European immigrants were the largest single group to settle in Winnipeg during this era. Although the majority of those people residing in the city continued to report British origins, their relative dominance in the city's demographic landscape eroded from nearly 84 percent of the city's population in 1881 to 67 percent in 1916. Other western Canadian cities experienced similar or even higher influxes of foreign-born residents during this period. However, Winnipeg was the only urban centre where Eastern European-born immigrants outnumbered those migrating from Britain.[15]

Religious affiliations reported by its residents also reflected changes in Winnipeg's demographic composition. Although Protestant denominations continued to predominate, residents claiming membership in Protestant churches dropped from 86 percent of the population in 1881 to 71 percent in 1916. Those reporting membership in Roman Catholic churches rose from 13 to 18 percent during the same period. However, the most dramatic increase occurred among those of the Jewish faith, whose numbers increased from 0.3 percent of Winnipeg's population in 1881 to over 8 percent in 1916.

As the city developed from its original configuration as a small, undifferentiated settlement, most members of the middle class, particularly those of British origin, relocated or settled in newly developed suburbs a short

distance south of the city's Canadian Pacific Railway yards. In 1916, for example, 86.5 percent of those residing in the city's southwest suburbs were
of British origin. In contrast, 61 percent of the residents crowded into Winnipeg's North End, which was situated north of the CPR yards, were of
non-British origin. Many of the remainder were English-speaking working-
class residents, most of whom had recently emigrated from Britain.[16] While
British immigrants were not generally labelled as "foreigners," their class
position was an important determinant of their place of residence.

Although social class shaped the development of Winnipeg's residential
districts, ethnicity and social networks based on language, customs, and
faith more significantly determined the city's residential patterns. The un-
stable "intersection of class and ethnicity" not only underlay the material
deprivation of Winnipeg's working-class and immigrant populations,[17] but
it also played a key role in positioning them as a separate race, particularly
the Eastern Europeans. Differences in language, social behaviour, dress, and
personal hygiene simultaneously constituted both the city's "white" Anglo-
Canadian middle class and its "not-white" working-class and immigrant
citizens.

Many middle-class western Canadians defined "whiteness" as being the
essential trait of those of British descent. In his infamous editorial of 13 May
1901, W. Sanford Evans of the *Winnipeg Telegram* explicitly linked "whiteness" with Anglo-Canadianism, stating that "the white people of Western
Canada" did not perceive "Slavonic immigrants" as "desirable settlers."[18]
Even among the more compassionate and well-informed members of Winnipeg's "charter group," the "immigrant problem" created deep anxiety.[19]
For example, J.S. Woodsworth, the superintendent of the All People's Mission, devoted his energies to working with new immigrants.[20] Although
sympathetic to their plight, he also believed that not all newcomers could
be assimilated into Canadian society. In 1909, Woodsworth systematically
described the "typical type" of immigrant by country of origin. In his hierarchy of suitable immigrants, he placed British- and American-born middle-
class immigrants at the top of the list. He characterized Eastern European
immigrants as being distinctly different and much less desirable "newcomers." He signified the differences between these two "races" not by morpho-
logical characteristics or skin colour but, rather, by language, behaviour, and
social station: "The ordinary Canadian [that is, a white Anglo-Canadian
male] ... classifies all men as white men and foreigners. The foreigners he
thinks of as the men who dig the sewers and get into trouble at the police
court. They are all supposed to dress in outlandish garb, to speak a barbarian
tongue, and to smell abominably." Woodsworth also described English
working-class immigrants in racialized terms. Irish, Scottish, and Welsh immigrants, he asserted, did well in Canada, but the "failures" of English cities
and the "culls from English factories and shops ... cannot compete with

other English-speaking people and often not with non-English, despite the latter's disadvantages in not knowing the language."[21]

Spatial, material, and "racial" divisions created two solitudes within the city. Winnipeg's North End was virtually *terra incognita* to the city's middle-class residents, who formed their perceptions of working-class and immigrant life in the city as much by prejudice as by reality.[22] Crowded into substandard housing and beset by many health problems, Winnipeg's working-class/ immigrant population was regarded with a combination of loathing and compassion by the city's middle-class Anglo-Canadian citizens.

Apprehensive of the potentially destabilizing impact that large numbers of "foreigners" might have on the city's social fabric, Winnipeg's political and social leaders embarked on a number of initiatives to assimilate them and "to make them ... good Canadians."[23] Assimilation is a contested term whose meaning shifts in relation to both time and context. In early twentieth-century Canada, assimilation was conceptualized by the dominant Anglo-Canadian culture as a process that compelled immigrants to conform to Anglo-Canadian beliefs, values, and customs and to adopt this "superior" way of life.[24] The establishment of institutions to care for the sick poor was an important component of middle-class efforts to assimilate Winnipeg's recently arrived immigrants. The Winnipeg General Hospital (WGH), founded in 1872, provided public wards for indigent patients.[25] The city offered organized relief, although apparently it was provided on a very parsimonious basis, as early as 1874. Other agencies devoted to the relief of the poor and the assimilation of the city's immigrant population included the All People's Mission, founded in 1892, and the Associated Charities, founded in 1908.[26]

Social reformers also identified the need to provide skilled nursing care to the sick poor in their own homes during this period. In 1897, at the urging of the Local Council of Women (LCW), Winnipeg's Anglo-Canadian citizens participated in the national debate regarding the proposed establishment of the VON to commemorate Queen Victoria's Diamond Jubilee.[27] Shortly after the *Manitoba Free Press* published the national VON proposal on 23 April 1897, deputations from the LCW appeared before the council and civic finance committee requesting that the city assist them in establishing a committee to "consider the best means of raising the funds necessary to carry out the scheme" in Winnipeg.[28] Despite the support of prominent civic politicians and citizens, the organizing committee encountered very effective opposition from local physicians. The establishment of an endowed visiting nursing order posed a real threat to western Canada's medical community. Many rural physicians could not attract enough paying patients to sustain themselves and their families, and even in Winnipeg ordinary "medical men" scrabbled to make ends meet. Subsidizing nurses to care for the poor, they believed, placed nurses and physicians in direct competition by sending

in "the assistant before the principal is summoned."[29] Instead, local physicians proposed that medical services should be subsidized: "If a doctor could
be subsidized with $300 to $500 they [the patients] could be treated on
paying a nominal fee."[30] Otherwise, young physicians could not expect to
earn a living, as Dr. Hutton argued at one of several public debates regarding
the VON.[31] However, regional ambitions also influenced the medical community's response. Local physicians asserted that they, rather than the
easterners, knew best what was needed in western Canada. "With our more
perfect knowledge of work in attendance on the sick," they pronounced,
"we feel sure that the scheme, as outlined in the announcement given to
the public, so far as Manitoba and the Northwest Territories is concerned,
will prove an entire failure."[32]

Regional priorities also underpinned the response of the local politicians
who opposed the VON proposal. In 1897, Winnipeg was still a fragile Canadian transplant situated on the edge of a vast, sparsely settled hinterland.
Its citizens were acutely aware of the city's tenuous position and of the need
to nurture its own recently established social institutions. Lady Aberdeen's
"ill digested"[33] plan was perceived by some as being a potential threat to the
proposed construction of a Jubilee Wing at the WGH. Local proponents of
this initiative feared that a simultaneous appeal for funds to support the
VON would hamper their fundraising campaign. "The citizens," argued
Alderman Alfred J. Andrews, the council's representative to the WGH Board,
"would require every cent to perfect the organizations they had already
started and which would fail if not aided at once."[34]

The VON proposal also undermined local efforts to consolidate the hospital's position as the region's leading medical institution. Twenty-five percent of the patients treated at the WGH came from outside the city limits,
but the hospital's capacity to respond to the steady demand for specialized
medical care was compromised by its precarious financial position.[35] Arguing
that an expansion of the WGH was a more effective way to meet regional
health care needs, Alderman Andrews stated that the facility merited the
wholehearted support of the community because its costs were significantly
lower than those reported by similar institutions in eastern Canada.[36]

Those opposed to the VON proposal moved quickly to consolidate their
position. In June 1897, the WGH's directors launched a public appeal for financial support for its proposed expansion.[37] To quell potential public criticism of their unwillingness to support the VON proposal, the hospital
directors also decided that "district nursing should be taken up by the hospital." Ida Memberry, a recent WGH training school graduate, was to work
"under the instructions of the medical superintendent and ... gratuitously
attend in their homes such patients as the city health officer certifies are
proper cases for her services."[38]

The successful campaign to expand the WGH and provide a local alternative to the VON effectively prevented the LCW from establishing a VON branch in Winnipeg, and the local organizing committee disappeared until 1901. From 1901 to 1905, despite the fact that nine local branches in eastern Canada operated urban visiting nursing programs, Winnipeg's local VON committee devoted its full attention to the establishment of cottage hospitals in rural Manitoba and the Northwest Territories.[39]

## The Margaret Scott Nursing Mission

Despite the significant local support that marked the establishment of a visiting nursing program in Winnipeg, the WGH's initiative failed to flourish, and in June 1901 the hospital discontinued the service.[40] Although the hospital did not explain its action, the facility's *Annual Report* of 1900 noted that when the district nurse went on leave for five months during the summer, there was not enough work to warrant hiring a replacement.[41] Other sources state that financial shortfalls led to this decision.[42]

The burden of providing care to the sick poor therefore fell upon Margaret Scott, a lay city missionary. Scott, who had been widowed at a very early age, moved to Winnipeg in 1886 where she found employment as a stenographer at the Dominion Land Office and later at a local law firm. A devout Anglican, Scott volunteered for Reverend C.C. Owen at the Holy Trinity Church, helping with his correspondence that was related to charity work. Owen encouraged Scott to leave her employment and devote herself to the care of the poor. In her new role, Winnipeg's "Angel of Poverty Row" visited the sick and delivered donated food and clothing to the needy. Scott had no formal nursing training but read widely to learn about how nursing missions, public health departments, charities, and social service agencies operated in other cities.[43] Believing that God would provide what was needed, Scott never accepted a salary for her work.[44]

Soon after the withdrawal of the WGH visiting nurse, Winnipeg businessman and philanthropist E.H. Taylor offered to pay the salary of nurse Elizabeth Lamont to assist Scott. In 1902, he persuaded City Council to pay half of these costs.[45] After Taylor's death in 1903, the city included the district nurse's full salary ($600 per annum) in the Department of Health's budget.[46] However, this arrangement also proved to be short-lived. Although many leading citizens insisted that Winnipeg was "a city in which poverty practically does not exist," a severe typhoid epidemic in the summer of 1904 necessitated the hiring of a second nurse to help Scott and district nurse Elizabeth Lamont with their work.[47]

Not surprisingly, the response to the typhoid crisis came from the city's evangelical Protestant women. In early May 1904, Mrs. A.M. Fraser invited "lady delegates from the Churches" to attend a meeting to discuss the establishment of a nursing mission to support Scott's work with the sick poor.[48] It would provide nursing care and health instruction, "above all, seeking with Christian influence to raise their moral tone to all that is highest and best."[49] On 12 May 1904, the Reverend C.W. Gordon and a "group of interested women" gathered at Fraser's home to discuss the proposal. Gordon's arrival at the meeting, it appears, was unexpected. The *Manitoba Free Press* reported the following day that he had apologized to those present, stating that "he had not understood that it was a ladies' meeting only."[50] However, his presence at the meeting signalled very powerful links between the MSNM's work with the sick poor and evangelical Protestantism. In the early twentieth century, Winnipeg was the epicentre of the Canadian social gospel movement, which articulated Christian faith in the language of social salvation and the attainment of God's kingdom on earth.[51] Gordon, better known by his pen name of Ralph Connor, was a nationally known leader in the social gospel movement, an ardent anglophile, and a passionate proponent of the assimilation of Canada's "foreign" population.[52]

The belief that Winnipeg's unique needs and demographic characteristics required a local solution underlay the MSNM's formation and its desire "to assist ... a different kind of poor than exists in many of the older cities of the Dominion."[53] At the MSNM's first public meeting, John S. Ewart, King's Counsel, was at pains to point out that Winnipeg had been the first Canadian city to pay a visiting nurse's salary out of civic funds. Further, he stated, only Toronto had made similar provisions by granting a local nursing mission $200 per annum to support its services. Thus, the proposed "expansion of old benevolence on new lines" asserted both the MSNM's unique local heritage and its linkages to "similar societies in other cities of the Dominion."[54] The mission's most enthusiastic advocates included prominent local clergymen representing Winnipeg's major Protestant churches. Several of their wives, including Mary Coombs (wife of Reverend George Coombs), Helen Gordon (wife of Reverend C.W. Gordon), and Alice Matheson (wife of Archbishop Samuel Matheson), served on the MSNM's Board of Management in its early years. As well, many of their congregations already supported outreach services within the city, including the All People's Mission, and were more than willing to support the MSNM's efforts to relieve the suffering of the poor and to mitigate the "immigrant problem."

Gender also played a role in the MSNM's founding. The seemingly effortless manner with which Winnipeg's visiting nursing service was transferred from the male-dominated WGH and city health department organizations to a voluntary women's association is an indication of the consensus on both sides that women were more suited to the business of providing visiting nursing services to the sick. In the wider efforts to protect the health of the city's citizens, men had other demands on their time and energy. For instance, in 1904, the male-dominated city health department, under the leadership of Dr. A.J. Douglas, focused on the construction of sanitary infrastructures, the cleanup of city streets, and the regulation of the food and water supply.[55] Providing direct care to the indigent poor was not yet part of the department's mandate. Transferring the city's visiting nursing program to evangelical Protestant women gave the responsibility for this work to those perceived to have the most appropriate skills and talents to execute it. The tact, sympathy, and innate godliness of the nurses and lay women associated with the mission, argued the physicians, clergy, and businessmen who publicly endorsed the plan, would do far more than provide much-needed nursing care to the sick. It would, in addition, elevate the physical and moral standards of "the foreigners" and forge a "closer relation between the churches and the homes of the ignorant poor in congested and unhealthy districts of the city."[56]

Armed with the support of civic authorities, the Protestant churches, and the business community, Scott's supporters quickly established the details to put the MSNM in place. In late 1904, it was formally incorporated, and "the ladies" took over the administrative responsibility from the former city district nurse, Elizabeth Lamont, and her assistant, Eliza Beveridge.[57] Margaret Scott assumed a somewhat ambiguous position within the MSNM's administrative structures. In 1904, she was named a member of the Board of Management, but by 1905 her position had changed to honorary life member, ultimately evolving to the position of honorary president. In 1907, Scott took up residence at the mission and continued with her own lay missionary work until her death in 1931.[58] The superintendent of nurses directly supervised the nurses and the services that they provided to the MSNM's patients. However, Scott's honorary status in no way diminished her influence over its work. The focus of the mission's nursing programs and the domestic arrangements within "the Home" at 99 George Street were, in large part, a direct result of Scott's recommendations to the board.

The MSNM accepted requests for visiting nursing services from a variety of sources, including other social service agencies, the health department, private physicians, and the families themselves. Since their mandate was to provide nursing care to the destitute, the nurses subjected every family they visited to a means test. The visiting nurse documented the number of family members, their ethnic origin, citizenship, years lived in Canada, religion, employment, income, and housing arrangements (including the presence of boarders). These particulars occupied the majority of space on the application form. She gathered sketchy information about the medical problem that precipitated the nurses' visit as well as the attending physician's name and information about any social assistance that the family might be receiving. Two different individuals completed many of the applications. The first was the visiting nurse, who signed as the "investigating nurse." Eliza Beveridge, who had succeeded Lamont as the MSNM's superintendent of nurses in 1905, completed the remainder of the form. Beveridge also evaluated the information and either approved or rejected the application. The most frequent reason for rejection was the discovery that the family could afford to pay for nursing services. In this case, they were referred to the VON or a private duty nurse for further care.[59]

The MSNM's physical location symbolized its function as both a provider of health care to the city's most destitute citizens and a rampart of Anglo-Canadianism in Winnipeg's "immigrant district." In the fall of 1905, the mission moved to its permanent headquarters, which was located a few blocks south of the CPR main line that separated the city's "unfashionable ... cluster of little black shacks" from the city's business district and the more distant southern suburbs where "the good folks of Winnipeg lay snug and warm in their virtuous beds."[60] At this location, on the physical and psychological margin between the city's Anglo-Canadian roots and its uncertain future, "the ladies" of the board were "at home" to their Anglo-Canadian supporters on the first Saturday of each month in order to interest them in the MSNM's work.[61]

The differences of class, faith, and ethnicity between the MSNM's Board of Management and the population that it served are striking. Between 1904 and 1921, the board was composed entirely of English-speaking Protestant women born either in Canada or Britain. In contrast, Eastern Europeans, Catholics, and Jews made up the majority of the MSNM's patients. Between 1904 and 1921, nearly 64 percent of those people visited by the mission's nurses were immigrants from non-English-speaking countries. Approximately 50 percent were Eastern Europeans. Thirty percent of the mission's patients were Roman Catholic and 19 percent were Jewish.[62] During this same era, Roman Catholics never represented more than 18 percent of the city's total population, and Jews made up only 8 percent.[63]

The husbands of the MSNM's board members represented the city's political, business, and professional elite.[64] Of the seventy-four women affiliated with the Board of Management between 1904 and 1921, seven were married to millionaires. In contrast, the overwhelming majority of the mission's patients were employed in unskilled and semi-skilled occupations, and most of the families lived in absolute poverty. Analysis of the financial information documented on the MSNM's application forms reveals that many of the applicants' reported annual incomes were only half of the amount necessary for a subsistence existence. They also reported significant levels of unemployment and underemployment.[65]

The MSNM played an important role in shaping the identities of the middle-class women who served on its Board of Management. In the late nineteenth and early twentieth centuries, friendly visiting in the homes of the poor was an accepted expression of female piety and charity. In 1907, board members formally adopted this approach to their charitable work and began to visit the mission's patients in order to "get in touch with the sick and poor."[66] It established a visitor's committee, and each month two board members visited selected patients, either at home or in the hospital. Unlike the practice that earlier visiting nursing associations in the United States and Britain had adopted, there is little evidence that MSNM board members regularly recommended nurses to visit individuals and families nor did they select patients for their visitors' committee.[67] Instead, they chose appropriate patients from a list that Eliza Beveridge provided. Language barriers limited the board's choices and their ability to interact with most of the mission's patients. Despite the fact that the majority of the patients were non-English-speaking immigrants, most of those identified in the minutes who received visits from members of the Board of Management had surnames suggesting a British origin.[68]

From the perspective of the board members, the goal of friendly visiting was to create sympathetic relationships between the recipients and the providers of charitable works, although little can be learned about the real impact that the friendly visiting program had on those visited. Sources providing insight into the patient's responses to these visits are not available. However, this work was profoundly rewarding to the women who served on the board's visitors' committee. Friendly visiting enabled board members to demonstrate to the city's impoverished citizens that their suffering had not gone unnoticed by the city's leading citizens.[69] Personal and spiritual growth were also valued outcomes of their charitable work. In her farewell address to the board, which was read aloud at the annual meeting since she was too ill to attend, Board President Georgianna Wood reflected on the personal impact of her work for the MSNM: "I can say with abundant joy and satisfaction that my connection with the Mission, and contact with Margaret Scott, has been in my life an inspiration and a great privilege, and has afforded me the opportunity of seeing ever near the heart of things both human and divine."[70]

Friendly visiting also gained the respect of fellow Anglo-Canadian Winnipeggers and consolidated the MSNM's status as Winnipeg's premier visiting nursing agency. The obituary of Mrs. A.F.D. MacGachen, a board member from 1908 to 1917, emphasized this aspect of the board's friendly visiting program: "She was especially loved for her interest and sympathy for the sick and poor of the city; and many homes were brightened by her frequent visits, which she paid in a very unobtrusive way."[71]

As white middle-class females ministering to ethnic and racialized "others" in their own community, Winnipeg's female social reformers had their own "mission" upon which they could bestow their religious fervour. Creating God's kingdom on Canadian soil enabled them to fully participate in the worldwide social gospel movement. It also gave them considerable personal and public freedom. These women managed the MSNM's programs and entered into co-operative ventures with other social service agencies, including those dominated by men. Board members moved freely in the political and public spaces of the city, including the city council chambers, the board rooms of local businesses, and even the streets of the infamous "immigrant districts" to pursue their charitable work. In so doing, they approximated the autonomy and social power enjoyed by their fellow unmarried female missionaries working in the mission fields both at home and abroad.[72]

## Assimilation and Health Education

Assimilation of "the foreigners" was an important component of the MSNM's work with the sick poor. In a city divided by ethnicity, faith, and class, Winnipeg's middle-class women were uniquely positioned to create assimilationist projects and to put them on the public agenda.[73] They conceived social reform work among the immigrants as a womanly calling because it emphasized education and conceptualized those who needed to be educated as childlike or dependent.[74] Although they could not interact directly with male immigrants – lest this activity lead to accusations of impropriety – middle-class women could and did organize projects to "uplift" immigrant women. However, the direct imposition of middle-class customs, values, and beliefs was likely to be met with resistance. More complete assimilation could be accomplished through moral regulation, which, in its most effective form, actively worked to have each individual internalize the discourses, practices, and standards of the elite.[75]

Foremost among the MSNM's normalizing projects was the imposition of Anglo-Canadian middle-class standards of personal and household hygiene in the homes of the city's working-class and immigrant families. The appalling living conditions, high rates of sickness, and high mortality rates observed in the city's North End were the result of a complex set of circumstances that included the lack of running water and sewer connections, substandard and overcrowded housing stock, low wages, and chronic unemployment and underemployment.[76] Although the city's middle-class reformers recognized that the material circumstances of immigrant and working-class families were part of the problem, the alleviation of poverty was not their focus. They identified education as being the more appropriate remedy for the problem. In 1911, for example, while discussing Winnipeg's very high infant mortality rate, the city's medical health officer stated that "we recognize that economic conditions are responsible for a large portion of the infantile mortality, but we felt that no matter how bad the economic conditions, a very large number of children's lives could be saved if the mothers only knew that in the care of infants what not to do is often more important than what to do.[77]

By focusing on the "ignorance" of the city's "impecunious strangers,"[78] the MSNM's founders and supporters defined the plight of the city's immigrant and working-class citizens as a moral problem.[79] Only the liberal application of the "gospel of soap and water" and instruction in "ordinary habits of cleanliness" could lift the shadow of death and brighten their lives.[80] Louise Minty, the MSNM's secretary, drew particular attention to the benefits of alleviating the physical and emotional suffering of the sick poor by providing them with health information that would enable them to help themselves: "Such people when discouraged were peculiarly liable to typhoid and often the homes were not models of cleanliness. Yet although in many cases those helped by the Mission were illiterate and sometimes filthy, they had hearts which grew sore at the sufferings of their little ones and which felt the keen pangs of bereavement ... The Mission did a great deal of good in teaching people the rules of nursing and hygiene and habits of cleanliness."[81]

This difficult and complex work was delegated to the MSNM's nurses, who had considerable experience in negotiating the social barriers created by language and custom. The nurses' presence in the home was, in effect, the embodiment of all of the agencies and individuals who had supported the MSNM and/or who had co-operated with it in providing services to poor and immigrant families. The nurses both modelled and deployed the "gospel of cleanliness," and their visits represented the impetus and inspiration for the physical and spiritual transformation of the family's home. As stated in one annual report, "many are the pitiful sights that meet their eyes; a cheerless home; cold, untidy and unclean; emaciated children; a delicate mother and in her arms a little sick child crying from the cold, no fire, no nice warm food, no anything to cheer the heart. But when the neatly uniformed nurse arrives all is quickly changed. A bright fire is soon blazing; the mother is made comfortable, and the wee baby is washed and dressed; warm food is prepared; the house is made tidy; tactful suggestions are given as to better modes of management, while many bright and encouraging words are spoken, elevating to higher things."[82] Public tributes praised the courage and persistence of the nurses who dedicated themselves to this work, which was described as "a heavy task" and "one of the noblest works of Christian charity done in the city."[83] They deemed the nurses themselves to be "Samaritans" to the sick, "always ready to go out when summoned, whether by day or night."[84]

The MSNM's work with women and children created many opportunities to pursue the assimilationist agenda of the city's middle-class social reformers. Postpartum visits by the mission's nurses, for example, were a helpful and often appreciated service. Yet there is little doubt that they encouraged the substitution of Westernized child rearing practices for those of the immigrant's Eastern European homeland: "We pass into the inner room where we find one of our nurses busy bathing and dressing the baby and making the mother comfortable for the day. The poor woman's eyes are sparkling as she gazes at a bright colored quilt sent her by the mission. She is Polish,

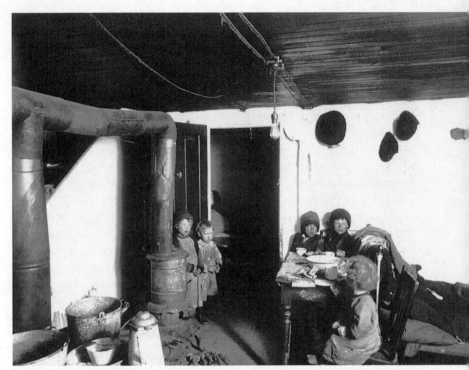

In 1916, J.S. Woodsworth commissioned this photograph, showing the interior of a slum home, for his book *(My Neighbour)* describing the work of the All People's Mission in alleviating the suffering of Winnipeg's destitute immigrants. Other social service organizations used similar strategies to elicit the charitable support of the middle class. However, these strategies also reinforced middle-class anxieties about the impact of unregulated immigration from non-British countries.
*Courtesy of Archives of Manitoba, Foote Collection 1492, N2440*

and cannot speak English, except to say, 'Tank you, tank you,' but her eyes show her pleasure. The baby, which had only been wrapped in dirty cotton rags before, is now washed and dressed in pretty baby clothes which nurse has brought with her. The mother and children look on admiringly. 'English baby,' the mother says and smiles."[85]

While working in the homes of the sick poor, the nurses embodied the social power held by the city's social reformers and the complex network of social service agencies that had been founded to work with Winnipeg's "less fortunate" citizens. Thus, whether they knew it or not, the nurses possessed considerable power over the families they visited. Their ability to scrutinize the living arrangements and financial circumstances of the MSNM's patients made them privy to information that might be of interest to other, potentially more punitive social service agencies. Destitute, recently arrived immigrants, for example, could be deported if their situation was reported to immigration officials. The nurses obtained and shared information with other agencies about neglected children, drunkenness, and marital infidelity. For example, the MSNM's case files in 1916 document that a police officer had discovered and reported to Children's Aid a mother whom he presumed too drunk to care for her children. Eliza Beveridge's subsequent investigation determined that the mother was fit to look after her family.[86] Although her assessment of the mother's competence might well be an indication of her sympathy and support for the woman, it also reveals the extent to which the city's health, welfare, and legal systems interacted to create a complex web of moral regulatory strategies aimed at the populations that the middle class sought both to assist and assimilate.

From its inception, the MSNM co-operated with at least seventeen other voluntary and governmental agencies.[87] This co-ordinated effort kept immigrants and the poor under the gaze of the city's social reformers. If the mission had been overtly oppressive, open resistance to its interventions might well have arisen.[88] However, given that its assimilationist agenda was contained within much-needed and often appreciated nursing care, the MSNM's efforts to shape the beliefs, values, and behaviours of the population it served were rarely publicly questioned.

Co-operation among the city's social agencies enhanced the degree to which moral regulatory strategies surrounded and penetrated the lives of immigrant families. In one example, the MSNM's nurses were summoned to care for a twenty-six-year-old male bricklayer who "seem[ed] not to have much wrong." They soon uncovered other information about this family's circumstances. M. Rodger, the investigating nurse wrote: "Woman has 3 husbands." Eliza Beveridge, after reviewing the case, added: "(married to 3) has lived with many men."[89] Two elements of moral regulation are evident. First, some of the information about this family was obtained from another agency. As well, the woman was not the individual requiring nursing care, and the man for whom the request had been made was not eligible to be placed on the MSNM's case load. Other cases also signal the mission's acute interest in the morality of the families its nurses visited. The 1918 case records document a husband's incarceration for indecent assault, which occurred at least five years prior to the MSNM's involvement with the family. In 1921, a case file contains details of a love triangle between a husband, his wife, and the wife's sister. The husband was described as being "on too intimate terms with the wife's sister who refuses to give him up."[90]

Inter-agency health care initiatives also sought to shape the behaviours of Winnipeg's immigrants. In 1911, the MSNM and the Winnipeg School Board co-operated to found the Little Nurses League. Miss Robertson, one of the mission's nurses, visited several schools in Winnipeg's North End to instruct school-aged girls about the basics of personal and household hygiene, including food preparation, infant care, and "how to guard against flies."[91]

Like similar programs in other North American cities, the league's other purpose was to encourage these students to teach other family members, particularly their mothers, about household hygienic practices. Thus, this program sought to impose middle-class domestic values not only on school-aged children but also on the adult members of their families. The manner in which the program positioned the school and school-aged children as normalizing agents within the family facilitated the broader agenda of assimilating the city's non-English-speaking citizens.[92] The program was deemed an outstanding success. In September 1912, the MSNM's board members were gratified to learn that, despite only a month of instruction, "the children had passed their first examination with surprising intelligence."[93] In an early example of the transfer of female-founded voluntary programs to the public sector, the school board undertook complete responsibility for the program in 1913 and expanded it to many other Winnipeg schools.

## The Winnipeg Branch of the VON

The VON also played a significant role in the development of visiting and public health nursing in Winnipeg. Indeed, in 1904, the VON's local Lady Minto Society might well have been the logical organization to take over and enlarge the city's district nursing program. However, as a result of the lingering impact of the 1897 debate regarding the merits of establishing a local VON branch, it was not requested nor did it offer to provide this service. Just prior to the 1904 public meeting at which the MSNM was formally organized, the Lady Minto Society's minutes document that a "lengthy" discussion of its "real work" took place. Ultimately, it was decided "that our efforts should, as in the past, be directed to providing the necessary furnishings for country hospitals."[94] The society's reluctance to compete with the work of the MSNM and the work of the revered Margaret Scott continued for several more years. In 1905, when the Central Board requested that a local branch be established in Winnipeg to supply district nurses for the entire West, the society did not immediately comply. Instead, it delegated two members to "obtain information relative to the scope of the Margaret Scott Nursing home and see if it would be feasible to form such an order without interfering in any way with it or other institutions of a similar character."[95] The society cautiously tested the waters six months later by employing a district nurse for one year.[96] Winnipeg's first VON nurse, Mary McCullough, arrived from Ottawa in December 1905.[97] Since there was a "decided antipathy to having the Victorian Order open a field of work in the city," the society made no public announcement of the nurse's presence in the city for eleven months.[98] Instead, it settled McCullough into a small apartment and privately introduced her to several local physicians.[99] Even though the experiment was so successful that it had to hire another nurse in the fall of 1906, the society continued to maintain a low profile.[100] It was not until December 1907 that it changed its name to the Winnipeg Branch of the VON.[101]

Like the MSNM, the VON's board was composed of women who represented the city's social and political elite. However, the VON and the MSNM differed in two important ways. First, the social gospel movement inspired the mission's work with the sick poor and attracted the support of evangelical Protestants. The VON was a secular organization. Second, unlike its locally inspired counterpart, the Winnipeg Branch of the VON deliberately cultivated the vice-regal connections that also characterized the VON's Central Board in Ottawa. The wife of the province's incumbent lieutenant-governor often served on the executive of the VON's Central Board, and, for the first several years of its existence in Winnipeg, the board held meetings at Government House. Although the province's lieutenant-governor also served as the MSNM's patron, the mission drew on the support of the city's religious leaders rather than its political leaders.

In order to avoid direct competition with the MSNM, the VON provided services only to those able to pay at least a portion of their nursing fee. It received requests for its services from a variety of sources but primarily from physicians and family members. As was the case with the MSNM, there is no evidence that board members sponsored or recommended patients on a regular basis. VON nurses made one visit to assess the family's health care needs and their ability to pay. They visited again only if the family physician requested and provided medical orders. Patients who were too destitute to pay the VON's nursing fees were referred to the MSNM.

Much less evidence of moral regulatory strategies is found in the records of the VON. No client files survive for the period under study, but the Central Board minutes and annual reports indicate that it focused far less attention on the "foreignness" of clients and the contrast between their standards of living and those of the city's Anglo-Canadian middle class. Instead, the reports and minutes of the VON's board emphasize its business-like practices, the educational standards set for the nurses it employed, and the many innovative new programs established in addition to the provision of bedside nursing care. Between 1925 and 1942, the VON operated child welfare clinics in the suburbs of St. James, Fort Garry, and East Kildonan. In 1922, it introduced a fee-for-service prenatal visiting program. The demand for this service was so high that it soon replaced individual home visits with group instruction at various locations in the city. As well, the Winnipeg branch was the first in Canada to offer an industrial (occupational health) nursing program. Between 1922 and 1929, it provided preventive and visiting nursing services to the employees of several large retail stores under an arrangement with the firms' owners.[102]

Although the VON's Central Board was apparently less interested in the assimilation of the city's immigrant population, it did establish one program that could readily be described as a project of moral regulation. This development occurred in the years following the 1919 general strike. Concerns about the true allegiance of the city's Ukrainian population pervaded Winnipeg's Anglo-Canadian middle class in the aftermath of this cataclysmic event. However, the MSNM and the VON responded to this potential threat to the city's civic order quite differently. The mission's records do not indicate that the general strike altered in any way their perception of the population that it served or the nature of its work. Indeed, the general strike merited only a few lines in both the board minutes and that year's annual report. From the MSNM's perspective, the major problem created by the strike was the difficulties with transportation, which resulted in the need to cancel one board meeting and recruit volunteers to drive the nurses to their home visits, since the street cars were not in service.[103]

The VON responded quite differently. Between 1922 and 1926, motivated by a belief that the city's Ukrainian population was a potentially seditious group, it provided maternal-child services to a group of Ukrainian women living in Winnipeg's North End. Describing it as a "counteracting influence" on the "communistic influence undermining Ukrainian society," the Central Board believed that the "Ukrainian Clinic" contributed to the maintenance of social order and the Canadianization of these immigrants.[104] However, discussions at the meetings of the board and Medical Advisory Committee revealed that the VON decided to take on this project only because the MSNM and other agencies were not responding to the perceived need for health care services within this specific population. At the VON's Medical Advisory Committee meeting of 27 March 1923, A.J. Douglas, the city's health officer, stated that "it was really the work of the Margaret Scott nurses, but they had been approached about two years ago, & as they had done nothing, the V.O. [sic] had decided to take up the work." As well, hoped-for hospital-managed clinics in the city's North End had failed to materialize, and the Federated Budget (the organization from which the United Way evolved in Winnipeg) was reluctant to become involved because of "the difficulty of the work being confined to one class, viz Ukrainians."[105]

For these reasons, the VON continued to operate the clinic despite its serious reservations about whether or not it was the appropriate thing for it to do.[106] When the clinic was first established, it collected no fees. However, in 1923, two board members recommended that the policy be changed. Both Mrs. Waugh and Mrs. Macleod "agreed that the patients looked well to do & able to pay a small fee, as they were getting a great deal for nothing," and they reminded the board that it was not the VON's policy to provide free services.[107] This sentiment was not entirely true. In several municipalities surrounding Winnipeg, the VON was providing free "teaching visits," child welfare clinics, and mother craft classes.[108] Insisting that the clinic's patients should pay for their health care services more likely signalled the Central Board's commitment to the principle of not pauperizing the poor and its desire to remind these "foreigners" that they were expected to make their own way in their adopted city. As a compromise, the board encouraged women who attended the clinic and who truly could not always afford to pay to sell embroidery and give the proceeds to the VON. This money was used to defray the cost of the clinic physician's salary.[109]

Throughout the clinic's existence, the VON's board vacillated in its support of the work and its opinion of the patients. In April 1925, for example, Mrs. Weed reported to the board that she had "gone to it [the clinic] prejudiced, but came away feeling that on account of these maternity cases & from the health standpoint it was worthwhile." Ten days later, she telephoned the board president stating that she had "revised her opinion" and felt that they must decide whether or not to offer services to a group of women who refused to go to the Winnipeg General Hospital for obstetrical care. In the summer of 1926, likely to the board's considerable relief, the clinic was closed. Maternal-child health care programs within the Ukrainian community were continued by "their own Mutual Benefit Society ... and by the outpatient department" of the newly constructed St. Joseph's Hospital, an institution that the city's Eastern European immigrant population had founded in the hope that their health care needs would be better served by members of their own community.[110]

## Conclusion

This chapter has argued that regional anxieties related to the assimilation of recently arrived immigrants from Eastern Europe shaped the organization and focus of early visiting and public health nursing programs in Winnipeg. A complex intersection of class and ethnicity simultaneously positioned the immigrant and working-class citizens of Winnipeg as "racialized others" and affirmed the Anglo-Canadian identities of the city's middle-class social reformers. The first organized response to the significant need for nursing services within Winnipeg's immigrant population emerged from male-dominated organizations such as the WGH and the civic health department. However, the MSNM, founded by the city's evangelical Protestant middle-class women, took on these responsibilities by 1904. As well as providing much-needed health care services in the home, the mission shaped its interactions with patients in ways that consciously sought to introduce middle-class, Anglo-Canadian beliefs, values, and behaviours to working-class and impoverished families. Although much less likely to interact with the city's most destitute residents, the VON, by founding and operating the Ukrainian Clinic, also consciously shaped its mandate to counteract the "communistic tendencies" of the city's "alien" population. Thus, both the MSNM and the

VON contributed to the Canadianization of recently arrived immigrant families, the maintenance of social order, and the early development of Winnipeg's public health and visiting nursing programs. The material and physical care provided to the "less fortunate," and the health education programs deployed in public schools and to new mothers, were convenient vehicles for the dissemination of multiple messages about the appropriate behaviour, attitudes, and beliefs expected of Winnipeg's "foreign" residents.

# 6

# "Suitable Young Women": Red Cross Nursing Pioneers and the Crusade for Healthy Living in Manitoba, 1920-30

*Linda Quiney*

Nurse M.R. Gant's report for the Kinosota Nursing Station in rural Manitoba on 30 September 1921 notes: "Had to go to a woman today who hurt her hand. She had rubbed it with skunk oil, covered it with burdock leaves, and then tied rat skin over that, and it had not been washed in a few years."[1] The outcome is not recorded, but the circumstances were far from unique. The station served a remote population, largely Métis, living in extreme poverty. Until the arrival of the Canadian Red Cross Society (CRCS), there had been no access to any kind of regularized health services in the region.[2] The nurse at the Fisher Branch Station, Edith Macey, also noted that she was required to perform major surgery on a cow and a horse, in addition to saving a flock of young turkeys with medication from the agricultural college. This last intervention saved the flock, earning a large donation for the CRCS and a turkey for Nurse Macey's Thanksgiving dinner.[3]

Nursing in the remote regions of rural Manitoba in the 1920s and 1930s was rarely dull, frequently unconventional, and demanded patience, perseverance, and a great deal of hard work. A special temperament was required to balance humour with a pragmatic approach to the unpredictable. Early in 1920, the Executive Committee of the Manitoba Division of the CRCS, which sponsored the establishment of the nursing stations, emphasized the need to encourage and develop nursing within the province as well as the "growing need" for additional services. The committee ruefully acknowledged that one critical problem was its "difficulty in obtaining suitable young women to take the training offered, from lack of means or lack of inspiration."[4] Consequently, attracting "suitable" candidates – women with the training, stamina, confidence, independence, and a sense of adventure necessary to face the challenges of unconventional nursing practice – became a matter of pressing concern for the division.

This chapter examines the goals of the state to ensure a healthy Canadian citizenry for the future, through the willing intervention of the CRCS and the work of the nurses charged with carrying out this mission, in the specific case of rural Manitoba in the 1920s. The conflicting realities of the nurses' experiences as "pioneer" health care providers in the remote nursing stations of Manitoba are explored in relation to the ideologies and expectations of nation building that were inherent in the CRCS' "Crusade for Good Health."[5] The chapter argues that regardless of the political agenda that underscored their employment, the outpost nurses of the Manitoba Division maintained their primary concern for the health and well-being of the people under their charge.

Part of the research for this chapter is based on personal documents, particularly those of Flora Hill and Margaret Litton, who were among the first generation of Manitoba's outpost nurses. While excerpts of the monthly reports compiled by several of the nurses are found within the records of the Manitoba Division's Nursing Committee, they are not always identified by name, and Nurses Hill and Litton left more concrete records. Hill's correspondence with the nursing commissioners in the 1930s, and Litton's memoir of her eight years as a nurse at the Fisher Branch Station, from 1922 to 1930, provide a more intimate and detailed insight into their relationships with the communities they served and the political interests that governed their role. Caution is necessary, however, since the correspondence of Hill is not complete, and Litton's memoir is subject to the limitations of memory and selective editing. Litton appears to have compiled her memoir long after her retirement from outpost nursing, and it is probably based on her monthly reports as well as on personal memories of the events she recorded and her impressions of the people with whom she lived and worked. Thus, memory is coloured by the passage of time, nostalgia, and the absence, deliberate or accidental, of pertinent detail. As such, while recognizing its value as a "first-hand" account of the time, we need to recognize its limitations as an accurate account of people and events. In addition, Litton left her work reluctantly, due to reorganization, but she makes no mention of this forced retirement in her account. Her negative feeling toward her retirement must be considered in the compilation of the document. Regardless, these personal documents offer invaluable windows into the distant era of Manitoba's pioneer outpost nurses.

## The Manitoba Nursing Stations
Following the First World War, the CRCS was transformed from a temporary wartime medical relief service for the military into a permanent peacetime civilian public health agency, rededicated to "the improvement of health, the prevention of disease and the mitigation of suffering."[6] The new CRCS was closely aligned with the national post-war agenda, enthusiastically promoting its new "crusade" for the improved health and well-being of

Canada's children.[7] As the spectre of social control hovered in the background, the concern to assist the government's goal to rapidly assimilate, or "Canadianize," new immigrant populations became a primary focus of the highly successful post-war Junior Red Cross school program. Directed particularly toward the children of Eastern European immigrants, these efforts served to motivate the CRCS to rationalize health services in rapidly expanding urban and rural centres across Canada, imposing a "civilizing" influence, particularly in the remote settlement regions of western Canada.[8]

In post-war Canada, increasing demands for improved health services and health education derived from a combination of social, economic, and health-related factors. The poor physical condition of wartime recruits, the recent influenza crisis, and alarming statistics on infant and maternal mortality compounded internal pressures, including the return of convalescent and disabled veterans, increased immigration, and the impetus to open up the West.[9] The CRCS worked closely with provincial health authorities to determine the needs of each region. It regarded nursing as critical to the restructuring of national attitudes toward hygiene, nutrition, and the "simple laws of healthful living" in order to help overcome deficiencies and guarantee a healthy and productive population for the future growth, prosperity, and defence of the nation.[10]

The growing concerns regarding health care and social services in Manitoba added to these problems. The influenza crisis had highlighted various inadequacies, and the provincial nursing associations as well as the CRCS cited the need for a reserve of emergency nursing personnel in both urban and new settlement regions, where provisions for general health care services were frequently non-existent.[11] In addition to implementing programs such as the Junior Red Cross and special services for veterans and their dependents, the new Manitoba Division of the CRCS gave special attention to the expansion of public health nursing, particularly in more remote and under-serviced areas.[12] Following the peacetime reorganization of the CRCS, provincial branches were given autonomy to control their own finances and consult with provincial health authorities in order to determine specific programs that would address regional concerns.[13] After 1919, the CRCS directed the main thrust of its programming toward the future, particularly toward the health of upcoming generations, since the society had adopted the late nineteenth-century reformist zeal that had characterized early public health activism. Delegates to the 1919 annual meeting of the CRCS went a step further, linking their efforts to the post-war ideology of citizenship and nationhood. Health education and public health nursing were ultimately endorsed by the governor general, as the representative of the state and the official patron of the CRCS, for "laying the foundations of a great nation such as Canada is bound to become."[14]

The nationalist rhetoric of the era and the optimism of the CRCS' new directive buoyed the Manitoba Division, which began to formulate its own provincial policies in 1920. One objective set out to increase the supply of graduate nurses through the support of existing training programs, with the goal of establishing a post-graduate nursing course in public health at the University of Manitoba.[15] The CRCS judged this program to be a priority in conjunction with larger, national initiatives to expand national public health services by developing graduate programs in designated centres across the country. By 1920, as Meryn Stuart argued, specialized training for nurses in Canada was fully recognized as a necessity for "the post-war work of re-construction and health education." University accreditation also had the potential to raise the status of nursing by identifying the nurse as a "profes-sional" public health worker.[16] The CRCS subsequently supported the estab-lishment of five university-based public health nursing programs, one on each coast and three in central Canada.[17] In 1920, however, a lack of programs still required public health nurses in Manitoba to complete their training outside of the province.

The most critical issue for the Manitoba Division, and for provincial public health authorities alike in the early post-war years, was the general lack of health services available to the province's more remote rural territories. These regions were defined by a mix of race, ethnicity, and economic diversity and were populated by new immigrants and untried, new war veteran farmers, as well as by long-term Aboriginal and Métis settlements. They had scant access to basic health or social services and endured much poverty and deprivation.[18] Kathryn McPherson has argued that nurses in the employ of public health agencies such as the CRCS were among the earliest of Canada's social welfare workers.[19] In the isolated regions of Manitoba in the early 1920s, the nurse's dual role of health care provider and social service worker was unquestioned.

Public health nursing was no less important in urban centres, but Winni-peg's Margaret Scott Nursing Mission had long provided auxiliary nursing services to the city.[20] The Manitoba Division agreed to fund two additional nurses for the mission and four additional nurses for the Victorian Order of Nurses (VON) in outlying areas, and further supported a province-wide program to establish social service departments in urban hospitals.[21] In the more remote regions, however, which lacked any existing service structures, the division consulted with the provincial health department and agreed to establish four nursing stations in the province.[22]

In 1922, G.J. Seale, commissioner of the Manitoba Division, described the situation in the remote regions as not conforming to "Canadian ideals" due to the lack of health services available to families struggling to bring order and productivity to the virgin territories.[23] The division's intent was to serve as a catalyst for establishing locally funded health services in these regions

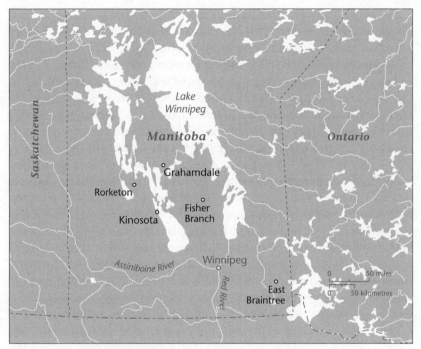

*Map 6.1* Canadian Red Cross Society outpost stations in Manitoba, 1920s
*Cartography: Eric Leinberger*

by supporting nurses' stations in the more isolated regions for a limited period of time. It was anticipated that within an agreed time frame, each district would begin to bring its nursing station under local management at the community's expense, and the division could then reallocate the funds to another needy district.[24] It established four stations between 1920 and 1922, and a fifth in 1924.[25]

A co-operative arrangement between the Manitoba Division and the provincial Board of Health determined that the society would cover the basic costs of maintaining the stations, including the nurses' salaries, the provision of necessary furniture and equipment, and all pharmaceuticals, plus medical and surgical supplies. The provincial authorities agreed to engage the personnel, determine the location of the assignment, and supervise and direct the nursing services, including any issue of discipline.[26] Planning moved ahead rapidly once the decision to initiate the nursing program was finalized, beginning with the establishment of station headquarters in the two initial districts to accommodate both a nurse's residence and a small emergency ward. A third "emergency post," which either of the nurses in the region could use as an overnight hostel, never materialized. Instead, the division established one station at Reynolds in a comfortable cottage, with walls of varnished wood and a fully screened veranda to protect against Manitoba's legendary mosquitoes. It contained five rooms with a water supply and telephone service, a three-piece bath, and indoor plumbing. The second proposed station in the Amaranth region was less promising. Asked to fund the construction of a suitable cottage, the community objected to the cost but agreed to donate labour if the Manitoba Division would provide the $1,500 for materials. The Division's representative, a nursing supervisor with the provincial Board of Health, caustically described a community eager for a nursing service but "unwilling to exert themselves" in helping to establish the facilities. The station was subsequently relocated to Kinosota, west of Lake Manitoba and thirty miles farther north than originally planned, but with "a much better prospect of co-operation." Established in a four-room duplex, the two rooms designated for the station, each measuring fourteen square feet, allowed for a modest hospital space on the lower floor and a residence above. The rooms had large opening windows to let in light and air, which was so essential to the contemporary ideology of the therapeutic environment, and water available in a nearby well, a wood-burning stove, and a properly maintained outbuilding for "sanitary convenience."[27] By the end of July 1920, the first two nursing stations were operational.

The caseload and hours of work steadily increased through the 1920s. Many factors contributed to the workload, including an increasing settlement, improved transportation, and the community's growing acceptance of the station nurse. The first two nurses in the program, Edith Frances Macey and Elva Gunn, were completely new residents in their communities. Over their first two months, each nurse treated just under 100 patients and spent almost 350 hours on duty. Only one-quarter of the patients came to the station so travel between the station and the patients' homes consumed the greater part of the nurses' time.[28]

By the spring of 1923, with four stations in operation, each nurse's caseload averaged 120 to 150 patients per month.[29] By 1929, with five stations in long-term operation, the demand for nursing service had increased steadily, although it varied by location, with East Braintree reporting 605 patients for the year and Rorketon reporting 1,393 patients. The passage of time had also resulted in a new classification system for "mileage" in the division's reports, indicating the increased pressure of development. Buggies and cutters were becoming the relics of an earlier era of district nursing, the automobile rapidly replacing them on new roads and highways. Nurse Flora Hill of East Braintree had the smallest caseload in 1929, but travelled a much greater distance by car than the other nurses over the year, covering 4,430 miles (6,900 kilometres). Nurse M.J. Robertson at Rorketon now treated the majority of her 1,400 cases at the station but still travelled nearly 3,000 miles (4,800 kilometres) to visit the others. Although by the end of the decade many patients now used their own vehicles to travel to the nursing station, the Nursing Committee concluded that nurses had covered nearly 14,000 miles in 1929.[30]

Kathryn McPherson argued that the urban private duty nurses of the era were "at best" the social equals of their patients and were generally assigned to cases from the middle and upper classes in rural Manitoba. The station nurse more often administered to families with meagre resources.[31] As an employee of the Manitoba Division and an agent of the provincial government, the station nurse provided a cost-free service for many patients who could ill afford a fee, had one been charged. The division nevertheless declined to characterize the outpost service as "charity." It expected its initiative to serve as an impetus to local organization and co-operation, to help develop a sense of citizenship and collective welfare. In assisting with "an ameliorization of conditions" by providing the services of a nurse, it hoped to demonstrate the value of having reliable and competent health care available in a locality. It anticipated that the community would begin to assume "a larger proportion of the responsibility" as conditions improved, allowing the division to gradually withdraw its support and "extend its benefits" to other districts in need.[32] The division's support was intended to be finite as the community developed a local system for covering the costs of the station. Within two years, however, it realized its expectations were overly optimistic and often unrealistic, given the demographic, environmental, and economic circumstances in the various districts. The Nursing Committee reported late in 1922 that the anticipated self-sufficiency of at least two of the four stations was "practically impossible of accomplishment" within the foreseeable future and, with considerable dismay, concurred that the work was developing along "purely charitable lines."[33]

Despite its original goal of self-sufficiency, the division agreed to assume full responsibility for the operation of the four original stations from the provincial Board of Health in 1923, continuing sole administration until 1928, when the province agreed to provide a grant of $500 for each station and $1,000 yearly thereafter. During the time that the Manitoba Division held full control, communities formed local nursing committees to help with the administration of the stations, with the expectation that they would provide a percentage of the upkeep. As Jayne Elliott noted, by 1923 the local Nursing Committee at Rorketon had guaranteed 15 percent of the operating costs of the outpost.[34] East Braintree was also able to contribute about 15 percent to the operating costs, but by 1929 the division had determined that $300 per station was a sufficient contribution, having long since abandoned expectations that the stations would be fully self-sufficient.[35] Although the national policy was to avoid the impression that the society was a "charitable" organization by encouraging self-sufficiency, every provincial division presented a unique set of circumstances. Elliott cited the Ontario Division's credo to "supplement not supplant," but even before the onset of the Depression, Manitoba's resources could never hope to match those of its prosperous neighbour.[36] Thus, from the perspective of the Manitoba executive, regular contributions by the committees were considered a success.

### "Suitable Young Women"

The Manitoba Division's call for "suitable young women" to fill the need for regularized health services in its remote rural areas reflects both the class and gendered expectations of the 1920s. It viewed its nurses as "model" citizens who demonstrated the characteristics of the "ideal" Canadian whom new immigrants, or even indigenous populations, could strive to emulate.[37] The division required more of these "suitable" nurses, however, beyond their training and social respectability. Work in this rugged environment among an ethnically and socially diverse population demanded a certain resolve and sturdiness that did not detract either from their femininity or their approbation. In 1920, the division was finding it difficult to fill this order, especially with the requirement that a trained and experienced "young" nurse had to be willing to undergo further training for this potentially difficult role. Nevertheless, one group of experienced nurses seemed ideally suited to the requirements – the veterans of the wartime Canadian Army Medical Corps (CAMC) nursing service.

As early as 1919, Jean Gunn, president of the Canadian National Association of Trained Nurses, had been pressing for the redirection of veteran nurses into public health work.[38] Gunn was well aware of both the national impetus to improve public health services generally and the CRCS' desire to be recognized as a critical component of these developments in order to justify its peacetime reorganization and, as Jayne Elliott has argued, to "enhance its reputation."[39] Gunn's concern was that the vacancies in public health nursing might be filled with less qualified women, such as the veteran wartime voluntary aid nurses.[40]

When the Manitoba program was initiated in the summer of 1920, Edith Frances Macey and Elva Gunn were the first two nurses to be assigned to a station.[41] Born in Saskatchewan, Macey understood the rigours of the western landscape, and as a normal school graduate she was also well prepared to take on the educational requirements of the job.[42] A 1908 graduate of the Winnipeg General Nursing School, Macey had six years of experience as a nursing superintendent at two western hospitals and three years of experience overseas with the CAMC during the war. Closely reflecting Jean Gunn's vision for a public health nurse, Macey also conformed to Meryn Stuart's profile of a CAMC nursing veteran – one who was well suited to the rigours of post-war public health nursing, having demonstrated courage, independence, confidence, and often ingenuity under wartime conditions of stress and hardship.[43]

Originally from Nova Scotia, Elva Gunn opened the new nursing station in Reynolds in July 1920. Like Macey, she also attended normal school prior to her nurse training at Montreal's Western Hospital. Graduating in 1911, Gunn worked for two-and-a-half years in private duty before taking a hospital post in Saskatchewan, but soon left for three years of overseas service with the CAMC. The Manitoba Division hired Gunn following her six months of hospital retraining at the end of the war. A three-week district nursing course at Winnipeg's Margaret Scott Nursing Mission further helped her prepare for her new role as the first station nurse at Reynolds.[44]

Margaret Litton arrived to take over the Fisher Branch Station from Macey in April 1922, just as the Manitoba outpost service was extended to four stations, with a fifth station in the planning stage. Recently arrived from Scotland, Litton did not exhibit the original profile of an outpost nurse, to which Macey and Gunn had so closely conformed. Trained at the Glasgow Royal Infirmary, she graduated in 1912 but took further training, first as a district nurse and then as a midwife. In the summer of 1921, Litton left Scotland for Montreal. Her memoir does not explain the reasons for her emigration, but by March 1922 she had re-qualified at the Winnipeg General Hospital and joined the Manitoba Public Health Service. For the next eight years, she served as the outpost nurse at the Fisher Branch nursing station, and finally resigned in 1930 to become superintendent of the Margaret Scott Nursing Mission in Winnipeg. Arriving after the Manitoba Division had dealt with its initial "growing pains," Litton was able to benefit from the experience and example of pioneers such as Macey and Gunn, who each moved on from their original postings to establish subsequent nursing stations. Litton and those who followed, including Flora Hill, were subsequently able to remain longer in their original posts and become well acquainted with the communities that they served.[45]

With the passage of time, CAMC veterans became less available as they married or otherwise retired from practice, but public health training was becoming more generally available to post-war graduates.[46] Thus "suitable" recruits, in Manitoba's case, were more likely to be women with prior public health training and experience, such as Litton and Flora Hill. Hill arrived in 1927 to take over the East Braintree station (formerly known as Reynolds), and moved on to the new Rorketon station three years later. A member of Kathryn McPherson's "third generation" of Canadian nurses, Hill was a 1924 graduate of the Winnipeg General Hospital.[47] Hers was a familiar career path of private duty punctuated by two brief periods of hospital nursing, but she lacked the opportunity for wartime nursing that helped to mould the character of her predecessors and that had helped to attract them to a rugged and independent life in Manitoba. Instead, a three-month assignment to the Fisher Branch station in 1926, while Litton was on sick leave, brought Hill to the realization that this was the career she wanted, and she "accepted with alacrity" when a post opened up at the East Braintree station in the spring of 1927. Retiring in 1938 to care for her ailing father, Hill characterized her work as both a great responsibility and a "great joy," never regretting "for one moment" her decision to join the outpost service.[48]

As a testament to the demands of "pioneer" outpost nursing in Manitoba, one of Litton's more memorable cases has earned a certain mythic status. In January 1925, a nineteen-year-old appendix patient needed hospital care. The Fisher Branch station was four miles from the farm and the boy had to be brought out by wagon-sleigh, but there was then a three-day wait for the train. Worried about the consequences of the delay, Litton convinced the local foreman of the Canadian National Railway to transport the patient, his mother, and herself by railway jigger to a station outside Winnipeg, where an ambulance would be waiting to take them on to the hospital. They travelled all night in a snowstorm, with the boy bundled in blankets and warmed with a charcoal brick, stopping only once at a train depot for a half-hour's respite. On the second leg of the journey, the gas-driven jigger broke down, and they subsequently exchanged it for another after the driver and the boy's mother had pushed it four miles down the track to the nearest train station. When they finally arrived at their destination, the doctor and ambulance had long since departed, but a taxi took the boy and his mother to the hospital. The local doctor, meanwhile, gave Litton a bed at his home. Although the patient had a "ruptured appendix with abscess and peritonitis," he was making a slow but steady recovery by the time Litton returned home two days later.[49] Although seemingly the stuff of Hollywood drama, such experiences were not uncommon in the undeveloped regions of 1920s Manitoba. Litton's memoir and other nursing reports are punctuated with similar harrowing accounts, and the railway jigger figures prominently in the early accounts of Canadian outpost nursing.[50] It is likely that not even Jean Gunn, in the security of her Toronto hospital, could have foreseen the "adventure" of outpost nursing in Canada's developing settlement regions in the 1920s.

## Work and Community

The Manitoba Division was not alone in providing much-needed medical and nursing services to its more isolated citizens. Jayne Elliott's study of the Ontario Division outlined an ambitious program with comparatively larger and better-equipped nursing outposts, of which thirty-one were in simultaneous operation by 1940.[51] Manitoba had neither the resources nor the population to match the Ontario program, and Elliott's description of fully functioning "hospitals," with a capacity ranging from nine to thirty beds, was far from the Manitoba model, which usually consisted of a tiny station housing one nurse and a wardroom for emergencies only.[52]

Yet it was not the interior space that shaped the lives of Manitoba's pioneer station nurses as much as the exterior environment of the regions in which they lived and worked.[53] Designated as "outposts" in the CRCS literature, the wardrooms, in reality, were primarily holding centres for patients waiting to be transported to hospital facilities in larger centres. Members of the local population frequently presented themselves for outpatient treatment, but the nurse treated the majority of her patients in their own homes after she had been summoned by telephone or messenger. A worried family member often travelled miles in from the backcountry to alert the nurse, having no other means of communication. The nurses each had a telephone line available at their stations, but in the early years these were most often used by the nurse to contact the regional physician. Few telephone lines existed beyond the boundaries of the larger town centres.

The Manitoba Division provided each station nurse with a designated district, ostensibly situated within a limited radius of 35 miles (56 kilometres) from her station. This boundary was somewhat illusory, as Litton wryly observed in her memoir of the Fisher Branch station, where "miles did not mean much, except mounds and cornerstones."[54] As Elliott observed, transportation in these remote regions of Canada was one of the greatest challenges facing the outpost nurses.[55] Although the reports from the Manitoba Division situate the Fisher Branch as being ninety-eight miles (160 kilometres) outside of Winnipeg, Litton's memoir cites a more realistic distance of 120 miles (190 kilometres), with train service available every four days. Until there were adequate roads and cars to drive on them, the train remained the most efficient means of transporting patients to the hospital.[56] In winter, the nurses relied on a horse and cutter, switching to a buggy for the rest of the year. Either way, transportation was limited by unpaved roads that were rife with ruts and potholes often filled with snow, ice, mud, or water, making a car useless. Often the nurse had to resort to a long, wet slog by foot through snow banks, brambles, or bog to reach a patient's home.

While the station nurse was primarily concerned about the physical health care of the community, she was also expected to be a social service provider, acting for the state under the aegis of the Manitoba CRCS. The provincial police summoned Nurse Gant in February 1922 to help investigate the case of an elderly woman "shut up in a chicken house" at a farm thirteen miles (twenty kilometres) from the station. When they arrived, the woman was indoors but barely clothed. With the help of the officers, she was bundled into some old clothing, including the officers' extra socks, and taken back to the station. Gant recounted the woman having "cried with joy" as she left her daughter-in-law behind, and following a bath, a meal, and a good night's sleep, she was transferred to the Portage Home for Incurables.[57] Early in 1925, Nurse Robertson was called on to mediate in the case of a thirteen-year-old girl who had run away from her stepfather's "ill-treatment." She found the child in a haystack on a neighbouring farm, sleeping between a dog and a pig for warmth. The nurse described the abuse as physical and reported that following "some persuasion I took her home, and the father (a Ruthenian) approached regarding the harsh treatment." The nurse expressed some uncertainty about the outcome in her report, but concluded: "I think everything will go satisfactorily."[58] Whether or not this situation was exactly as it was interpreted is impossible to determine, but Robertson had no evidence or authority to remove the child from the home and could act only with the resources available.

Recent scholarship confirms that outpost nurses were frequently required to take on far more responsibility for the diagnosis and treatment of patients than they would have been permitted in a more urbanized locality, with physicians and hospital facilities in close proximity.[59] An analogy can be drawn to the conditions confronting military nurses in stationary hospitals close to the combat zones of the First World War. They frequently cite examples of hospital personnel, confronted with thousands of wounded coming in directly from the field of battle, being required to perform tasks usually assigned to those with more training and authority. Similar situations occurred in the hours and days following the Halifax explosion of December 1917.[60] It is not surprising, therefore, that veteran CAMC nurses were recognized as ideal candidates for outpost nursing. It is also perhaps the reason why these veteran nurses were drawn to work demanding independence and resourcefulness and why they were not easily deterred by either the physical or emotional demands of the work.[61]

By 1922, however, the Manitoba Division realized that some medical situations were "beyond the limitations of the nurses' training, or the responsibility [they] could be fairly asked to assume." Initially, the Manitoba Medical Association agreed to support voluntary medical clinics at the stations, but this solution proved inadequate, and a full-time itinerant physician was subsequently named to visit the districts on rotation. Unlike the nurses, who could not accept any fee for their services, the doctor was to receive a nominal fee for his services from those patients who had the means to pay.[62] The doctors were not only in the employ of the province, but also worked on a fee-paying basis in their private practice in this pre-medicare era.

Throughout the 1920s, despite the positive community response to the outpost nurse, there were inevitably indications of friction, often between the nurses and the local nursing committees. Flora Hill, who had been the nurse at East Braintree since 1927, was transferred to Rorketon as a result of a general reorganization following the death of Nurse Gant in 1930. In 1931, a disagreement arose over Hill's request for vacation time. The secretary of the local Nursing Committee complained to the provincial commissioner that it would be inconvenient for Hill to take her leave in the summer, since the local women liked to use the station as a rest stop when they came into town. The commissioner had little patience with this argument, following a similar complaint against Nurse Robertson at Grahamdale. He chided the local secretary for regarding the station as a convenience stop rather than a vital health care centre, noting in a memo to the provincial Nursing Committee that impending maternity cases were already forcing Hill to divide up her August holiday. He was particularly sympathetic since Hill had been previously forced to take two weeks of sick leave in May when she "was on the verge of a nervous breakdown."[63]

Hill's correspondence at the time demonstrates her own frustration with the local committee, which may have contributed to her problems. The committee had previously complained about a four-day leave that she had taken following a dental clinic, and although Hill had left her assistant to take messages and was prepared to return if any urgent calls had been relayed, nothing of note had occurred. She was further criticized for leaving a committee meeting to tend to a patient. Hill had also suffered an angry response from a patient's husband when he was asked to settle his account for the doctor's eighteen visits and became affronted by the apparent insult to his ability to pay. She was upset by the man's unreasonable response and elicited the support of the provincial Nursing Committee, declaring: "My work is everything to me, and I do not want to hurt the Red Cross cause, so tell me if I am really in the wrong." The chair of the Nursing Committee, Mrs. Speechley, replied that Hill was correct in asking for payment from the husband on the doctor's behalf.[64] As with other nursing services, the division did not want the impression of "charity" to accrue to the organization. Although it covered the nurses' start-up salary, the community was to supplement it, where possible, using support from the local community in the expectation that it would eventually assume full responsibility. The physicians, as private practitioners, relied on fees even though the province provided some support. In this pre-medicare era, however, many physicians still balanced the needs of their less affluent patients against the larger fees charged for their wealthier clientele.[65] Apparently, the problem was resolved, since Hill remained at Rorketon until 1938. It is notable that during this time the division severely reduced the salaries for station nurses following the onset of the Depression and lowered the top salary of $135 per month prior to 1930 to $105 by 1938. It cautioned that there was no guarantee against further reductions, since salaries depended on the results of annual campaigns and, at the time, surplus funds were in short supply.[66]

Nurse Gant also experienced problems with her local committee at Alonsa. Mrs. Speechley, however, was less sympathetic in this instance, noting "much friction" in the region and citing the "nurse's attitude toward some of the

Alonsa people" as the cause of some ill feeling. Although she noted that Gant was "greatly beloved by the very poor," Mrs. Speechley observed that Gant did not get on well "with certain people" in the town, likely the more affluent residents who sat on the local committee. Mrs. Speechley, however, knew where the funds came from and regarded this local Nursing Committee "as really energetic and public-spirited, several grades above the average personnel."[67] Gant's response is not recorded, but Mrs. Speechley herself abruptly severed her connection with the Manitoba Nursing Committee in 1931, taking "a well-deserved holiday."[68] General discontent and uncertainty likely ensued with the onset of the Depression years. When Gant died suddenly from "acute nephritis" in June 1930, it prompted a general reorganization of the nursing assignments. Gant's temporary replacement, Miss D. Cox-Smith, proved so popular with the people of Alonsa that they requested that she remain.[69] Margaret Litton resigned her post because of the reorganization, but the majority of the nurses appear to have weathered the period of change and discontent. The reassignment of personnel may have quelled some of the friction, and despite the uncertain finances of the Manitoba Division during the Depression, the nurses remained in regular employment. Notwithstanding the occasional upset, the overall relationship between the Manitoba nurses, their clientele, and the local committees appears to have remained relatively congenial into the 1930s.

In many ways, the community functioned as an extended family, with the nurse, local townspeople, farmers, and homesteaders in the outer regions coming together to mark notable dates and events or to take a leisurely break from their labours. Litton's assistant frequently organized a collegial meal and game of bridge for the nurse with the local schoolteachers. The outlying farmsteads were also a regular source of sustenance, where the nurse could depend on a cordial welcome upon an unannounced appearance for a meal, combining her work with her social life. Litton noted how the doctor's monthly calls throughout the district frequently served as an excuse to organize social encounters, often combining tooth extractions, tonsillectomies, and maternity cases on the same rotation. On these occasions, Litton would inquire where the doctor "would like to go for supper?" and select a nearby farm, where two new places would quickly be prepared.

Through the winter months, the local Nursing Committee for the Fisher Branch station also organized fundraising events such as parties, concerts, and dances, and in the summer there would be picnics and a sports day. During one of these events, Margaret Litton met her future husband, Bill Hodgins, a local businessman and president of the local Nursing Committee. In 1926, the committee also raised funds to buy Litton a second-hand Chevrolet that was a great boon both to the nurse and her aging horse, although the road conditions still made winter driving impossible on the back roads.

The car provided further opportunities for socializing, as the car owners gathered on summer Sundays on the shore of Lake Winnipeg to wash their vehicles and picnic on the beach, to drive out to one of the farms after supper, or to gather round the organ and sing, frequently concluding the evening with tea at the outpost station.[70]

## Community, Class, and Ethnicity

Margaret Litton's brief but detailed account of her experiences as a station nurse demonstrates how intricately her social life was woven into the fabric of her working life. The division's hierarchy always regarded the Fisher Branch station as the "jewel in the crown" of the five outposts, and the successful fundraising ventures illustrate how much the local community valued the nursing service. Fisher Branch catered to a clientele that was more prosperous and settled than the other regions and much more socially cohesive, serving a large British and francophone farming and business population. The Manitoba Division considered "the Branch" to have status above the other stations, which catered more to the needs of Eastern European immigrant, Aboriginal, and Métis settlements.[71] The province had grown to a population of more than 460,000 by 1911, which, fuelled by the railroad and the developing wheat economy, had gradually relocated to the Prairies from southwestern Ontario. These new Manitobans had a varied mix of British, francophone, and Eastern European ancestry, who settled on the farmlands or developed satellite business ventures in Winnipeg, Brandon, and other rapidly urbanizing centres.[72]

Like much of early post-war Canadian society, Manitoba was also caught up in the labour turmoil that accompanied the return to peacetime conditions. A number of factors contributed to the discontent simmering beneath the surface as Canadians readjusted to a new post-war economy and social structure following the upheaval of the war.[73] The sudden demobilization of thousands of veterans, some permanently disabled physically or emotionally, was compounded by disorganized resettlement programs and often inadequate support to assist in the readjustment to civilian life. Able-bodied men eager to return to productive lives often found the initial peacetime provisions for work and housing lacking. A rush to claim the as yet undeveloped farming regions, which were available for returning veterans through government loan schemes, exacerbated these problems in Manitoba. The initial demand overwhelmed the claims' procedures, and while ultimately successful over the longer term, the resettlement process proved particularly challenging for new farm families with scant experience of rural life.[74] As labour unrest swept across the country in the aftermath of war, it brought work stoppages and strikes to industrialized centres such as Winnipeg. The problems of rapid wartime industrialization, with unhealthy factory conditions and housing shortages for workers and their families, aggravated the discontent. Following the war, frustration and anger culminated in six angry and violent weeks during the Winnipeg general strike in the spring of 1919.[75]

At the time, much of the labour unrest was perceived as emanating from the large influx of Eastern European immigrants into the regions around Winnipeg. This immigrant population became the subject of particular distrust in the wake of the strike and was feared to harbour much of the same revolutionary tendencies that had fuelled the 1917 Bolshevik revolution in Russia. The division's executive echoed these sentiments, characterizing "all of their ideas [as] the reverse of those which are common to a democratic country."[76] The fear of the immigrants' revolutionary ideas garnered great mistrust in the West but was equally unsettling for business and political leaders nationally. It was not coincidental, therefore, that beyond the health care benefit gained by extending CRCS services to the more remote western and northern regions of Canada was the "civilizing" influence it would have on the settlements. The CRCS literature clearly outlines the expectations of the nursing outposts, echoing the philosophy of the previous century toward Native populations with regard to the need to "assimilate." The desired result was to "Canadianize" the Eastern European immigrants through acculturation, with the nurses serving as both educators and models of the Anglo-Protestant, middle-class way of life.[77] The society had reason for optimism since, unlike the Aboriginal communities, this was a "white" community whose children attended local schools.[78]

The 1919 general strike was a flash point in Canadian labour politics, and scholars still debate the relative influence of ethnicity on the violent culmination of the dispute.[79] The CRCS literature reflects the tone and attitudes of the time from the perspective of its entrenched Anglo-Protestant, middle-class base. In the early 1920s, the provincial executive heralded the advent of the Manitoba outposts as having brought "Angels of Mercy" to the region, who "by example and advice proved a potent force along the avenues of education, citizenship and material progress."[80] While the CRCS' seaport rest centres on the east coast of Canada may have been the "first step in assimilating the immigrant," the western outposts and their nurses were considered by the society to be ongoing role models, ready to guide the newcomers toward the "Canadian" way of life. The immigrants from Russia and bordering regions such as the Ukraine posed particular problems since they had suffered from totalitarian regimes that undermined their trust in authority. The CRCS saw itself, through the agency of its outpost nurses, as a neutral, non-threatening organization that was able to provide a service "of the utmost benefit to the State."[81] The underlying discourse firmly expected that the leadership of the outpost nurses would help stem any subversive tendencies and would mould the immigrant communities into "good citizens" possessed of the proper Canadian values of civil order.

Thus, the Manitoba Division's lack of confidence in the nursing station's ability to become self-sufficient stemmed equally from racial and class stereotyping. It considered that the primarily Eastern European population served by the Reynolds station, in particular, would continue to suffer from the legacy of its former "paternal government," which would render it incapable of understanding the expectations of working collectively within the community to fund its own local services. It expressed even less confidence in the abilities of the Métis population to completely fund the Kinosota station or even contribute in a small way. The Nursing Committee did concede, however, that had either group been able to overcome its inherent social and cultural inadequacies, the extreme poverty of the local population would "render it impossible" for either station to become self-sufficient for "many years to come." It also expressed a grudging optimism regarding the prospects of the "rising generation" of immigrant children who might eventually assume responsibility for the local nursing station, due to the "superior opportunities for education" in their adopted country. It did not hold the same optimism for Métis children. Only at the Fisher Branch station, which served a mixed francophone and anglophone clientele, did it hope for a "satisfactory conclusion." Based on these projections, the Nursing Committee at that time advised against extending the nursing program beyond the initial four stations.[82]

Regardless of these gloomy prospects, the Nursing Committee still characterized the project as a success in its early years, acknowledging that the program was achieving its primary goals and noting that "lives are being saved" and standards of "health, hygiene and sanitation" were improving.[83] The committee credited this outcome directly to the intervention of the station nurses and viewed the advent of the station nurse as a progressive step toward nation building. The following year it had even more reason for optimism when the Reynolds station disproved the initial pessimism of the Nursing Committee's judgmental stereotyping. The local community raised $185 in support of the station, of which nearly half came from the Ruthenian women in the district. Based on this funding, the medical officer for the division projected that the Reynolds district could now "undertake to defray" about 12 percent of the operating costs to meet the immediate needs of the station.[84]

Before these "suitable" women could begin their work, the division had to organize the sundry details of uniform and housing. The CRCS insignia was selected for the nurse's uniform rather than the emblem of the Manitoba health authority, out of concern that some Eastern European immigrants might view a state employee as a threatening authority figure or as an interfering government public health inspector.[85] The provincial police were also wary of this anticipated hostility and were "instructed to constantly keep the nurses under their watchful protection," further reflecting the attitudes that regarded the outpost nurses as contributing a much-needed "civilizing" influence on the rural regions of Manitoba in the 1920s.[86]

Although the nurses' reports to the Manitoba Division provide more information about their patients' domestic circumstances than about their ethnic or racial backgounds, the nurses' own Anglo-Saxon middle-class perspective cannot be denied. The racialized attitudes of the larger Canadian society of the era permeate the division's records.[87] Nurse Dempsey noted a confinement case in which a Russian mother was pregnant with her sixteenth child, but having her first experience with a trained nurse, "she had many surprises." In February 1927, Nurse Robertson described a call to a Ruthenian concert, where a dispute over "home brew" resulted in one of the participants requiring seven stitches. Seeing a positive side to the situation, the nurse concluded that by calling upon her nursing services, the patient was consciously "strengthening the Red Cross in the district" and introducing her skills into the Ruthenian community. Litton also noted an elderly Ruthenian man who declared: "English people are best and we Ruthenian people come next, but Red Cross people are best of all." Since he held considerable "power" in the district, Litton believed he could influence the "thought of all the foreign-speaking element." While her inherent Anglo-Saxon ethnocentricity is clear, she also considered his response as a "breakthrough" in a cultural community that had initially been wary of the division's intrusion.[88]

While Litton may have believed that she represented the CRCS as an agent of "Canadianization" within the community, her memoir offers little in judgmental commentary. She was fulsome in her praise of the "spotlessly clean" condition of the Ukrainian homes and actively worked to learn some of the language of a culture she obviously admired. She also noted how tragedy had resulted from one family's Ukrainian Christmas traditions, when hay and grain brought into the house as part of the celebrations had led to a fire that claimed their three children.[89] As noted in the work of Ina Bramadat and Marion Saydak, by integrating health workers into developing regions, the CRCS was effectively creating "medical missionaries."[90] These nurses and physicians were disseminating the normative ideals of the Anglo-Saxon middle class with regard to the expectations of proper hygiene and household management, a message that could be argued as having a gendered application since mothers were seen as the purveyors of domestic health care practices. Litton was not an unwilling participant in this distribution of "proper" domestic health and hygiene education, which would undoubtedly require some adjustment in cultural domestic arrangements.

In late 1923, Nurse Glenn at Grahamdale recorded the death of a child from a "septic throat" that had led to a chest infection. She blamed the father, who refused to leave the child at the nursing station for treatment. Describing the little girl as "delicate" with a "very poor physique," the nurse's final notation provides some indication of her thoughts, noting that the family "live thirteen miles out – German." In this instance, Glenn had not insisted that the child be left in her care or called on the local doctor for support, although she clearly thought the father was in the wrong and attached significance to his ethnicity. Similarly, Litton did not hesitate to dictate her instructions to the son of an elderly woman from the local reserve. Having discovered that the family had "turned her out owing to her age" and left her to die outside, Litton "made someone take her in" and wrote to the absent son to come home "at once and look after her."[91] In this example, Litton once again assumed the role of social service worker for the CRCS, using her apparent authority to rectify a situation that was as much a domestic issue as one of health care. She was also assuming something of the "missionary" attitude in her outrage at what she appears to have perceived to be a cultural practice. Yet poverty figured just as prominently as race or culture in the nurses' critical appraisal of domestic arrangements, rendering class an equally broad issue in the CRCS' "crusade" for a healthy citizenry.

The Manitoba Division's Nursing Committee gradually eliminated the categorization of patients by race or ethnicity from the monthly station reports through the 1920s, possibly reflecting a maturing of its sensibilities. It remained cognizant, however, of its role in the process of assimilation favoured by the state, as well as of its need to raise the domestic standards of the newer settlement regions in the West to reflect the expectations of the Anglo-Saxon middle-class core of Canadian "identity."

## Conclusion

The "suitable" women who first brought organized health care services to Manitoba's remote settlements in the 1920s, like the legions of other provincial CRCS nurses across Canada, should be considered pioneers in their field.[92] It was their responsibility to carve out a style of public health nursing that conformed to the needs of a rugged and diverse population and to the demands of the challenging environment in which they all lived and worked. They also had a political responsibility, charged with carrying the CRCS banner and the crusade for "healthful living" into regions yet to be conquered. The state burdened the nurses with its expectations that the CRCS would aid in the construction of a national identity, cultivating a sense of community, responsibility, and citizenship among a diverse population of new immigrants, native peoples and Métis, established farmers, and new homesteaders. The station nurses confronted these challenges, ultimately developing a deep sense of commitment and concern for the communities in which they served. Guided by their training and experience, nurses in the Manitoba Division made a home for themselves among the people, becoming a part of the social fabric of the rural settlements. They entered a world full of hope and uncertainty, coloured by the varied experiences of veteran soldiers, British and francophone settlers, new immigrants leaving war-torn homelands and harsh political regimes, and long-time Aboriginal and Métis settlements still adapting to strangers in their midst.

Looking back on the problems of the war era, Canadian authorities at all levels of government recognized that competent and reliable health services were an essential component in the quest for the productive, prosperous, and cohesive growth and development of western Canada in the 1920s. Still in the shadow of the recent war and coping with the labour unrest that followed in its wake, Canada's elite and elected leaders also saw the wisdom in striving to cultivate a nationalist spirit among all citizens, old and new. These goals demanded a strong and healthy population, whatever its origins, ready to work and to stand and defend the nation if called upon. The CRCS was determined to be worthy of the trust that it had inherited during the war through its new peacetime mandate, which, by promoting the progress of the nation through the health of its citizens, fulfilled the larger goals of the international organization to promote peace through good health.[93] The Manitoba Division's station nurses, although few in number, were an essential component of these goals. Despite the division's initial misgivings that the CRCS' crusade for "healthful living" could not be mounted in the untamed regions of rural Manitoba in the 1920s, "suitable young women" were found, who more than met the challenge.

**Acknowledgment**
The author gratefully acknowledges the generous support of this research from the Hannah Institute for the History of Medicine through Associated Medical Services, Inc., Toronto.

# 7
# The Call of the North: Settlement Nurses in the Remote Areas of Québec, 1932-72

*Johanne Daigle*

During the Depression of the 1930s, the Québec government sent nurses into remote regions of the province, which had been newly opened by colonization, and charged them with the task of providing health care in small communities called settlements. This solution, intended to be temporary and deemed "reasonable" in light of the absence of doctors and the poverty of local populations, was systematized under the government-organized Medical Service to Settlers (MSS).[1] Once the Depression had passed, the health department extended the service beyond the settlement territories and maintained it until the early 1970s. The administrative records of this service, however, give only a vague idea of the experiences of the nurses in the field. In this chapter, I will focus on the perceptions of the nurses themselves as they lived and worked in these often isolated environments.

Recent historiography includes a number of studies associating the development of nursing services with the involvement of the government in the public health field and the settlement of remote regions that had no medical services. In an essay summarizing nursing care in outlying areas of Canada, Dianne Dodd, Jayne Elliott, and Nicole Rousseau wrote of a vast enterprise to create health care positions in the remote regions of the country from the 1890s to the 1960s, which was given added impetus by the First and Second World Wars.[2] The same scenario was repeated in many different locales. Popular agitation, generally orchestrated by women, was followed by greater public sector participation. The case of Alberta during the settlement of the West is particularly well documented.[3]

I believe, however, that the unique aspect of the Québec nursing service is the substantial support that it received from the provincial government at the very beginning of this traditional clergy-organized nationalist settlement project. This chapter illustrates how, in the context of the Depression, the resurgence of the discourse calling upon French Canadians to move to the "North" to preserve the "race" justified the expansion of existing efforts to provide public health services to the poor populations who had responded to the settlement appeal. Few studies have highlighted the role of health care in this nationalist ideology. The "medical aid" provided by the nurses, often sought by the priests, turned out to be just as important to the maintenance of the populations as that provided by the clerics (if not more so). Historical studies and the MSS archives, including annual reports and correspondence, support this view.

Nurses working in isolated areas all faced similar circumstances: the distance from other medical services, the difficulties with transportation, the poverty of the populations served, the priority given to maternity care, and so on. The use of nurses in isolated health care stations raises the obvious question of why the decision was made to dispatch young single women to work and live under such conditions. For the early decades of the twentieth century, Meryn Stuart made a convincing argument that the involvement of women in moral, social, and religious reform movements shaped the professional identity of Canadian nurses.[4] Traditionally, charitable works for the poor had made women the front-line dispensers of care for the ill in the community.[5] Like Kathryn McPherson, I believe that the training model in force up to the Second World War, which combined Christian concepts with the organization of scientific and medical services, provided nurses with legitimacy and sufficient knowledge (if not always the practice) to provide basic care independently.[6] In the case of the Hôtel-Dieu Hospital in Montreal, I observed that the nuns offered an independent model of nursing practice to the lay students they trained.[7] Denyse Baillargeon demonstrated that nurses working in urban working-class communities between 1910 and 1970 helped to mediate medical knowledge for their patients, which led to the eventual medicalization of maternity in Québec.[8]

The polysemous notion of isolation provides an organizing framework for understanding the experiences of nurses working in remote areas. Their working and living circumstances were connected to the cultural and social relationships between women, space, and isolation. Sara Mills has illustrated how, in general, women both enjoyed greater freedom and had more responsibilities in the colonial setting.[9] According to Mary Jane McCallum, the paradigm of isolation, which she noted was everywhere in the public health journals between 1910 and 1970, promoted increased medical supervision by the public authorities at the same time as it offered adventurous practitioners an opportunity to extend themselves. The notion of isolation, as illustrated in Marita Bardenhagen's study of bush nurses in Tasmania, combined geographic, professional, personal, and social aspects.[10] In analyzing the spatial configuration of the nursing stations in the Ontario Division of the Canadian Red Cross Society between 1922 and 1945, Jayne Elliott showed how the multiple uses of the interior space (hospital and community services, lodging for the nurse, hostel for occasional visitors, and so on) shaped and sometimes constrained the conditions under which nurses practised and lived as they disseminated new rules about hygiene and health to isolated populations.[11]

Relationships between nurses and their patients in remote areas took place in what can be considered "contact zones," the useful expression Myra Rutherdale and Katie Pickles coined to designate spaces in which people from various origins interacted.[12] The need to collaborate, even within unequal relationships of power, sometimes influenced nursing practices. Although Judith Bender Zelmanovits concluded that nurses posted to the Canadian North from 1945 to 1988 were agents in the medicalization of childbirth and ultimately contributed to the process of change in traditional practices, she noted that some nurses earned the respect of their communities by working together with local midwives.[13] Laurie Meijer Drees and Lesley McBain observed that nurses working in northern Saskatchewan in 1930-50 were not very involved in the social life of the Aboriginal communities, but they dispensed care without regard for the government's preference that their services be reserved only for status Indians.[14]

This rich historiographic context reveals a number of similarities with the nurses working for the MSS in Québec. I suggest that, in general, the presence of nurses in the colonization projects mediated the isolation of the "settlers" by obtaining for them extended health care services that not only facilitated necessary hospitalization but also provided varied health and social assistance. And by experiencing the isolation of the populations they served, the nurses mediated their own situation by adapting their way of life and professional practice to the local context. At the same time, however, I believe that using the concept of contact zones provides the best insight into the wide diversity of perceptions that the nurses held on their experiences.

Interviews made it possible to document this hypothesis. My sources are drawn from interviews conducted with forty-eight former nurses, part of a large body of oral studies produced under our direction in the early 1990s.[15] These accounts are based on the nurses' "settlement" experiences and represent a diversity of practice environments (grouped in the four main remote zones of Québec and located on maps in the appendix: Abitibi-Témiscamingue; Bas-Saint-Laurent, Gaspésie, and Îles-de-la-Madeleine; Saguenay and Lac-Saint-Jean; and Côte Nord), different lengths of service (from a few months to more than forty years), and several periods (most are from the 1930s to 1950s, but some extend into the 1990s). The analysis of these accounts was completed in three ways. I compared the nurses' accounts, which were reconstructed from within their life stories (1) with each other, (2) with MSS written sources, and (3) with the relevant historiographic and historical contexts.[16] To these accounts, I added several that had been written by nurses who published their memoirs. I am aware that these personal sources are subjective and that perceptions may have been altered or transformed from a distance of several decades. On the other hand, the depth and breadth of these interviews offer a coherent picture and demonstrate the similar experiences of the nurses.[17]

This study is divided into two parts. The first part describes the particular historical context that resulted in the institution of this unique nursing service in Québec during the Depression of the 1930s, and it discusses its relationship to settlement models developed elsewhere. The second part illustrates the conditions experienced by the nurses in remote regions of the province and their perceptions of isolation, which were centred on themes that have also been documented for other nursing services: the poverty of the local populations, the organization of the dispensary/residence, and the difficulties of travelling to "go to the sick people."

## Necessity Obliges: The Organization of a Nursing Service

The idea of using nurses as substitutes for doctors to serve isolated and generally poor populations was not new.[18] The experience of the First World War had given Western leaders a sense of what made nations strong: the size and state of health of their populations. A number of countries substantially increased their allocations to public health, following the US example of the "New Public Health," which was targeted mainly at mothers and young children and intended to reduce infant mortality. During the interwar period in Canada, government interventions into health care increased, and the number of nursing staff rose. With few exceptions, however, nurses did not obtain legal authorization to act as midwives, and Québec was no exception.[19] Beyond the nationalistic concern with preserving the "national momentum," liberal ideology maintained its fierce opposition to the nationalization of medical care and contributed to limiting the government's role to one of emergency and necessity.[20]

In Québec, the issue of infant mortality had a particular connotation due to the fact that this scourge was more virulent among French Canadians and was associated with perceptions of their inferior position in society. Before he became director of the provincial Departments of Hygiene and Public Assistance in 1922, Dr. Alphonse Lessard publicly discussed this viewpoint: "When English immigrants arrived here, without big families but armed with capital ... our people, having nothing, little education, with little or no direction with regard to the necessities of their many children in terms of hygiene, unfortunately lost a too considerable portion of the large families that had been granted to them."[21] A large part of the French Canadian medical community and the broader clerico-nationalist elite agreed with this rationale.[22]

## "The Call of the North": A Nationalist Solution to the Economic Crisis

Proud of the fecundity of French Canadian women, which was seen as a distinctive trait, as a hope for national survival, and even as an essential point of reference, the clerico-nationalist elite made motherhood more than an ordinary metaphor or obligatory example for the nation. It considered mothers to be the guardians of the "race" in both the biological and the cultural senses of the term. In Québec, religious and nationalist ideology assigned to mothers the mission of maintaining a high birth rate and transmitting patriotic values to their children. These values, which were under attack by rising waves of industrialization and urbanization, were articulated through Roman Catholicism, the French language, family traditions, and rural roots.[23] The solution, which was considered typically French Canadian, was colonization.

The call for colonization, which reached back to the English conquest of 1760 but which had only received a response beginning in the 1830s, became more insistent in the 1880s, when massive emigration to the United States raised fears for the survival of the French Canadian "race." Settlement took on an identitary dimension that the bard of Québec colonization, Curé Antoine Labelle, best expressed: "We, the children of the North, we, the founders of this future empire of North America, we, the men chosen to renew in America the glorious and famous feats of old France, we must conquer, over the English philistines, this land of America through our vigour, our fertility, our skill, and with the help from on high that is granted to us so aptly to realize these great dreams."[24]

The Depression brought this ideology back into fashion by reigniting the dream of national conquest. Denouncing the insufficiencies of the materialistic and individualistic liberal system for which French Canadians, more imbued with family and community values, were paying the price, nationalist clerics and militants proposed a program of "social restoration" by attracting attention to social problems and the duties of the provincial government.[25] "Let us take back the land!" cried the economist Esdras Minville, giving new impetus to the settlement movement, after a century of inactivity, as a solution to the economic problems of French Canadians.[26] The nationalist ideology, bound by the definition of space, was based, as in the past, on the mythical image of the "North" (this space was, in fact, the "Little North" or the "Second North," as opposed to the "Far North" or "North of the North"), which "connected the idea of survival to that of being rooted in the northern soil – the only space, in fact, that was not yet threatened by the English presence."[27] Attaching isolation to this image produced a powerful metaphor, according to which French Canadians would be sheltered and protected, have their traditions brought back to life, and prosper by having many children to increase their population size.

At first, the northern regions of Québec – these undifferentiated stretches of land – were given place names: Côte-Nord, Lac-Saint-Jean, Abitibi, and so on. Yet the North was still seen as "the end of the world."[28] Writer Arthur Buies, a fervent propagandist of settlement, illustrated this notion well in

1900: "We had scaled the last foothills of the Laurentians ... Now appearing before us, in its fierce virginity, was the North, the immense and still forbidding North, enclosed by no borders and bounded only by the impossibility of living in these regions where the land refused to produce ... Before us, as far as the eye could see, now extended this profound North, seen up to then as impenetrable, this protective North, now forbidding to all save the French Canadians, and which would become the inviolable rampart of their nationality."[29] Though obsolescent, this mythic discourse was to serve as the basis for the domestic settlement plan, led this time by the government. It was suddenly seen as a viable solution, even the most profitable one, to the economic crisis. However, aside from this discourse, the propaganda designed to convince settlers to move to new lands was no different from that in old English and American pamphlets. As Serge Courville has shown, this propaganda vaunted the advantages of the new lands with concrete examples, emphasizing the employment and settlement possibilities for immigrants while minimizing the obstacles in the field, and maintained that success depended on work and perseverance.[30] Thus, the myth of the North, to use Christian Morissonneau's expression, was founded on Quebecers' consciousness of "a hope."[31]

## A Partnership Settlement Model: The Respective Roles of Church and State

There are few recent studies on domestic colonization. For Québec, the phenomenon is generally interpreted as a conservative enterprise undertaken by a traditional society that was having difficulty adapting to modernity, as a utopian search for recovery and independence that was bound to end in failure, or as a solution designed essentially to resolve economic problems, particularly in unemployment.[32] According to Courville, the settlement model used within the province was in fact inspired by British "home colonization," which consisted of settling the plateaus as colonies to contain surplus populations from the lowlands.[33] In the second half of the nineteenth century, the government based this model on a mixed economic system, often agroforestry. It ceded public lands to settlers at a low price, while forestry companies enabled the settlers not only to sell their production of timber but also to work on the companies' sites during the winter.[34] Paradoxically, however, the definition of the term "settler" remained linked to that of "clearer of land" in Québec.[35]

Traditionally, the government left the settlement initiative to the clergy, simply providing funding for surveying, road construction, and railways. Starting in the mid-nineteenth century, settlement societies took charge of selecting the recruits and sending them to the land. The true agent of civilization in the middle of the forest was the priest. The most famous missionary-colonizer was Curé Antoine Labelle, who moved to Saint-Jérôme, north of Montreal, in 1868. He visited ministers' offices to obtain funds and services, founded dozens of parishes, brought in religious communities, and orchestrated a vast propaganda campaign by giving sermons and writing newspaper articles. In the field, he was relentlessly active, whether he was ensuring that a chapel-school would be built at a modest cost or distributing "provisions and advice, recipes and seeds."[36] Premier Honoré Mercier's Liberal government finally appointed him deputy minister for settlements in 1888.

On the local scale, the church, and especially the presence of the priest, constituted the nucleus around which parish life gravitated. Concretely, the role of a missionary-colonizer, as described in a report on agriculture, immigration, and colonization in 1868, was related to that of an entrepreneur: "To encourage the settler, share his suffering, instruct him, direct him, dispense to him the assistance of religion, and assist him in his illnesses ... oversee the construction of religious buildings and the opening of roads, interpose himself between the settler and the department of lands or large landowners; supervise operation of the municipal law; as needed, he must be notary, doctor, postmaster, justice of the peace, etc."[37] The extensive material assets from which the religious authorities benefited explains why, as Yves Frenette put it, "the parish framework gave the migrant an identity and a sense of security and belonging in a foreign environment."[38]

When the governing Liberal party encountered the Depression, it supported the settlement movement by defining new rules, primarily through the Gordon (1932-34), Vautrin (1935-37), and Rogers-Auger (1937-41) plans. The federal government initiated the Gordon Plan with the participation of the provinces and municipalities. The plan was aimed essentially at the urban unemployed and those forced to live off charity, and it left the selection of recruits to the provincial "return to the land" commission and the diocesan settlement societies. Starting in 1932, a thousand families were sent to far-flung regions, most to Abitibi-Témiscamingue and some to Bas-Saint-Laurent (the lower St. Lawrence) (see Map 7.1).[39] Since no plans had been made to provide health care, the provincial Hygiene Department stationed a few nurses in the most populous settlements to avoid hospitalization charges, which the Department of Public Assistance paid for indigent settlers – of whom there were many, it seems – who fell ill.[40]

The missionary-colonizers charged with accompanying the first groups of settlers were quickly overwhelmed. Under the Gordon Plan, a number of would-be settlers arrived in the Auclair settlement in 1932, most of them unemployed people from Quebec City, Montreal, Trois-Rivières, Hull, and other cities (see Map 7.2) . If one is to believe Father Léo-Pierre Bernier, who accompanied them, this population was "embittered by lack of anything to do and by privations, in most cases," and he called them "pseudo-settlers" to distinguish them from settlers "in good faith."[41] Only once their first rudimentary cabins had been built did the men receive permission from the

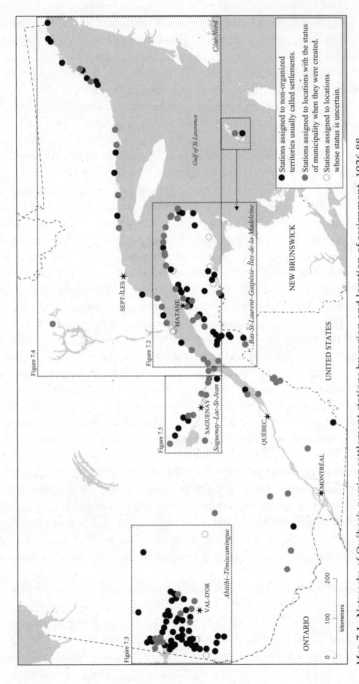

*Map 7.1* Networks of Québec's nursing settlement stations by region and location of assignment, 1926-88

*Cartography: Centre interuniversitaire d'études québécoises, Université Laval*

The legend reads:

● Stations assigned to non-organized territories usually called settlements.

● Stations assigned to locations with the status of municipality when they were created.

○ Stations assigned to locations whose status is uncertain.

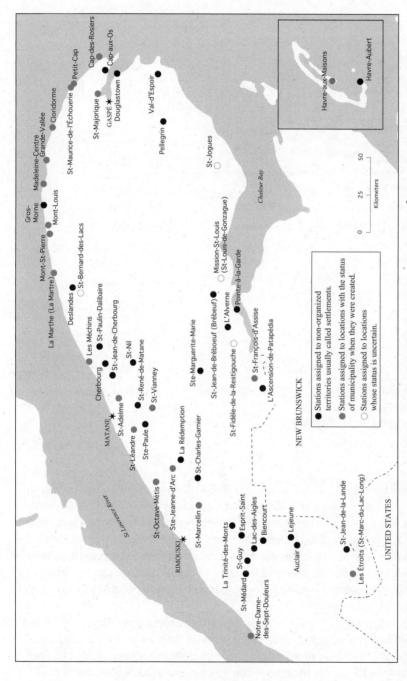

Cap-des-Rosiers
Cap-aux-Os
Petit-Cap
Douglastown
GASPÉ ★
St-Majorique
St-Maurice-de-l'Échouerie
Cloridorme
Grande-Vallée
Madeleine-Centre
Val-d'Espoir
Mont-St-Pierre
Gros-
Morne
Mont-Louis
Pellegrin
La Marthe (La Martre)
St-Bernard-des-Lacs ○
St-Jogues ○
Deslandes
St-Paulin-Dalibaire
Les Méchins
Cherbourg
St-Jean-de-Cherbourg
St-Nil
Mission-St-Louis
(St-Louis-de-Gonzague) ○
St-René-de-Matane
Ste-Marguerite-Marie
Pointe-à-la-Garde
St-Vianney
Chaleur Bay
St-Adelme
MATANE ★
St-Jean-de-Brébœuf (Brébœuf)
L'Alverne
St-Léandre
Ste-Paule
St-François-d'Assise ○
St-Fidèle-de-la-Restigouche
L'Ascension-de-Patapédia
La Rédemption
St-Octave-Métis
Ste-Jeanne-d'Arc
St-Charles-Garnier
NEW BRUNSWICK
RIMOUSKI ★
St-Marcellin
Esprit-Saint
La Trinité-des-Monts
St-Guy
Lac-des-Aigles
St-Médard
Biencourt
Lejeune
Notre-Dame-
des-Sept-Douleurs
Auclair
St-Jean-de-la-Lande
Les Étroits (St-Marc-du-Lac-Long)
UNITED STATES
St. Lawrence River

● Stations assigned to non-organized
   territories usually called settlements.
● Stations assigned to locations with the status
   of municipality when they were created.
○ Stations assigned to locations
   whose status is uncertain.

0    25    50
Kilometers

Havre-aux-Maisons
Havre-Aubert

*Map 7.2* Locations of Québec's nursing settlement stations, Bas-Saint-Laurent and Gaspésie–Îles-de-la-Madeleine regions
Cartography: *Centre interuniversitaire d'études québécoises, Université Laval*

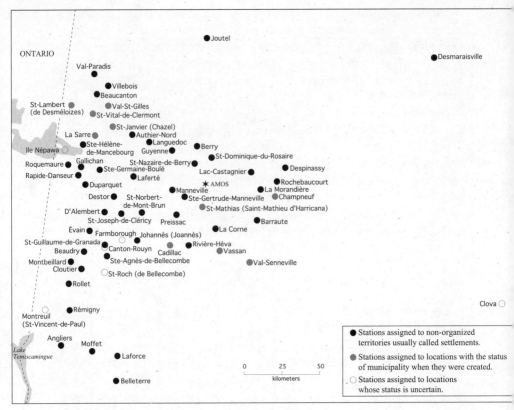

*Map 7.3*   Locations of Québec's nursing settlement stations, Abitibi-Témiscamingue and surrounding regions
*Cartography: Centre interuniversitaire d'études québécoises, Université Laval*

missionary to bring their families. Transportation by train with their personal effects was provided free of charge. Another priest described his disappointment when he arrived in Rollet at the same time: "We had to live in a rudimentary house, without electricity, with no conveniences at all, in this desolate environment. Even the most courageous were shaken to the depths of their souls" (see Map 7.3).[42] The move to the settlement lots was done in a makeshift manner, which he believed explained the high abandonment rate of these settlers.[43]

The Vautrin Plan, which was a provincial settlement plan adopted in 1935, was intended mainly for landless farmers and their sons. With a substantial budget of $10 million in a time of economic crisis, the government of Québec took responsibility for the cost of constructing roads, churches, and schools; provided for settlers public works, the funding of which normally devolved to the municipalities; and offered more generous premiums than in the past for clearing land, building houses, preparing land for cultivation, and other activities.[44] Starting in 1935, parishes grouped their new settlers by parish or region of origin and assigned them lots along the same concession roads in the settlement in the hope that this would make it easier for them to adapt. When they arrived at their destination, representatives of the Ministry of Settlement supervised the groups of settlers. For their health care needs, Dr. Alphonse Lessard made provisions within the Vautrin Plan to use the services of nurses for the most populous settlements: "Here as elsewhere, the women settlers give birth and need services on this occasion; here as elsewhere, there are accidents; here as elsewhere, there may be epidemics or pulmonary diseases, diseases that require emergency care."[45] In spite of the urgency and necessity invoked, the government of Québec agreed only reluctantly to create a nursing service for the settlers after unsuccessfully attempting to entice young physicians to move to the new settlements.[46]

A third settlement plan, the Rogers-Auger Plan, aimed to consolidate the gains that enabled settlers to be resettled on deserted lots and granted certain facilities for acquiring animals and farm equipment.[47] In spite of everything, government assistance was insufficient. In the Bas-Saint-Laurent and Gaspé regions, the situation was just as difficult. Father F. Casey of Saint-Jean-de-Brébeuf told his bishop about the misery of his parishioners in the fall of 1938: "I have just given away my slippers, pants, and jackets" (Map 7.2).[48] In Gaspé-Nord, according to reports, "all the settlers, with few exceptions, are forestry workers." In Gaspé-Sud, the situation of the disillusioned young fishermen forced to live in the forest was deemed "even worse." In Bonaventure, direct assistance had to make up for a lack of income in many cases, despite the premiums.[49]

The settlers were felt to have a particular mentality associated with the frontier spirit or the pioneer front. "Isolation and the relative difficulty of access to institutional services led to the development of a sense of inventiveness in the face of the challenge of starting over at zero," noted a writer on the pioneers of Abitibi-Témiscamingue. It was also recognized that in pioneering areas where populations from various origins came together, "there are no set structures ... When one moves to a new country, one is ready to become a new person." The presence in Abitibi of illegal settlers (squatters) at the edges of mining operations, with names such as Roc d'Or, Paris Valley, and Hollywood, attracted "gamblers, bootleggers, prostitutes, and adventurers of all species," which contributed to this spirit of independence in the temporary absence of social control.[50]

The proponents of settlement felt that women were essential to the success of the project: "In a new land, a woman is as valuable as a man for her work and industry."[51] Women who chose to follow their husbands to a pioneer front may have represented a variety of situations, as shown in the oral inquiries conducted for the Abitibi-Témiscamingue region: "Some women, already with children, looked forward to starting again from scratch; others, especially those who were leaving established family networks 'down south' or in town, feared the remoteness and the lack of services and consumer goods ... Some shared their husband's taste for adventure and starting over. Nevertheless, for women at home, *isolation remained the main dread.*"[52] This isolation was a reminder of the fact that "men left in the fall for the work sites and the women stayed alone with the children and [had] the barn chores to do."[53]

### The MSS: Organization of a Nursing Service

The solution of sending nurses to serve populations that were remote from all health services was first used in Québec in 1926 in locations that were home to indigent, isolated communities on the Côte-Nord (see Map 7.4).[54] In addition, the desire to reduce infant mortality, a particularly devastating scourge in Quebec, had given rise to a string of initiatives in the 1920s that formed the skeleton of a provincial public health system extending beyond the municipalities and targeting care to mothers and children in rural areas. The government also increased its social assistance program to cover part of the hospitalization costs for indigents.[55] The settlement region par excellence during the Depression, Abitibi-Témiscamingue, with a birth rate of more than fifty births per 1,000 people and a large population of indigent settlers, provided the best justification for this initiative (Map 7.3).[56]

After much reluctance and trial and error, the solution that was adopted and systematized to serve the new settlements consisted of assigning nurses to the population of a given territory. Their mandate was the same as that set out for nurses who had been sent to the first settlements opened under the Gordon Plan. Under the mandate that the director of the provincial Department of Hygiene gave to the Auclair Plan in January 1933, the nurses found themselves entrusted with the entire responsibility for providing health care: "Until a physician has settled in the territory that has been assigned to you, you shall have the latitude to provide the required medical care to the population, attend childbirths, and follow the cases of each patient in such a way as to supply as complete a medical service as possible. However, if a special case of exceptional seriousness arises, you will have to use your good judgment and agree with the interested parties or the community's priest to call for a doctor."[57]

This broadened mandate, which was designed over the objections of physicians to limit the hospitalization of indigents, left much initiative and responsibility to nurses in the field. The department added more details to the regulations adopted by the MSS in 1936. One major change was the use of forms for hospitalizations, on which the nurses had to enter a probable diagnosis. Another included a directive to the nurses to make weekly reports

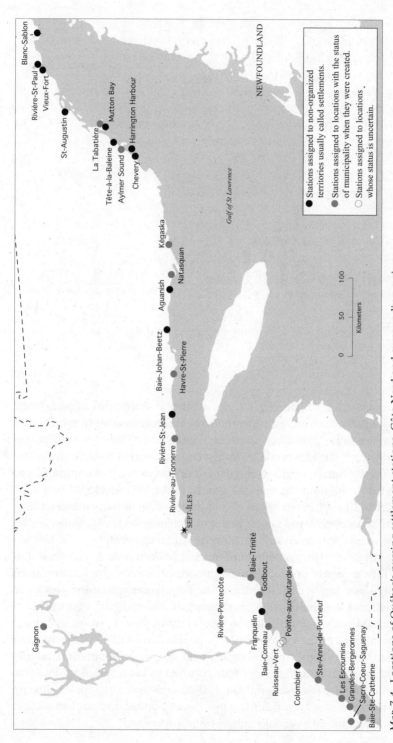

Map 7.4  Locations of Québec's nursing settlement stations, Côte-Nord and surrounding regions
Cartography: Centre interuniversitaire d'études québécoises, Université Laval

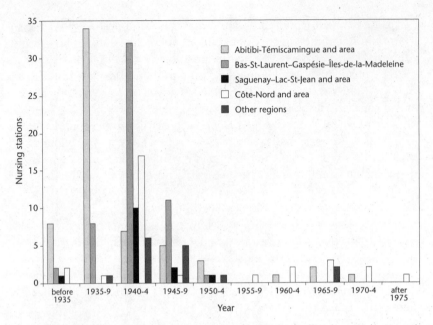

*Figure 7.1*   Distribution of settlement nursing stations in Québec by region covered and period of creation

of their activities, which ranged from assisting at childbirths to performing small surgeries, from extracting teeth to teaching maternal and baby hygiene, and from holding dispensary hours to making home visits and distributing medications.[58] The MSS produced its first annual report in 1944. At this point, the nurses' postings, which were meant to be temporary, had multiplied and extended throughout the outlying regions as the MSS developed over time (see Figure 7.1). Although it was officially reserved for non-organized territories (the settlements), the service had been extended to small municipalities that were too poor to assume their health care responsibility.

The criteria for the assignment of nursing stations, which were set out in 1936 for the newly opened settlements, were based on the distance from hospitals and physicians, the size of the population and of the area to be covered, and the ability of the local people to maintain the basics of a dispensary (water, telephone, and so on).[59] For the Rollet station, the nurse who was already in place had to serve a population of 1,200 people in a territory extending eight to ten miles (thirteen to sixteen kilometres), mainly on county roads (Map 7.3). Her transport had to be provided by a private individual under contract, and she had to draw water by bucket directly from the river and live in an "inappropriate" house. Her settlement was thirty-five miles (fifty-six kilometres) from the hospital.

The government report emphasized that this was a posting "for a physician" and noted the presence of a resident priest. The nurse in Rochebaucourt, for her part, served a small population of 550 inhabitants over a distance of six miles (ten kilometres) to the west and the same distance to the east (Map 7.3). It was suggested that she travel on foot or rent a horse-drawn carriage. Her residence, an "inappropriate settler's house" since the dispensary was still under construction, had neither running water nor a telephone. This settlement was forty-seven miles (seventy-five kilometres) from the closest hospital. These examples reveal difficult situations faced in these small communities and the necessity invoked by the government to justify the nurses' services.

Government authorities attempted to limit the nurses' activities from the very beginning by asking them to distinguish indigents from the people who were able to pay for their care in order to obtain reimbursement for the cost of medications that the nurses had defrayed.[60] The directive was practically impossible to apply. Not only were settlers confused with who was considered an indigent in the eyes of the province but also not all indigents were settlers, due to the very fact that many remote and disadvantaged communities, as well as settlements, had acquired or were going to acquire the status of municipality, an ambiguity that favoured increasing the number of nursing stations.

Between 1926 and 1988, the government created 174 nursing stations in the province as a whole (Map 7.1). Of this number, it placed seventy-one in small communities that were already organized into municipalities, which, if one includes the twelve stations whose status was uncertain, equalled 44 percent of the total number of stations. Add to this number the thirty-eight stations that it continued to maintain in communities after they were municipalized, and it equals a total of 109 nursing stations (or 67 percent) in organized territories. To start, this network followed the corridor of settlement territories created during the Depression. However, the vast majority of stations opened in municipalized communities that were created after the Depression ended – that is to say, after 1939 – with the greatest expansion occurring during the Second World War, due to the lack of available doctors. Following the lead of the federal government, the provincial leaders felt impelled in this apparent period of prosperity after the war to guarantee access to care to all citizens, regardless of where they lived. The network of settlement nursing stations in Québec was, to our knowledge, of a scope unequalled anywhere else in Canada or even Australia.[61]

The basic model for this large network of nursing services required hands-on involvement by the provincial government since it had conceived of the idea of moving disadvantaged populations to remote communities without health services. Although the government initially intended to supply nurses only to settlements in their colonization project, this new discourse of the state on increasing access to health care provided opportunities for other remote communities even in municipally organized areas, which they soon widened to their advantage. These communities, facing the same problems of isolation and lack of physician services as the settlements, often success-fully argued for a nursing station as a reasonable solution to problems of distance, medical need, and poverty. Nevertheless, over the years, the MSS retained both its original name and its primary mission of helping women in childbirth, perhaps because it drew its legitimacy from one of the major symbols of the French Canadian nation. And so it fell to the government to maintain a service that was intended to be temporary and to try to prevent its expansion.

## Nurses and Isolation in the "Contact Zones"

> As for myself, the North called out to me, I felt boiling within me the tumultuous blood of the ancestors who discovered the continent and the builders of the country, and I responded in a single bound: "Abitibi, I am coming."
> – Rocabérant Berith, *Les tribulations d'une jeune infirmière chez les pionniers de l'Abitibi*

From the start, the nurse quoted in this earlier passage said she was touched by the "call of the North," which she associated with the pioneer front. Once she arrived, she listed the many problems, including a lack of water, a lack of electricity, which only came in the 1950s, intense cold, and, especially given the distances and the difficulty of travel, the isolation. While many nurses related to the concept of "the North," which was broadly dissemin-ated in discourses on the settlement project, they also experienced the same sorts of problems associated with living in isolated and poverty-stricken communities as other community members did. Some nurses, evoking the borderline or even the extreme situations linked to the early days, recalled a sense of freedom and independence, courage, and self-sufficiency. Others observed that the cold, isolation, absence of conveniences, difficulty of travel, and lack of services in the field, when combined with poverty or personal deficiencies, engendered only misery.

### Isolated Populations to Serve: Omnipresent Poverty
The settlement stations were not all similar in profile, as we have seen. Some served communities of 2,000 people, while others served only 550. The dis-tance to the hospital or to a doctor, the distances that were necessary to travel and the means of transport, the natural geographical features of the area (mountains, watercourses, and so on), and the mentality of the populations

served varied, according to the accounts of the nurses stationed in these remote communities. Despite these differences, however, the poverty of the population in each territory was a constant factor in their memories. The presence of the nurses and the skills that they brought worked to mediate the isolation imposed by colonization on these poor communities by providing at least some form of health care. At the same time, however, the nurses viewed the people they served from different perspectives. Although some felt close to the people, mentioning that they were united and shared a sense of commonality, others expressed reservations, either because they found "hard cases," a large population, greater isolation, people whom they believed could not take care of themselves, or communities that they felt were closed to outsiders.

The nurse stationed at st-Norbert-de-Mont-Brun in the mid-1930s explained that "the women of this era showed exceptional courage, since they left for the unknown in the hope of starting their very own household" (Map 7.3).[62] The nurse in Rochebaucourt opined that "here, poor people have an advantage over poor people in town, since they have space. Almost all of them have a house" (Map 7.3).[63] Another nurse in the Abitibi region in the late 1940s analyzed the situation as follows: "Everyone had come from outside, so it was like people arriving in a foreign country, they were far from their loved ones, and so they formed a big family."[64] There were similar accounts from other regions, such as the one from a nurse at L'Anse-Saint-Jean in the 1930s: "Everyone was very nice to me ... and they always tried to make me as comfortable as possible when I left in the cart; they heated bricks to put at my feet so I wouldn't be cold" (see Map 7.5).[65] When she arrived in Côte-Nord in the 1970s, the nurse at La Tabetière was struck by the fact that "people were really very reasonable, very well disciplined" (Map 7.4).[66]

The opinions expressed by the nurses reflect not only the characteristics and attitudes of the people in their community but also their own motivations. In her memoirs, Marguerite Turgeon, who was stationed at Berry (Saint-Gérard) in 1935, related: "I dealt with good people, and people were very religious, with the faith to move mountains. They were poor but very generous and very helpful. Everyone helped each other, and doors were never locked" (Map 7.3).[67] Another nurse, looking for a personal commitment in the late 1940s, recalled: "The people of Quebec, when you talked about Abitibi, it was very special, very remote, people didn't live like everyone else, it was poor, but it grabbed me, and I said, I'll go there as a missionary. I was disappointed when I arrived in Amos, the beautiful town ... then I arrived at my settlement and my pretty little house ... It was marvellous."[68] Although one nurse expressed her initial disappointment with her posting, she ended up living in her dispensary in Abitibi for forty-two years: "They hadn't told me how miserable I would be there ... because probably I wouldn't have gone. I went like an innocent."[69] Another nurse, stationed

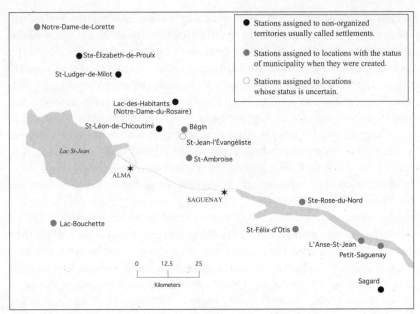

*Map 7.5*   Locations of Québec's nursing settlement stations, Saguenay–Lac-Saint-Jean
*Cartography: Centre interuniversitaire d'études québécoises, Université Laval*

in Bas-Saint-Laurent is now more critical of the poverty she found then: "To see them suffer, I suffered with them because it wasn't normal that people, in communities like that, that they had no more help, no more assistance ... then, to see the lack of interest of our political leaders ... It was unimaginable, it was unacceptable."[70]

Other nurses, however, remembered making harsh judgments and revealed unpleasant realities. The nurse stationed in the Abitibi-Témiscamingue region in 1936 analyzed the situation in the following way: "There were people who went hungry, who lacked ... most of them lacked initiative ... They were people who had lived in the city, who had been on unemployment, and they were a bit discouraged ... There were exceptions ... but lots of them lacked initiative."[71] The nurse stationed at Beaucanton in 1942 offered the following explanation: "No one was rich, but there were poor ones, some were very poor, and it was by their own fault that they were poor ... because they hadn't been able to manage their affairs" (Map 7.3).[72] A nurse stationed in another settlement in Abitibi at the same time related that along two county roads "it was as if everyone who had arrived together, who were related, were, you might say, of the type who had no plans [lacking judgment], the only ones in the entire parish. They all married each other, cousins, abortions, and then miscarriages, and then ... always hard up ... they had nothing, they farmed nothing."[73]

One nurse found it difficult to conquer the mistrust of the population that she served in the Saguenay region during the 1950s: "It was a very closed community and they had a hard time accepting strangers ... so it took me a year to get through, but once I was accepted ... I came ahead of the priest" (Map 7.5).[74] The situation in Côte-Nord was considered more difficult, and the people poorer, than on the south shore of the St. Lawrence River. As one nurse who worked in the area during the 1960s and 1970s commented: "The mentality was pretty tough in that neck of the woods, you know."[75] A nurse stationed in the Bas-Saint-Laurent area and serving several communities, most of them now closed, noted that "there were truly poor people. We called it St. Nothing." She felt, looking back, that "these were parishes that had been opened by priests who knew nothing ... they were errors of course."[76]

The nurses frequently referred in their remembrances to housing that was particularly deficient due to the poverty of the communities that they served. During the Depression and even into the 1940s, one nurse noted that many homes were log cabins: "They had one room and a wood stove, and the floors were on dirt; they were very, very cold houses before other houses were built ... one small window, just single-paned glass, and it was very cold."[77] The outhouses were outside. This situation existed in both Abitibi and Bas-Saint-Laurent. One nurse recalled a family that "was so miserable it was terrible ... you could see daylight through the walls [of the house] ... I had asked the farmers' wives to send wool blankets and tried to explain that they should put mud in the walls."[78] As the nurse at Sainte-Paule recalled, many people lived in very poor housing conditions even into the 1960s: "About 10 percent of these women lived in almost, in hovels, you might say, the snow came in in the wintertime because the doors and windows were in such a bad state, and often the house was full of brats, the floors were covered with bread crusts, and the linoleum was dirty" (Map 7.2).[79]

Given such living conditions, it is hardly surprising that almost all of the nurses in our group mentioned that they gave away medications from time to time, since many people did not have the money to pay for them. Although some noted that the local populations were heavily indebted to them, others saw things differently. The nurse stationed at Bégin expressed a fairly widespread opinion among the settlement nurses: "I was no business woman. It wasn't a matter of making us rich, not at all" (Map 7.5).[80] Aside from donating medications, it was not rare for the nurses to donate various basic goods to their community. One nurse stationed in Bas-Saint-Laurent from 1936 to 1976 recalled: "I left with things to eat, bread, I made my bread ... in the spring, when people didn't have the means to buy oats, to sow oats for the animals ... I asked the government for oats ... One time I was able to get school supplies ... I gave school supplies for the children ... I asked for money from the government for the poorest people who were starving ...

or potatoes for seeds."[81] Despite the different interpretations that the nurses gave it, living in proximity to such poverty was certainly a motivation to act beyond their habitual caregiving role, following the example of the missionary priests.

### Isolated Living in the Settlement: The Nurse's Dispensary-Residence

The housing conditions of the nurses also contributed to the isolation that they experienced in the settlement. The first dispensaries built in settlements created during the Depression were hastily erected cabins that were not much different from those of the settlers. Even the government authorities admitted that the only thing house-like about the dispensaries built by the Ministry of Settlement before 1937 was their name.[82] In her memoirs, Marguerite Turgeon described her dispensary in Saint-Gérard-de-Berry as a two-storey house without a foundation, with a double-box stove and a potbelly stove attached to a single stovepipe, and with no bathroom, running water, or electricity. She used straw pallets as mattresses for the beds and quickly learned, by observing the settlers, to melt snow and collect rainwater for her domestic needs and to set snares so she would have something besides sauce to eat.

It took a long time before housing conditions for both the nurses and the local residents improved significantly. Without electricity, wood stoves and hand washers were still in use in Abitibi in the early 1950s. In the middle

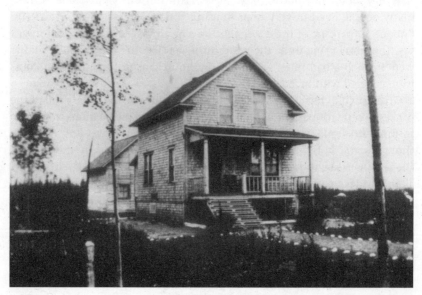

Blanche Pronovost's dispensary at Villebois, Québec, before it burned (c. 1936-38).
*Courtesy of the National Archives of Québec in the area of Abitibi-Témiscamingue, Rouyn*

of the decade, the nurse at Île-aux-Grues, which was not one of the main peripheral regions because it was an island and thus quite isolated, reported: "For a mattress we had straw, so we changed the straw every two or three months. There was no question of radio, because there was no electricity, and there was no question of a bath, so you always washed with cold water" (this station is located outside of the major remote areas, on an island close to Quebec City).[83] For years, the settlement nurses had to learn to operate the gas pump, light the stove, and chop their wood. In addition to combining their working and living spaces, these women also had to host visitors. They may have provided welcome company to the nurses, but they undoubtedly entailed extra work. The nurse in Beaucanton recalled: "Most often, it was government employees or surveyors who came and had no place to stay, so they came to sleep in the dispensary. It was almost like a hotel, I had to keep something for them to eat ... there was no other place to go."[84]

Other nurses who considered themselves less lucky had to live for a time in a presbytery or a settler's house or share the schoolhouse with the teacher or share a house with the representative of the Ministry of Settlement. Some, especially in small towns, rented a house or sometimes a trailer. The nurse in Saint-Mathias-de-Bonneterre in Estrie, which was southwest of Montreal and outside of the main peripheral regions, lived with the local schoolteacher. She observed: "We were at very, very, very close quarters ... there was a small kitchen, and a very small bedroom, I had to open my bed, open the wardrobe door to open my bed every night, it was truly unpleasant to live like that ... if patients wanted to see me, they had to disturb the class to come in ... it was really not adequate."[85] Nevertheless, nurses were happy simply to have a place to live, especially during the Depression. One recalled: "I didn't die, since I ate pea soup, pork rinds, and beans like everyone else."[86]

For a few nurses, the beauty of the setting where they found themselves compensated for the nuisances of everyday life. Some provided romantic descriptions of the natural landscapes and the communities where they were stationed. One nurse explained that she was enchanted by the Abitibi region: "The landscape, the sky, the lakes around, the colour of the air."[87] Another described her idealized vision of the place in the late 1940s: "In the evening, I remember, I had ... a wood stove that smelled good and crackled, moonlight, and big fields with a glistening crust as far as the eye could see ... I was all alone, but I told myself if I were a millionaire it couldn't be more beautiful."[88] Another nurse remembered: "I took lovely trips. You know, when a little snow has just fallen ... I was on a reservation, and they made this trail. The spruce trees were loaded down [with snow] and it was very beautiful; a pretty bit of sun shone through. It was clear, clear; it was beautiful, beautiful."[89] In the Gaspé region as well, nurses recalled their emotions. One who was stationed there in the 1950s noted: "The landscape was so beautiful. We had five lakes."[90]

Whether they retained a romantic vision or a rawer version of their stay in a settlement, almost all of the nurses remembered the omnipresent cold, either in their dispensary-residence or during their travels. One nurse who was stationed in Bas-Saint-Laurent in the first half of the 1960s stated: "What I found hard there was freezing in the winter in the dispensary, which was very poorly insulated."[91] Such an experience was more common when new settlements were opened. It was so cold, as Marguerite Turgeon described her dispensary, "that the knots of the wood popped out and I had to use cotton batting to fill the holes."[92] Many noted that their dispensary was not insulated against the cold. One specified that "when I woke up in the morning it was as cold as -30 to -40 F. And when I breathed out, it steamed just as if I was actually outside." Under these conditions, it was not rare for the water in the dispensary to freeze.[93]

Since they had to go out often, notably to attend childbirths, and could not predict how long they would be away, a number of nurses remembered that they had found it difficult to reconcile the use of wood stoves with the impossibility of making sure that they would be monitored for long periods of time. The result was that they returned to icy dispensaries from trips to care for sick people. Their travels also exposed them to the cold. One nurse posted in Gaspésie in the early 1940s exclaimed: "Oh, my dear, I was cold, I was cold, oh my gosh, once I was on horseback in the settlement, they were ... old horses that could not move forward ... my legs were so cold ... when I got home I lay down on the bed, exhausted ... when I woke up ... I took off my stockings and there were blisters ... Oh, but I was cold" (Map 7.2).[94] Another nurse, in Deslandes during the 1950s and 1960s, recalled one experience of going to attend a childbirth during a snowstorm: "I will tell you that I was scared that time of dying, of dying of cold" (Map 7.2).[95] Consistently recalled in the nurses' memories, the cold speaks to the aridity of the remote regions of Québec, but it also evokes and contributes both to the imagery of "the North" and to that of the isolation.

### Isolation: Difficulties Encountered in "Going to the Patients"

Isolation was a complex phenomenon encompassing a sense of cultural, psychological, and professional insecurity. It was symbolized by the most visible factor – the means of transport – which was a leitmotiv in the memories of people who experienced the beginnings of settlement. The nurses reported that they suffered from "being shut in, not being able to go out"[96] and of feeling trapped "almost like prisoners."[97] The nurse stationed in Saint-Mathias-de-Bonneterre explained how she felt: "[I] wasn't bored when I could go out, but if the road was closed because of a storm, oh, then I felt really bad ... I was bored, I felt trapped, I felt like my wings were clipped."[98] For others, such as the nurse stationed at L'Anse-Saint-Jean in the 1930s, isolation meant "being far from civilization ... being far from my social life."[99]

Isolation also meant, as one of the settlement nurses clearly put it, "the weight of being a nurse. This status lasted twenty-four hours a day, and sometimes it was a heavy load."[100] Not being able to share her experience or get away when she felt the need was a source of stress for one nurse in Côte-Nord in the 1970s and 1980s: "You have working relationships that are ... it's hard, you feel isolated. You know, in the city, if you're not at work, well, you go to a restaurant, you can go out and eat, whereas here ... "[101] Another nurse in the same region at this time, however, saw things differently: "I organized meals at home, and also people in the place invited us over a lot, a lot, a lot, and so we were carried along, we lived life intensely, we shared things with everyone else. So I didn't have the feeling of being alone."[102]

In comparison, a few nurses were struck by the isolation of the families that they served. One nurse in the Abitibi region in the 1950s recounted that, even at the time of her interview, what hit her was "the prodigious isolation of the families, the women who were living near a little lake ... so far from their neighbours ... and they were alone, and then their husbands left ... [A woman] made signals, for example, to the neighbour, who was far away, and whose house she could barely see. She said, 'if I need help, I'll put a red rag on the clothesline ... and you'll send your oldest kid' ... This isolation was inhuman."[103]

Almost all of the nurses in our group shared this isolation with the women in their territories when they went out to attend a childbirth – which was the primary reason for their being in the settlement – during the winter when the roads were closed and most of the men had gone to work as lumberjacks. Almost all of them mentioned experiences linked to snowstorms, which they associated with the difficulties and dangers of transportation. They remembered images of horses that could not go forward anymore, of walking long distances, and sometimes even crawling, freezing in the bitter cold. One nurse stationed in Gaspésie recounted not being able to send a patient to hospital for a cut on his leg during a snowstorm: "So I stitched it up. And it healed well."[104] For another nurse in the same region, whose dispensary was located thirty miles (forty-eight kilometres) into the woods, this insecurity proved unbearable: "In winter, it [the road] wasn't even open the first three years, and that's why I quit."[105] The nurse in La Marthe related that even in the 1950s, "when there were storms, I couldn't go out with my car, eh, so I felt trapped because I felt far away ... and I told myself that if something happened to me, you know, if something ... I really felt insecure then" (Map 7.2).[106] When it was stormy, the population also felt this insecurity. "The people were anxious," explained one nurse who was stationed in Bas-Saint-Laurent.[107] Their remoteness also led to professional insecurity. A nurse posted to a location accessible only by train explained: "No, ma'am, it was not rosy, because, I'll tell you, there were times when my heart was in my throat ... you made the patient comfortable ... We were lucky if we had something to provide relief with."[108] For one nurse posted in what she thought was the last village before James Bay, it was "the outer limit of civilization."[109]

## Conclusion

When universal health and social assistance programs came into effect in the 1960s and 1970s, the necessity of maintaining nursing services, though they were highly valued by the communities, seemed to have passed. The nurse in Vassan who lived through this transition recalled: "There was propaganda that had it that women who gave birth at home – they were settlers, you have to say the word, [and] it was as if they were people who felt more backward than others – said ... we'll go to the hospital" (Map 7.3).[110] In the vernacular of the time, the term "settler" came to have a pejorative connotation. As Morissonneau recalled, "'settler' now meant peasant, ignoramus, uncivilized man, even woodsman."[111] The provincial government adopted a policy of systematic elimination of settlement stations. It abolished the MSS and the Ministry of Settlements in 1962 and transferred the supervision of the 110 remaining nursing stations to the health unit authorities. This service, in turn, was dismantled in 1972. A few stations, however, had to be maintained, and new ones opened in communities that were totally deprived of access to health care services.

As I highlighted at the beginning of this chapter, the uniqueness of the MSS project lies in the church/state partnership model for the settlements, which was instituted in the context of the economic crisis of the 1930s. In directing the movement, the state conferred legitimacy upon the traditional clerico-nationalist project of reclaiming the "North," an isolated territory deemed an appropriate space for regenerating the French Canadian "race." Making French Canadian mothers, with the propensity to give birth to many babies, responsible for the transmission of nationalist values was at the heart of this project. Health care, especially concerning maternity, thus acquired a status that was as important as, if not more important than, that of religion.

Although the settlement movement began to fade once the Depression passed, the nursing service that had accompanied the movement underwent unprecedented expansion, spreading to small, isolated communities, including those that were organized into municipalities and those that were not. Hundreds of nurses responded to the "call of the North," which, when combined with the appeal of the "pioneer front," placed them on the front line in situations of urgency and need. A nurse who worked in the 1960s remembered that "what I liked the most was to see that I could provide a service to people who didn't have any way to find it farther away ... no means of transport, no money."[112] In my opinion, this was the essence of the issue. I believe that the presence of nurses among local populations mediated the settlers' isolation from medical services by providing a wide range of health care services and facilitating hospitalization. Faced with widespread poverty and the absence of other resources, many nurses took it upon themselves to offer services of all sorts, despite the constraints that the government imposed. They helped to provide a modicum of security in the face of suffering, illness, and other vicissitudes of life, especially among women facing childbirth, which comprised their primary mandate. Centring my discussion on the idea of isolation has allowed me to explore from different perspectives the impact of the remote nature of settlement work on the social and professional experiences of these women. Examining the oral histories of the nurses who lived and worked in these isolated postings brings the "contact zone" of interaction between settler community and nurse into sharper focus and makes a vital contribution to the administrative record of the colonization project in the province.

### Acknowledgments
Please note that all text and quotations have been translated by Käthe Roth. This research has been undertaken in collaboration with Nicole Rousseau, professor emerita in the Faculty of Nursing, Laval University.

# 8

## (Re)constructing the Identity of a Red Cross Outpost Nurse: The Letters of Louise de Kiriline, 1927-36

*Jayne Elliott*

If Louise de Kiriline is known at all among historians of Canadian nursing, she is best remembered as the nurse that Dr. Alan Dafoe placed in charge of the Dionne quintuplets, the tiny babies born in a small village south of North Bay in May 1934. Their seemingly miraculous survival ignited national and international attention during the dreary Depression years. De Kiriline remained with the Dionne babies for only their first year, but her name has become securely linked with the "famous five," albeit overshadowed by the name of their more famous physician. The fame that de Kiriline derived from her position during this critical period in the lives of the quintuplets rests primarily on her identification as the quintuplets' chief nursing care-giver. Drawn to this "friendly Red Cross nurse," the press at the time clamoured both for news of the babies' progress and for information on the background of the woman who clearly reigned over their care.[1] When de Kiriline later parlayed her experiences into a book, she herself claimed that her authority on the quints arose from her relationship to the nursing profession. "I wish every Canadian nurse to feel that this record of the nursing of the Dionne quintuplets is her own record, the honour and fame of which belongs to our profession alone," she wrote in the preface. "For it was on the groundwork of its training and teachings that we, the nurses of the babies, individually met with such unbelievable success."[2] Not surprisingly, then, present-day historians have also focused solely on de Kiriline's identity as a nurse in her relationship to the Dionnes.[3]

Dafoe's request that de Kiriline take charge of the quintuplets interrupted a much-anticipated leave of absence from her work as an outpost nurse with the Canadian Red Cross Society (CRCS). She was part of a growing contingent of outpost nurses employed by the Ontario Division and other provincial divisions of the society, which after the First World War had begun to supply and staff medical outposts for people in outlying districts that had little or no access to basic health care and medical services.[4] Prior to the birth of the Dionne babies, de Kiriline had spent six years as the sole nurse in the village

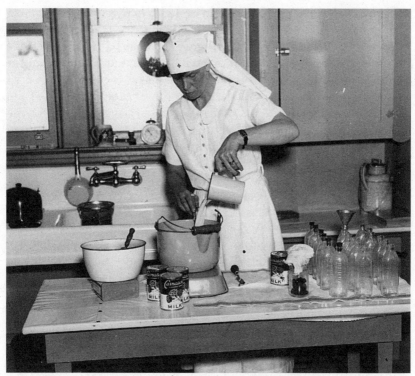

Photographers were fascinated with the attractive, intelligent, and approachable Louise de Kiriline, charge nurse of the Dionne quintuplets.
*Courtesy of Library and Archives Canada, 1993-199, File 4, 2000813819. Reproduced with the permission of the Minister of Public Works and Government Services Canada, 2007*

of Bonfield, a tiny French Canadian community that was thirty kilometres south of North Bay. She was not a typical Ontario Division outpost nurse. While 85 percent of the division's outpost nurses employed during the interwar years were young, single, and Canadian-born, this thirty-three-year-old widow, who had trained at the Red Cross hospital in Stockholm during the First World War, had arrived from her native Sweden only shortly before being hired on with the organization.[5]

Despite her years working for the division and the legacy of her involvement with the quintuplets, which has fixed her identity in historical accounts, I argue that nursing was only one aspect, albeit an important component, of de Kiriline's self-identity. As Canadian historian Joy Parr pointed out, we often "lose sight of the 'multiple determinants' that constitute any individual's social position ... and also of the ways in which social identities are simultaneously formed from a multiplicity of elements."[6] At the same time that de Kiriline established herself as an outpost nurse, she was also a daughter, a recent immigrant, and a self-supporting single woman in a northern Canadian environment – identities that often assumed greater importance in her life than that of a nurse. This chapter thus considers the construction of these other identities and the specific and historical contexts of gender, race, class, and region out of which these various social positions were made. While an understanding of these other factors adds richness and depth to our knowledge of this woman beyond her involvement with the Dionne quintuplets, it also reminds us, as nursing historians, to pay attention to what identities beyond that of their professional identity nurses considered important.

### Letters and the Construction of Identity

This discussion is based primarily on a collection of private letters, which forms part of a larger archived deposit of papers covering de Kiriline's life well into her later years. De Kiriline wrote frequently to her mother, Hellevid Flach, back home in Sweden. The correspondence under study in this chapter is composed of 198 letters that begin shortly after her arrival in Canada in 1927 and end ten years later as she was settling into her own home following her retirement from nursing.[7] Her future plans to "to write about my life … amongst the French Canadians" may help to explain why they have survived.[8] Most of these letters are written in Swedish, and because I have translated only sixty-five of her letters (from 10 June 1927 to 20 July 1929) to date, this article is a preliminary investigation or a work in progress. I have also included, however, twenty-eight letters that de Kiriline wrote in English, a language that she knew and began to use when she acquired the use of a typewriter during her year with the Dionnes.

As one set of authors has admitted, reading other people's mail continues to fascinate researchers.[9] Letters offer an immediate perspective on actions and events, which other sources written years later may lack, but, as historians and scholars from other disciplines have pointed out, they are not produced without reflection. Particular attention has been paid to the question of identity formation in historical personal correspondence. Rebecca Earle, who views letters as "key cultural sites for the construction of the self," suggested that writers may have used them to create "fictions of the self."[10] James How argued, however, that rather than creating "alternate" selves, authors writing close friends and relatives were more interested in "providing an arena within which already known 'selves' can speak and act."[11] Most relevant to my study of this letter collection is the research that has been undertaken on immigrant letters. Historians have recognized the importance of this correspondence for immigrants in maintaining contact with distant loved ones as well as in the negotiation and production of relations between them. "Letters mattered," David Fitzpatrick argued, not only because of their function in sustaining communication between immigrants and those they left behind but also "because they were potentially an effective instrument for defining and modifying human relationships."[12] At the heart of immigrant correspondence, David Gerber contended, was the attempt to hang onto a coherent self-identity, an awareness of the self as an individual that is forged over time through dynamic and multi-faceted relationships with others.[13] Emigration and the stresses of resettlement that disrupted these relationships threatened the familiar ways through which individuals formed their identity. In demanding personal reflection and an implied conversation with the intended reader, letter writing helped to continue the production of these "narratives" of self. Our understanding of the formation of de Kiriline's social identities in and through her letters must therefore be situated within the context of her need to highlight, above all else, her continuing commitment to nourish an intimate relationship with her mother and to remain a "knowable" person to both her mother and herself. "There was perhaps nothing more important to write about," Gerber argued, "than those who constituted to varying degrees one's most significant others; they were in one's memory and thus constant companions throughout life."[14]

## Background

Louise Flach de Kiriline was born in 1894 in Svensksund, 200 miles south of Stockholm. Her Swedish father and Danish mother each had connections to royalty in their respective countries. Sixten Flach was a good friend of one of the Swedish king's sons, and Hellevid Neergaard enjoyed a friendship with the four daughters of the crown prince of Denmark, which was close enough that one of them, Louise, became a godmother to her first-born daughter. The young Louise Flach spent her early years in relative ease, educated by governesses and enjoying the rhythms of life on a prosperous farming estate. Her father's premature death when she was in her late teens ended this idyllic period, and she moved into an apartment in Stockholm with her mother and younger sister following the sale of the family estate. Despite the reduced circumstances of her family, her mother arranged for her presentation at Swedish court at the age of eighteen.[15]

Apparently inspired to enter nursing through the noblesse oblige of her Aunt Jana, Louise Flach gained admittance in 1914 to the Red Cross Society's School of Nursing in Stockholm. After completing her training toward the end of the First World War, she obtained a position at a Danish prisoner-of-war camp. There she met Gleb de Kiriline, a White Russian army officer, whom she married in 1919 despite objections from her family that he would be unable to support her. She followed him to his posting at Archangel, but a short time later they were forced to flee when the Bolsheviks overran the town. Captured soon afterward, they were taken back to Moscow, where his incarceration separated de Kiriline from her husband. She never saw him again. While she attempted to find him or gain news of his fate, she spent

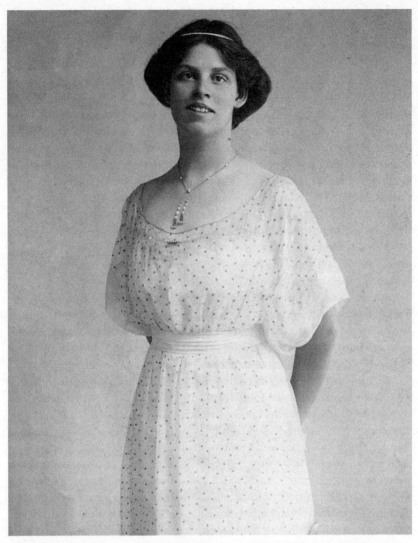

Louise Flach in 1912 at the age of eighteen. Her mother arranged for her presentation at Swedish court, and her second godmother took Flach on an extended visit
of "extravagant opulence," introducing her into Danish high society.
*Courtesy of Library and Archives Canada, 1993-199, File 2, 2000813819. Reproduced
with the permission of the Minister of Public Works and Government Services Canada, 2007*

several years in Russia nursing at a children's hospital and then working
with the Danish Nansen Relief Expedition, finally accepting that he had
been executed.

   After returning to Sweden in 1924, de Kiriline initially welcomed the security and ease of her home after the privations of Russia but soon found

herself restless and discontented.[16] Her restlessness resonated with that of other women who had experienced life on the front lines of war. Author Sharon Ouditt suggested that repatriated voluntary aid nurses typically became irritated by what they saw as the trivial nature of everyday life.[17] De Kiriline herself later admitted that she had been "experiencing life in the raw and I felt there was too much artificiality, too much dishonesty" when she returned.[18] She complained that when she attempted to talk to her friends and relatives about what she had been through, there came "upon the faces of my listeners ... such a look of flatness and indifference that I felt as if a thick wall had risen between them and me."[19] As the nurse who replaced de Kiriline at the Bonfield posting observed, "Sweden looked very tame after caring for 10,000 starving Russians."[20]

Although she remained in Canada until her death in 1992 at age ninety-eight, it is unclear whether or not de Kiriline had initially planned to make this country her permanent home. Considering emigration, however, was not surprising for a Swede. Historian H. Arnold Barton has argued that leaving for North America had long been a "safety-valve" for Swedish men and women during the transition from agriculture to industrialization, at first for the landless and the poor but later for forestry and industrial workers. Most migrants had made their way to the United States, but Swedish emigration to Canada had picked up considerably once the completion of the railway opened up the Canadian frontier in the late 1900s. Few Swedish families remained untouched by "America fever," and the increasing mobility of early twentieth-century emigrants meant that news of conditions in America became more widespread. Barton noted that the First World War marked the end of the "dynamic" period of Swedish migration to North America, but a steady trickle of people still made their way across the Atlantic.[21] De Kiriline could hardly have failed to be aware of this phenomenon; others have argued that the size and rate of Sweden's emigrating population profoundly affected political, social, and economic agendas at home.[22] Her choice of Canada as her destination, she maintained, was due to a chance meeting in Russia with a downed English aviator fighting with the British expeditionary forces. Having previously spent thirteen years farming in Saskatchewan, he "with the eloquence of eager enthusiasm ... filled [her] ears with fascinating tales of a far-off country of the gods – Canada" and piqued her curiosity to see "if [her] picture of Canada carried a good resemblance to the original."[23]

## Nursing Identity

De Kiriline forged her identity as a nurse out of a combination of her belief in the superiority of her education, her depth of background experience in the war, and a strong confidence in the practical fundamentals of nursing routines. As historian Meryn Stuart has pointed out, returned military nurses who had been forced to rely on their own initiative had often gained confidence in their judgment and skills.[24] Although de Kiriline had never been a military nurse, she had experienced many of the conditions of wartime nursing when she worked in the prisoner-of-war hospital after her graduation. Like many former First World War military nurses, de Kiriline rejected the confines of a hospital setting.[25] When she discovered Ontario's CRCS outpost nursing program, she decided that working at a small medical outpost was "the very thing for me."[26] Time spent in the emergency department caring for patients with serious injuries had been her favourite part of training, and, by its nature, outpost nursing had potentially similar opportunities for varied and challenging work.[27] During a period of boredom at the Haileybury outpost, she complained that it was "perfectly ridiculous" that there were four nurses for only ten beds. She was much happier when accident victims from the lumber camps had been admitted. "You know that it is certainly my strong point, the outpatients' department with wounds and infection and things like that," she reminded her mother.[28]

De Kiriline seems to have taken in stride challenges brought by the unknown. Wanting to upgrade her obstetrical nursing skills, she had taken a short course in July and August 1927, working on the maternity floors at the Toronto General Hospital. Believing that "two months [training] was dangerously short to learn to be a delivery nurse," she suffered from much the same anxiety as other nurses in outlying districts with little extra obstetrical training during her first confinement on her own in Bonfield.[29] Nonetheless, she was relieved and pleased with the part she had played in its happy outcome: "I successfully delivered her without a tear. The little girl cried briskly right away, for which I breathed thanks to God. The whole thing was over in 10 minutes with scarcely a drop of blood ... At 6:30 I was home again with the mother and child washed and everything done according to the rules. So what do you say! I feel quite proud."[30] Subsequent births appear to have caused her no great concern and merited only a brief mention when they interrupted sleep or work schedules.

Setting up the public health program in her district elicited much the same response. The Ontario Division had initially intended to hire trained public health nurses for its outposts and, indeed, several of its nurses had received formal public health nursing training through the year-long certificate program that had been available since 1920 at the University of Toronto.[31] De Kiriline's entire formal education in public health, however, consisted of observing district nursing work in Toronto for a two-week period immediately before taking up her position in Bonfield. Nonetheless, three weeks after her arrival at the outpost, she appears to have been ready for the challenge of instituting a typical CRCS public health program. "My work here is more social than medical care," de Kiriline wrote her mother:

I visit the schools, 13 in number ... hold lessons with [the children] in hygiene ... Then I visit their homes, to see what conditions they live in, obtain tax relief for the family when the breadwinner is disabled from the war or through sickness or death, get those with tuberculosis to the sanatorium ... Visit the pregnant mothers ... deliver them here when necessary to teach them how they should look after and feed their babies etc. etc. [I] hold well-baby clinics where the mothers can come and weigh their children, clinics for tonsils, dental clinics ... home nursing classes for ... mothers and their girls where I teach them how one should look after the sick, how one puts on a bandage, a wrapper, how one baths a baby, how one prepares babies' food etc. etc. ... Furthermore, I have and am forming where I don't have, a committee and subcommittee for the Red Cross where they collect money for the poor and the crippled etc. So when you imagine that I have an area 2 square mil [twenty square kilometres] and about 1,200 inhabitants, you can understand perhaps that I don't have time to be idle. To organize in such a place where no such work has been done before amongst the people, where one considered such work as good as impossible, you can probably understand it is more than interesting.[32]

She believed she had impressed her supervisor during a visit six months later, when, as she put it, the supervisor "exclaimed the whole time in different keys and asked if she could send me some foreign students to show them what a Canadian outpost is now."[33]

De Kiriline based her nursing identity in part on her feelings that her nursing education and practice were superior to that of her Canadian colleagues. In general, she considered that the quality of nurse training in Sweden exceeded that obtained in Canada. "The Canadian nurse ... with what I have seen so far ... is quite far under our Swedish Red Cross educated nurses in a great many ... quite fundamental things," she wrote.[34] Nursing at the Toronto General Hospital was "not entirely fine Swedish nursing," and she felt that patients at the Sabbatsberg Hospital had been "considerably better nursed and everything was proper."[35] She criticized the basic techniques of nursing practice in the little hospital at Haileybury, believing that dry sweeping in the presence of tuberculous and cancerous patients was not "the most hygienic" way to clean the floors.[36] She noted at the Kirkland Lake hospital that her colleagues washed patients "nearly everyday over the whole body but they would never dream to wash them clean on their backsides." She was scornful of them cleaning bedside tables "three times a day with a wet cloth" while leaving a thick layer of dust on the window frames and lamp shades.[37]

Another issue that was very important to her was whether physicians should be allowed to make rounds on their own and to discuss patients' conditions with only the patients. "The doctors go around without the nurses, find out what has happened from the patients themselves instead of the nurses and write their orders in a book, which is all well and good, but how can it inspire the nurse with interest when she does not get the opportunity to communicate her observations with the doctor?" she wondered.[38] De Kiriline had valued her emergency nursing experiences during her training precisely because she believed that sharing responsibility with doctors encouraged a more egalitarian relationship.[39] Indeed, she and her "kindhearted" local physician in Bonfield, Alan Dafoe, enjoyed feelings of mutual respect, and despite faulting his aseptic technique, she lauded his interest in the local residents and his skill in diagnosis. She was also proud that Dafoe would not accept any other nurse to take charge of the Dionnes, "thinking me so very efficient," and was delighted that "the little country doctor that I privately always thought a very great deal of [had become] world-famous."[40] Nonetheless, as a nurse schooled in the traditional, hierarchical culture of the hospital, she recognized the limits of this relationship. "He was so good in helping you," she admitted in an interview years later, "[but] he was very particular about what a nurse could do and how far she could go and that she wouldn't overstep into the doctor's realm. Of course, I understood him in that ... and we worked very well together."[41]

The annual reports of the Ontario Division of the CRCS for the years 1928 and 1929 outline the scope of de Kiriline's practice at the beginning of her work in the Bonfield community (see Table 8.1). Little in her letters home suggests that she did not feel competent in her nursing work. Although the statistics indicate that her first six months started off slowly, by the end of September 1928 she was complaining to her mother about "how horribly busy" she had been setting up her school program and examining youngsters so "rowdy" that half had been sent home to await her visit. She had also organized her first tonsil clinic, for which she and her housekeeper had prepared everything from "vomit bags out of newspaper" to the food for the physicians, the outpost nursing supervisor, and other volunteers helping at the event. In October, she held a baby clinic and a teacher's meeting and, for several weeks in December, battled "influenza and lung inflammation" during long days out in the community. She herself succumbed to the illness the week before Christmas.[42] By the end of 1929, we can trace increases in all aspects of her work.

Nonetheless, although few personal sources such as these letters exist for early outpost nurses, in the end they are only marginally useful to understand the role of an outpost nurse and the development of her practice during the interwar period. Although de Kiriline continued to write occasionally about patient illnesses, accidents, and the medical treatment and nursing care she provided, she most often mentioned her nursing work as an excuse to her mother for not writing sooner. De Kiriline often subsumed her nursing

*Table 8.1*

**Bonfield outpost statistics, 1928-29**

|  | (May) 1928 | 1929 |
| --- | --- | --- |
| Patients admitted | 0 | 2 |
| Hospital days | 0 | 5 |
| Outpatients | 30 | 134 |
| Home visits | 400 | 1,038 |
| Home confinements | 2 | 16 |
| School visits | 12 | unknown |
| Children examined | 236 | 1,269 |
| Clinics held | 1 | 5 |
| Clinic attendance | unknown | 108 |

Source: *Ontario Division Annual Reports* 1928, 32; 1929, 18.

identity under news about family and friends, in particular, news about her sister and brother-in-law whose two young children were growing up without her. We gain information as well on the weather, her housing, her pets, her clothing, and the various social activities in which she took part – all of the mundane items of emigrant writing that, until recently, historians considered trivial and frequently condensed or discarded in letter collections.[43]

It is perhaps only logical to suggest that de Kiriline recognized the limits of understanding and interest that her mother, with no medical background, would have taken in the details of her nursing practice.[44] Nonetheless, if Gerber's theoretical understanding about the fundamental purpose of immigrant letters is taken seriously, it was precisely these routine and ritualistic bits that provided the foundational framework through which de Kiriline and her mother maintained their familial relationships.[45] De Kiriline's writing of her own social engagements and the interest that she continued to take in her family and in her mother's activities back home formed a long-running, intimate conversation between a devoted, loving daughter and a mother who cared about her. This correspondence thus served as a means through which these relations could be sustained and nourished. However, not only did they function as a constant reminder of the mother-daughter relationship, but they were also integral to de Kiriline's reassurance that the separation imposed by her move to Canada, and the new experiences she encountered, had not changed her core identity. Her letters illuminated the gendered, classed, and raced identities out of which she had formed her own self-awareness, and the undoubted sharing of many of the same perspectives on her social positioning allowed her to remain "knowable" to her mother.

### Gender, Race, Class, and Region: The Making of a Social Identity
De Kiriline's hard years in Russia at the end of the First World War had probably strengthened an already strong streak of independence, a characteristic

of which her mother was possibly only too aware.[46] Demonstrating that she was comfortable with the challenges of an autonomous professional practice at an outpost, as well as with the independent lifestyle that accompanied it, de Kiriline was able to reassure her mother about her continued well-being. Her letters reveal, however, that both the idea and the experience of independence was a constructed part of her social identity. Authors Bettina Bradbury and Tamara Myers observed that identities are often "conceptualized as sets of understandings that are ... negotiated, performed, and reshaped collectively and individually in the unequal social and class relations of daily life ... As historians, we seek to determine how they were made in specific historical contexts and through particular relations with various 'others.'"[47] While de Kiriline appears to have slipped easily into building her life as a single woman on her own in a northern region, she was also aware of the gendered limits of feminine respectability as well as of her social positioning as a white middle-class member of a desired and welcomed immigrant population. This is not to argue that she did not push against these boundaries at times, but it is through her descriptions of her social activities that we can see her negotiating ideas of gender, race, and class both in constructing these identities through her new experiences and, perhaps most importantly to her, with her mother.

More appealing than the $75-$100 per month salary that the Ontario Division offered de Kiriline for her position in Bonfield was the subsidized accommodation in a converted home as well as the procurement of domestic help that was available to an employee of a provincial nursing station. It was also an option likely beyond what most self-supporting women could have afforded during the interwar period. De Kiriline's descriptions of her home were reassuringly domestic. Although she had initially hesitated when she first viewed the outpost building in Bonfield – "it was quite charmingly situated but remote and without running water or electricity," she wrote – she was soon delighted "to have my own little house and home which I can style ... as I please."[48] In many of her subsequent letters, she outlined in some detail the many domestic touches she employed to help her settle comfortably into her new home. She cleaned and painted and arranged her furniture, decorating the rooms with the few possessions she had brought with her and with the linens and pillows that her mother sent over from time to time. She planted a garden and wrote satisfyingly of the harvested fruits and vegetables put away for the winter. Although she sometimes laughed at her own culinary mistakes, she proudly introduced her young housekeeper and friends to Swedish cooking. On the whole, she told her mother, "my [domestic] learning has not been in vain although it probably seemed hopeless [to you] many times."[49]

Outpost nursing by its nature demanded a certain freedom of movement and dress that pushed at the boundaries of early twentieth-century feminine respectability.[50] This independence, especially during the interwar period, elicited close surveillance from members of small communities in which outpost nurses lived and worked, partly because of their "on-call" nursing responsibilities and partly because they were young single women on their own in a male-dominated northern environment often considered rough and slightly dangerous. As Tasmanian historian Marita Bardenhagen has suggested, bush and other outpost nurses were one of the first sets of rural women to have access to cars, but communities who maintained ownership over these vehicles also tried to control the movements of the nurse.[51]

In areas with roads, it was not unusual for outpost nurses to acquire cars for use during summer months, and, indeed, not having a car in their districts soon became a detriment to nursing practice.[52] The Ontario Division's office in Toronto facilitated de Kiriline's purchase of her own car soon after her arrival in Bonfield. Although physicians or other community members often taught outpost nurses to drive, de Kiriline had already acquired this skill, and she was able to make the ten-hour drive back from Toronto with her older model Ford roadster.[53] She relished the freedom the car gave her. Not only did a motor vehicle make it easier to reach her patients in the surrounding district, but it also made it possible for her to escape the confines of the village for the larger city of North Bay.

Like many other outpost nurses in the winter, de Kiriline used a dogsled on many of her visits to patients. She eschewed more common arrangements made by many of her colleagues, however, who were driven on their missions by village men with their own teams. Instead, she had decided to have her own team of dogs. As she wrote to her mother, "I'm going to get a real Eskimo dog, that is, a husky, from a doctor in North Bay and will then travel with a dogsled. Can you see me traveling in that outfit with my delivery kit in front to [a] delivery?"[54] Subsequent letters often expressed the fun she had in acquiring her dogs, training them, and learning to drive the team herself. The proprietor of Bonfield's general store contended that everyone rushed to their windows when she went by; thus, travelling unaccompanied on her calls ensured the villagers' attention to her whereabouts.[55] Rarely failing to mention de Kiriline and her dog team in articles, the press also appeared intrigued with her method of getting around her district. Since travelling by dog team was not unusual for men in a small snow-bound community in northern Ontario, intense interest in this activity was stimulated by the feminine imagery of the "good angel" juxtaposed with that of the more masculine endeavour of dogsled driving.[56] As one reporter commented, "Her tall, boyish figure, wrapped in a heavy fur coat, a fleece-lined leather helmet pulled down over her ears, her hands and feet encased in warm woollens and high boots, has become a well-known sight as she has gone about the countryside on her errands of mercy on a sleigh pulled by her faithful husky 'Bucky;' or as she has walked the streets of North Bay with

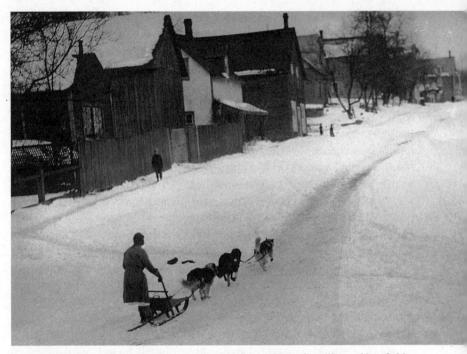

Louise de Kiriline and her dog team were a familiar sight in the village of Bonfield in the early 1930s. Other outpost nurses usually relied on local men to take them by dogsled, but de Kiriline insisted on assembling her own team and learning to drive it herself.
*Photo from Louise de Kiriline's biography,* Another Winter, Another Spring: A Love Remembered *(ISBN 13: 978-0920474-42-6, © 1987). Reprinted with permission of the Dundurn Group*

her mannish stride."[57] De Kiriline herself intimated that she was well aware of the limits of appropriate dress, and humour may, in part, have been a way to deflect her mother's potential criticism of her behaviour. Meeting one of the division's directors with her dogsled at the station, de Kiriline wrote that "[the supervisor] was delighted with me and my outfit, said she never saw anything so Canadian. Yes, my dear, in sweater, leather coat, leggings and moccasins, I am a vision."[58]

From all accounts, de Kiriline was outgoing and sociable. Playing bridge and dancing were among her favourite activities, and she often supplied her mother with detailed accounts of the parties to which she had been invited. Three months after her move to Haileybury, for example, she wrote that she had "entered right into society ... and am invited out ... almost every evening ... Everyone is so hospitable towards me and I feel so at home."[59] After a successful tea party attended by women from both Bonfield and North

Bay who composed the local CRCS outpost committee, she assured her mother that she had had "many invitations from people in North Bay so I'll have to really start getting into society."[60]

What constituted acceptable "society," however, was shaped by a combination of her perspectives on race, class, and gender. De Kiriline's ability to involve herself in "society" might have been hampered by her status as a new immigrant, but as a white Swedish migrant who spoke both English and French, she claimed membership in a privileged racial group. As noted earlier, Swedes had left their homeland for North America throughout the 1800s, although it was not until the early 1900s that Canada began to attract them in larger numbers. The 1931 census indicates that the Swedish population in Ontario, for example, had grown by 50 percent over the previous decade, with the majority of the 10,000-plus Swedes located in the north of the province.[61] The Swedes were considered a desirable group. As one American official proclaimed in 1888, "no immigrants of today, in both faith and works, so closely resemble the sturdy pilgrim fathers of New England as the Swedes."[62] De Kiriline, too, recognized these sentiments, telling her mother that "the Swedish are respected here." She believed that a "well-organized emigration of educated farmers would be a godsend for Canada," and, in her opinion, Swedes were far more acceptable than the "mostly middle-European rabble who fill up to 40 percent of Canadian jails."[63] As Canadian historian Karen Dubinsky has noted, anxieties about increasing criminality and sexual disorder in northern Ontario at this time were being fuelled by the political radicalism of large numbers of what were considered "undesirable" immigrants, especially single male Ukrainians, Italians, and Finns who were drawn to the mining and lumber camps.[64]

Being raised in privileged circumstances and having enjoyed close connections to both Swedish and Danish royalty undoubtedly informed de Kiriline's perspectives on class, easing her relationships with some and contributing to a sense of social distance from others. Only the rare person exhibited what she considered an adequate amount of refinement and culture, although she acknowledged that Canada was a young country and thus had not had the opportunity to acquire the same traditions and cultural background as Sweden.[65] As was typical of many outpost nurses who were invited out by the wives of local clergy and school principals, de Kiriline found much of her social interaction among the educated professionals that she chanced to meet. Bridge parties and dinners to which she was invited took place in the homes of engineers or mine managers stationed in the towns. Grace Morgan was a schoolteacher from North Bay with whom de Kiriline often stayed overnight on her days away from the outpost in Bonfield.

Other relationships, however, proved more difficult for her. She had been slow to warm up to her nursing colleagues and their social activities at the

Haileybury outpost hospital and was relieved to find that at her next posting in Kirkland Lake the "girls" there were fine, ladylike, and with good
upbringing. "It feels comfortable to be with your own class again," she declared, "because no matter how kind and nice the girls were in Haileybury,
they remained "maids."[66] As many outpost nurses discovered, one of the
unique requirements of their work involved winning the trust and respect
of local residents. Once installed in their outposts, all of the nurses had to
establish both professional and social relationships with the people in their
towns and villages. De Kiriline reserved her greatest disdain for the French
Canadian villagers in her local community. She wrote to her mother, betray-
ing her feelings of social aloofness, that they were not at all "chic" but "were
on a somewhat lower level than handyman Larson in our home village in
Sweden. The most refined family was the post master so you can imagine
the rest."[67]

Public health officials had often used assumptions of gender solidarity to
exhort outpost nurses to make friends with the local women, whom they
considered prime targets for the programs that the nurses offered. Indeed,
the success of an outpost nurse was sometimes measured by the willingness
of the local women to seek out her assistance and follow her advice.[68] Yet
de Kiriline appeared to find relationships with women particularly difficult.
After a month of her obstetrical course at the Toronto General Hospital, for
example, she wrote that "it was starting to be boring being kept with women,"
and although she enjoyed playing bridge, she "was not very fond of solely
women's parties."[69] The Ontario Division expected its outpost nurses to associate closely with local branches, but such meetings with "the old women"
in Bonfield, whom de Kiriline describes as "quarrelsome," were tedious to
her, reflecting the often complicated interconnections between both class
and gender. It was very "effective," she remarked with some condescension,
when "she pacified them with tea and soda crackers as they expected."[70]

Whatever de Kiriline's personal thoughts were on the social attributes of
the villagers, however, she did not shy away from public activities that increased her contact with others in the community. Despite her awareness
of the apparent lack of interest in her arrival in Bonfield, she nonetheless
seemed to believe that she would eventually win the residents over. She
worried a little about her first home visit, recognizing, perhaps, along with
many country physicians, that first impressions were very important in establishing a practice in small communities.[71] She went to church: "Catholic
of course but what does it matter, I didn't intend to be Catholic but I think
in any case I should go partly for the people's sake and not the least for my
own."[72] She was flattered by opportunities that placed her in a position of
authority in the community when, for example, the parish priest asked her
a few months later to give a lecture after the service on hygiene and the
prevention of sickness.[73] And if local residents sensed de Kiriline's aloofness,

they nevertheless sought out her nursing services – the number of her home confinements, in particular, increased steadily throughout the years. Still, not all were ready to accept her into the community. Almost a year after her arrival in Bonfield, she was heartbroken over the death of one of her sled dogs. "Can you imagine something so horrible but my little Dixie was poisoned last Sunday and died," she lamented to her mother. Since this incident was the second time an attempt had been made on the lives of her dogs, "it is evidently someone who harbours a hidden enmity towards me."[74]

## Conclusion

CRCS rhetoric during the interwar period constructed a particular identity for its nurses, a somewhat "exaggerated version of Victorian social deference," which bordered on what nursing historian Kathryn McPherson has described as the ideal of early twentieth-century feminine professionalism.[75] Tending to subsume the individuality of its nurses, the society viewed them collectively as modest foot soldiers in the crusade for good health or as angels of the North inspired to serve through the call of a missionary spirit.[76] The concept of modest, maternal, or submissive feminine respectability that this imagery invoked undoubtedly helped to legitimate the presence of outpost nurses as single females working on their own in primarily male-dominated districts. Moreover, suggesting that its nurses remained within the bounds of appropriate contemporary feminine behaviour was undoubtedly a wise strategy for the CRCS, which was itself an organization dependent on public good will for both its reputation and financial viability.

Louise de Kiriline's letters provide a rare opportunity to get behind this kind of public projection, and the images that emerge have very little to do with the constructed imagery that the CRCS projected about its outpost nurses. De Kiriline gave little indication that she considered herself "called to serve" in isolated northern communities. Cosmopolitan, self-assured, and strong-willed, she already possessed a wealth of lived experience and was attracted to the outpost program precisely because she believed it offered opportunities for personal autonomy and professional advancement. Nursing with the outpost program in Ontario offered her the kind of professional independence she had become used to and in which she strongly believed was desirable for nurses. Although CRCS officials assured official medical associations that the society's nurses always worked *under* a physician's supervision, de Kiriline always contended that relations between doctors and nurses should be more egalitarian. "Why should the nurse, a very highly trained nurse, not be considered exactly on the same level as the doctor?" she asked.[77] Fulfilment for her was found in meeting the challenges of her own personal standards in nursing practice. Years later, she admitted that it was "the work, the performance, knowing that you [could] do these things and that [you handled them] better and better."[78]

While she appeared to be competent and conscientious about her work, de Kiriline's letters suggest that her engagement with nursing seemed more a means to an end. As other authors have pointed out, the nature of the occupation provided both the respectability and the economic conditions through which single women (or women without other means of support) could support themselves at a time when a professional identity for aspiring middle-class women was not assured nor entirely accepted.[79] Outpost nursing with the Ontario Division also offered de Kiriline a home "of her own" and an adventurous lifestyle that suited her personality. Yet she was able to project enough of the ideal of what was considered appropriate feminine behaviour to be cloaked in respectable femininity, a protection that allowed her to attain the freedom and independence that she desired. It is interesting to note, however, that when de Kiriline left her professional duties at the end of the Dionne infants' first year of life, nursing as work disappeared entirely from her letters.[80] Although some evidence suggests that the skills of those nurses who remained in their outlying towns and villages continued to be valued long after their formal "retirement," and although some scholars have called for a broader reconsideration of how a professional nursing identity connected to nurses' domestic lives, de Kiriline herself no longer identified herself as a nurse.[81]

The project of this chapter has been to suggest that nursing was only a part, and at times only a small part, of de Kiriline's self-identity *even as* she continued to work as a nurse. A reading of her letters highlights other social positions that often appear to assume more significance in her life. De Kiriline's correspondence reveals constructions of identities organized around her status as an immigrant woman trying to build a new life in a new country on her own and as a daughter with strong ties to her family back home. Her letters must be read within the context of the important role they played in maintaining a close relationship with a loved one. The particular perspectives on gender, race, and class that they illuminated functioned as markers of familiarity in the ongoing conversation she maintained with her distant mother. At the same time, the significance of these other identities to de Kiriline herself reminds us, as historians, to consider other factors beyond that of a professional nursing identity in reconstructing nurses' lives.

# 9

# University Nursing Education for Francophones in New Brunswick in the 1960s: The Role of Nuns, Priests, Politicians, and Nurses

*Anne-Marie Arseneault*

This chapter explores the controversy surrounding the establishment in 1965 of the École des sciences hospitalières at the newly founded Université de Moncton in Moncton, a community in the southeastern section of the province of New Brunswick. The nursing school emerged out of major educational and administrative reforms introduced by the provincial government in the early 1960s as well as from pressure by the New Brunswick Association of Registered Nurses (NBARN). The establishment of this school, however, led directly to the termination of the baccalaureate nursing program that a congregation of religious women, the Religious Hospitallers of Saint Joseph, had earlier initiated at the Collège Maillet in Saint-Basile in the northwestern part of the province. The Religious Hospitallers of Saint Joseph had a long history of delivering health care in northern New Brunswick, and they directed several diploma nursing programs at their hospitals. After founding the Collège Maillet in 1949, they continued to be involved in the higher education of francophone women. The Hospitallers were thus important contributors to both education and the local economy in the region. Their baccalaureate nursing program had been in operation for only four years, but the transfer of the program at the Collège Maillet to the Université de Moncton signalled the beginning of the increasing secularization and centralization of education in New Brunswick. It heralded as well the demise of the powerful and autonomous role that religious women and men had played in higher education in the province.

As Helen Mussallem stated in her research on nursing in Canada during the 1960s, nursing education should be studied within the broader context of the general educational system.[1] Louis J. Robichaud, the young Acadian premier who was elected in 1960, placed great emphasis on his government's responsibility for social reform, ethnic equality, and harmony, and many of the surveys that he instituted formed the basis of what became known as his Equal Opportunity Program.[2] The eventual establishment of the baccalaureate nursing program at the Université de Moncton was facilitated particularly by the recommendations of the Royal Commission on Higher Education, which was the first commission organized under Robichaud's mandate.[3] Furthermore, for several decades, national and provincial professional nursing groups had been proposing substantial changes in nursing education.[4] Major changes in the health sector with the advent of hospital and medical insurance, coupled with the development of the health care infrastructure, also had important implications for nursing education in the province.[5] The following discussion examines the beginning of French university nursing education in New Brunswick. It is based on government records and correspondence between individual members of religious congregations and the administrators of existing universities and colleges involved in the discussions about the baccalaureate programs. I also refer to the minutes of the NBARN taken in 1961-65, the history of these two higher educational institutions, as well as interviews with a Hospitaller involved in both of the nursing programs.

## Educational Reform in New Brunswick

Health care and education in New Brunswick were caught up in the general tumult of social and political change that took place during the 1960s, and events related to the founding of the École des sciences hospitalières at the Université de Moncton were influenced by these major transformations. Determined to improve the decentralized and costly public administration system in the province, the New Brunswick government requested two major royal commissions to examine higher education and the administration of government services. Initiated in 1961, the Royal Commission on Higher Education, which was presided over by John Deutsch and thus known as the Deutsch Commission, was the first major undertaking of the thirty-four-year-old premier, Louis J. Robichaud.[6] Premier Robichaud believed it was necessary to begin by transforming the education system for both the francophone and anglophone linguistic communities.[7] Inequities had existed between the provincial university (the University of New Brunswick) and the other institutions, but all of the higher education institutions in New Brunswick were suffering from insufficient funding and demands for increased enrolment. This situation threatened all students in the province, particularly, the French-speaking students.[8] One-third of New Brunswick's population was (and still is) French-speaking Acadian, a group that forms a specific minority in the Maritime provinces.[9] Prior to the 1960s, religious orders were responsible for the administration of all of the French higher-education institutions. In the northern part of the province, the Eudist congregation administered the men's universities – the Université Saint-Louis in Edmundston and the Université du Sacré-Cœur in Bathurst. In the south, the Saint Croix fathers directed the Université Saint-Joseph in Memramcook. The Religious Hospitallers of Saint Joseph operated one of the three women's

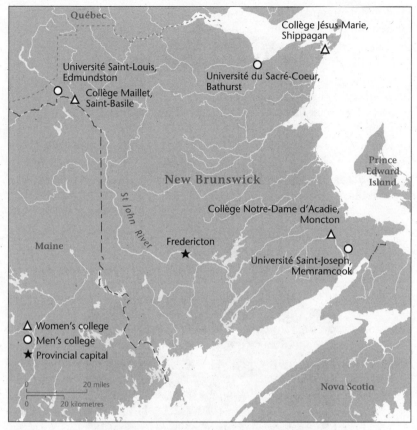

*Map 9.1* Francophone colleges and universities in New Brunswick, 1960
*Cartography: Eric Leinberger*

colleges, the Collège Maillet in Saint-Basile, which was also in the north near Edmundston.[10]

Premier Robichaud influenced the deliberations of the Deutsch Commission in several strategic ways. He handpicked John Deutsch as chair of the commission, and he named another friend, Judge Adrien Cormier, as a member.[11] Both Robichaud and Judge Cormier had studied with the Eudist fathers at the Université du Sacré-Cœur in Bathurst. Robichaud admitted later that he knew Judge Cormier would be favourable to his position. Robichaud was also an intimate friend of Father Clément Cormier, a Saint Croix father and president of the Université Saint-Joseph in southeastern New Brunswick.[12] During their studies at Laval University in Quebec City, both men had been students of Georges-Henri Lévesque, whose ideas had inspired the "Quiet Revolution" in the province of Quebec.[13] It has been said that the vision of the Deutsch Commission was essentially that of Father Cormier,

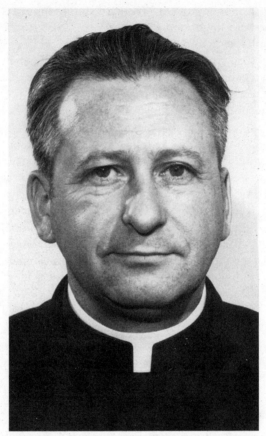

Father Clément Cormier, first director of the École des sciences hospitalières at the Université de Moncton. Close friend of Premier Robichaud and keenly interested in nursing education for francophones, Cormier had an enormous influence on the establishment of the school of nursing at the Université de Moncton.
*Courtesy of Centre d'études acadiennes, E36, 457B*

even though he was not a formal member of it, but Premier Robichaud also followed the evolution of the work of the commission very closely.[14] Several years later, he stated that unbeknownst to his own cabinet members, he had held secret meetings with members of the commission.[15]

In 1962, Premier Robichaud also initiated the Royal Commission on Finances and Municipal Taxation, which was known as the Byrne Commission in honour of its president, Edward G. Byrne.[16] Prior to this time, social assistance had been the responsibility of municipalities, counties, and charitable groups, and wide variations existed in education, health care, and welfare services. The Byrne Commission's report, published in 1963, proposed uniformity and increased efficiency for the province's administration system in order to aid economic growth.[17] The Byrne philosophy of equalizing opportunities for both linguistic communities contributed to the increasing government intervention in the delivery of public services.[18] The recommendations of the Byrne Commission led to the development of the Equal Opportunity Program, for which the premiership of Louis Robichaud is best known. The economic development of New Brunswick, the provision of greater social justice, and the centralization of public service administration were the prime objectives of this program, which had major effects on health care, education, social services, and the justice system.[19] Robichaud's vision of rationalizing services in the province was made clear in a speech at the Legislative Assembly in 1965, when he argued that "we must begin to think and act like a province with a population of 600,000 rather than continue to isolate ourselves according to economic advantages that derive from an outdated geographic regionalism ... Our loyalty towards our human community can only make sense if [it is] in accordance with our loyalty towards our province and nation."[20] His arguments against regionalism had a profound impact on higher education in New Brunswick, including nursing education.

A third development also played a significant role in the history of university nursing education for francophones in New Brunswick. In 1961, the federal government commissioned a survey of the state of health care services in Canada. One of the recommendations of this Royal Commission on Health Care Services, or the Hall Commission as it was more commonly known, was the establishment of ten new university nursing programs in Canada, including one at the Université de Moncton.[21]

## The Push for Reform in Nursing Education

Up to and including the 1960s, several studies on nursing education had identified major deficiencies in North American nursing education programs, which traditionally were offered in hospital schools. Examining public health nursing education was the original mandate of the 1923 Committee for the Study of Nursing Education in the United States, but instead the committee found that there was a need for an overall study of nursing education. Its recommendations included the call to assist schools to improve standards, to discontinue the exploitation of students as cheap labour, to make nursing schools independent of hospitals, and to push for university-based nursing programs.[22] In Canada, the 1932 report by George Weir, which the Canadian Medical Association and the Canadian Nurses Association had jointly commissioned, exposed major problems in nursing education and service. A key outcome of this report was the recommendation that nursing schools become educational institutions financed by funds allocated to education.[23] Helen Mussallem's 1960 study of nursing education in Canada, *Spotlight on Nursing Education,* was originally planned to determine if nursing schools were ready for accreditation. Her research found that little progress had been made since the Weir report and that only 16 percent of the schools would have met the proposed accreditation criteria. She recommended studying ways of upgrading the whole field of nursing education. In another survey undertaken for the Royal Commission on Health Services in 1964, she recommended introducing nursing education into the post-secondary education system and developing two types of programs: a university and diploma program.[24]

In New Brunswick, a survey of nursing education by Alice Wright for the federally sponsored Health Survey of 1951 assisted the NBARN to push for reform. Her report recommended broader content for nursing education programs and the creation of a baccalaureate program at the University of New Brunswick in Fredericton, the capital of New Brunswick.[25] E. Kathleen Russell, who was retired from the University of Toronto's School of Nursing, published a study of nursing education and nursing service in New Brunswick in 1956, a survey that stimulated reflection in general on nursing education in Canada. The recommendations of the Russell report included the creation of schools of nursing separate from hospitals and specifically called for a baccalaureate nursing program at the University of New Brunswick, which was eventually established in 1958. At the time of Russell's survey, there were fourteen nursing schools in the province: seven French schools administered by religious congregations, five of which were directed by the Religious Hospitallers of Saint Joseph, and seven secular schools for English students.[26]

## Nursing Education at the Collège Maillet
The Religious Hospitallers of Saint Joseph have a long history in New Brunswick. They arrived from Montreal in 1868 in Tracadie, a town in the northeastern part of the province, to care for victims of leprosy. Contributing to the economy of this region, they established educational institutions and hospitals, nursing schools in their own hospitals, and nursing homes and sanitaria for tuberculosis patients. In 1949, they established a college for women, the Collège Maillet in Saint-Basile, and, among other courses, offered a teacher-training program for religious sisters and a classics program for other women.[27]

In mid-1961, Sister Rhéa Larose, an educator and the director of the college who became a mythical figure in the region, proposed the creation of a baccalaureate program for registered nurses through a four-year basic program at the Collège Maillet.[28] This program was approved by the administrators at the Université Saint-Louis in nearby Edmundston, to which the college was affiliated.[29] Aware of the survey undertaken by the Deutsch Commission, Sister Larose proposed this course, even though she knew that Father Cormier wanted to include a nursing school and a medical school at the new university that he wished to establish in the city of Moncton. Under the leadership of Sister Larose, the Hospitallers presented a brief to the Deutsch Commission on 12 December 1961, requesting that the nursing programs at the Collège Maillet be maintained.[30]

The report of the Deutsch Commission was made public in the late summer of 1962, although its recommendations were widely known even as the Hospitallers were presenting their brief in December 1961. Calling for "a fundamental concentration of efforts," the report strongly recommended the creation of the new Université de Moncton as the only French higher-education institution in New Brunswick.[31] The men's universities were to become colleges affiliated to the Université de Moncton, while the women's colleges were affiliated to the men's universities. The Collège Maillet would therefore remain under the supervision of the Université Saint-Louis and was thus not directly affiliated to the Université de Moncton. The preliminary report of the commission also stated that the academic senate of the newly created university had the authority to decide the fate of existing programs, "it being understood that the courses now being offered in the three affiliated colleges will be permitted to continue."[32] The Hospitallers were convinced that they would be able to maintain the nursing programs that they had initiated.

### The NBARN

Under the direction of its leader, the NBARN played an active role in the development of university nursing education for both anglophones and francophones in the province. Katherine MacLaggan, the director of the School of Nursing at the University of New Brunswick, was president of the association between 1962 and 1964.[33] She knew Father Cormier well even before the Deutsch Commission was created, since he had been a member of the committee that had studied the feasibility of a nursing program at UNB.[34] As a result of his knowledge of nursing education, MacLaggan had invited Father Cormier in 1960 to attend a conference given by Mildred Montag, a well-known American nurse leader in education, and to discuss nursing education in New Brunswick. At that time, Father Cormier had told MacLaggan that he wished the Hospitallers to direct the nursing program that he wanted to establish at the future Université de Moncton.[35]

It was clear before the publication of the Deutsch Commission's report that the Robichaud government would implement its recommendations, but Father Cormier later admitted that one of the most delicate tasks was to bring the regions and the women's colleges to accept the "concentration of efforts."[36] Immediately following the report's publication, MacLaggan wrote a "nice confidential letter" to Father Cormier.[37] In it, she suggested that the baccalaureate nursing program for francophones be offered in Moncton and also recommended that the Hospitallers be invited to administer the program.

In July 1962, however, Sister Larose and the Hospitallers requested that the NBARN approve the four-year baccalaureate program at the Collège Maillet, which was scheduled to commence two months later.[38] The NBARN immediately evaluated the program and refused its approval due to a lack of human and clinical resources.[39] It also proposed that the administrators of the college wait for the provincial government's official reaction to the findings of the Deutsch Commission. Furthermore, it also suggested that the Hospitallers meet with Helen Mussallem, who was conducting a study of nursing education in Canada for the Hall Commission, and wait for her recommendation. Although a letter signed by Sister Larose in January 1963 informed the NBARN that the meeting with Helen Mussallem was no longer "opportune," it stated that "we have accordingly postponed all further activities and [have] decided to remain in "the statu quo" [sic]."[40] The members of the NBARN executive committee thus understood from this last statement that the Collège Maillet had abandoned its proposed baccalaureate program.

Nonetheless, in September 1962, the Hospitallers initiated their baccalaureate program and admitted students.[41] At the same time, they were well aware of the threats from the new Université de Moncton to their institution and its programs. Between 1962 and 1965, the Hospitallers at the Collège Maillet and at the provincial council of the religious congregation undertook a robust campaign soliciting support for the maintenance of their nursing program in Saint-Basile. They met with Premier Robichaud and other influential persons. In his history of the Université Saint-Louis and the Collège Maillet, author Jacques-Paul Couturier described the letter-writing campaign and the Hospitallers' numerous encounters with provincial and community leaders, including Bishop Gagnon of Edmundston, a senator, members of the Chamber of Commerce, several politicians including mayors, and members of the Legislative Assembly of New Brunswick and the Canadian House of Commons.[42] The Hospitallers believed that the college was a vital institution in this part of the province and that local officials wished to protect the program and keep students in the region.

## The Nursing Program at the Université de Moncton

The Université de Moncton was officially created in June 1963, and Father Cormier became its first president.[43] As the Deutsch Commission had recommended, nursing was among the specialized programs the university would offer to the francophone population. One of the first items on the agenda of the academic senate, therefore, was the controversy surrounding the nursing program at the Collège Maillet and the proposed program for the Université de Moncton.[44]

According to Couturier, the perseverance of the Hospitallers in their efforts to maintain the nursing program at the Collège Maillet provoked an "imbroglio," the first crisis of the new university.[45] Most members of the academic senate agreed that the nursing program should be offered in Moncton, and Father Cormier reiterated his suggestion that the Hospitallers nominate one of their sisters as director of the Moncton program. The Senate committee that was formed to study the situation recommended in 1964 that the program at the Collège Maillet continue for another year, which would allow the college the opportunity to study the recommendations of the Hall Commission on nursing education and to arrive at an agreement with the NBARN about the status of the students registered in its program.[46] An entente with the association was essential since the graduates of an unapproved nursing program would not be permitted to write the professional registration examinations.

In January 1964, however, the NBARN was surprised to learn that the four-year baccalaureate program had been inaugurated at the Collège Maillet in 1962, in spite of the NBARN's previous refusal to approve it. In a letter dated 7 February 1964 to the provincial superior of the Hospitallers, the association informed her a second time that it refused to approve the program and warned that students from the college would not be permitted to write their professional exams.[47] The Hospitallers were advised to transfer their students to a three-year diploma program or to the program proposed for Moncton. On the same date that this letter was written, the secretary of the NBARN, in order to accelerate the creation of the school of nursing at the Université de Moncton, wrote to Father Cormier suggesting that "perhaps a statement of intent would rule out the precipitate or ill-advised actions by others."[48]

Even as these events were unfolding, the Hospitallers had selected in September 1964 Sister Jacqueline Bouchard, one of their own, as the director of the school at the Université de Moncton.[49] Sister Bouchard was a thirty-one-year-old nurse from the Edmundston region who had recently obtained a master's degree in nursing from the Catholic University of America and was a faculty member at the Collège Maillet. As she was establishing the school in Moncton, the Senate of the Université de Moncton requested that she study the nursing education requirements for the francophone population of New Brunswick.[50] Sister Bouchard presented the recommendations of her report to the Hospitallers before presenting them to the Senate. She recommended discontinuing the program at the Collège Maillet because of the limited resources and wanted the Hospitallers to determine the status of their students.[51]

Not surprisingly, these proposals displeased the sisters and the other supporters of the program in Saint-Basile. In a letter to Sister Bouchard, the provincial superior of the Hospitallers stated that Sister Bouchard did not have complete knowledge of the events and that she had failed to obtain a broad picture of the situation.[52] Sister Bouchard replied that the documents

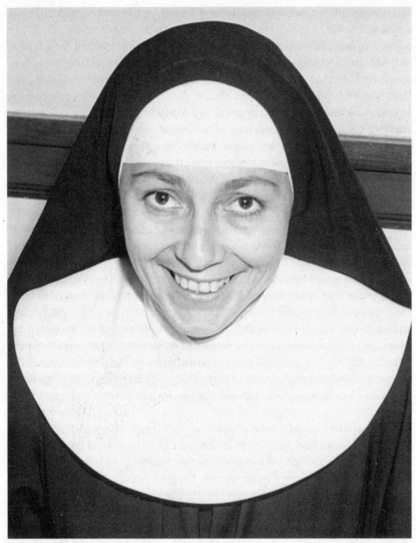

Sister Jacqueline Bouchard, first director of the École des sciences hospitalières at the Université de Moncton. When the new university's Senate asked her to study francophone nursing education, she defied her own religious congregation, the Religious Hospitallers of Saint Joseph, to recommend that the Hospitallers' four-year baccalaureate program be closed.
*Courtesy of Centre d'études acadiennes, E41557*

she had studied did not favour the Hospitallers because they had clearly demonstrated that the Hospitallers had chosen to put in place a program that the NBARN had not approved. Furthermore, they should have carried on only with the post-diploma program and waited until the Deutsch Commission had released its recommendations before initiating the four-year baccalaureate program.[53]

Sister Bouchard's superiors at the Hospitallers asked her to modify her recommendations to the Senate of the Université de Moncton to make it clear that they consisted only of her personal opinion and were not intended to commit the college, or the congregation, to her proposals.[54] Sister Bouchard nonetheless submitted her report to the Senate in June 1965 without modification.[55] After a last appeal from the director of the Collège Maillet, the Senate adopted Sister Bouchard's recommendations, which resulted in the termination of the four-year nursing education program at the Collège Maillet.

### The École des sciences hospitalières at the Université de Moncton

The École des sciences hospitalières at the new campus of the Université de Moncton received its first class of fourteen students in September 1965.[56] Even before this program was established, the university's Senate had decided in 1964 to award the baccalaureate degree in nursing to two students of the Collège Maillet.[57] According to Sister Bouchard, this was an important concession made by the university to the college. In 1969, the year of the first graduation, funds obtained from the federal government helped to construct a building to house the school.[58] That same year, the name of the school was changed to the École des sciences infirmières to reflect the integration of health promotion and community health into the program.[59] The loss of the word "hospitalière" in the name of the school, even if it did not refer specifically to the Hospitallers, did make less visible the role of the sisters in the development of university nursing education for francophones in New Brunswick. Sister Bouchard was director of the school from 1964 to 1971, and she began a second mandate in 1976 when she was no longer a Hospitaller.[60] Two years later, she died tragically in an airplane crash. In recognition of her vital role in nursing education in New Brunswick and at the university, the school of nursing named its building in her honour.

### People, Place, and Context in Nursing Education in New Brunswick

Politics, the push to develop higher education, especially for the francophone population, and health care services determined the fate of the Hospitallers nursing program. The roles of strategically placed individuals within these areas, however, were also significant. In opposing regionalism, Premier Robichaud believed that centralizing public administration and concentrating resources were essential for the economic development of the province. He admitted during an interview in 1998 that had the Deutsch Commission not recommended an Acadian university such as the Université de Moncton, he would have found a "subterfuge," in other words, a reason to set aside its report.[61]

Robichaud's relationship with Father Cormier, in particular, also directly facilitated the implementation of the project. Father Cormier shared Robichaud's vision for the province and for education. As president of the Université Saint-Joseph in Memramcook near Moncton, he was in a good position, politically and geographically, to influence the establishment of the new university in Moncton and to substantially modify the mandates of the two men's universities administered by the Eudists. Father Cormier's early interest in nursing and medical education deserves further study, since his notes and papers reflect his thoughts on nursing education and the quality of nursing education programs formed nearly two decades before the establishment of the nursing school at the Université de Moncton.

Even before Katherine MacLaggan became president, the NBARN had been a major force in the development of university nursing education for both the French and the English. Aware of the need for nursing education in the province, from the surveys that had previously been undertaken, the association strove for many years to increase the quality of nursing education in general. As its president, MacLaggan actively promoted university nursing education for the francophone population, and she was aware of the political issues related to the restructuring of higher education in their institutions. Her numerous conversations over several years with Father Cormier, even before the Deutsch Commission was created, and their common vision for nursing education greatly facilitated the establishment of the nursing program at the Université de Moncton in 1965.

The role played by Sister Jacqueline Bouchard during the final year preceding the opening of the school in Moncton also cannot be underestimated. As a young nurse and Hospitaller, she had taught at the Hôtel-Dieu Hospital diploma program in Edmundston and at the Collège Maillet. While colleagues lobbied to maintain the nursing program at the college, she took positions that required courage and determination. Nuns were required to defer to the decisions of superiors, and "no one would dare to question the judgement of mother superior." [62] She nevertheless resisted the pressures exerted upon her by her religious superiors as well as by supporters mobilized in the lay community. In opposing the continuation of a program not approved by the NBARN, she firmly believed she was protecting the integrity of nursing education.[63] Furthermore, she agreed with Premier Robichaud, Father Cormier, and Katherine MacLaggan about the need to centralize resources and avoid the duplication of services.[64] Even if Sister Bouchard's career in university nursing education was relatively short, her efforts at a crucial time marked the history of nursing education in New Brunswick and at the Université de Moncton.

The secularization of higher education profoundly affected the Religious Hospitallers of Saint Joseph and other women's and men's congregations involved in higher education. With the increasing social needs of the 1960s, it was difficult, if not impossible, for religious groups, male or female, to maintain their autonomy, programs, and services.[65] The struggle of the Hospitallers, the Eudists, and their supporters against the provincial government's efforts to centralize higher education and particularly to transfer the baccalaureate in nursing program to the Université de Moncton, awakened rivalries that played out regionally between the university and the colleges.[66] The Saint Croix fathers in the south, for example, often had direct access to the decision makers and were closer to the policy makers than were the Eudists from the northern part of the province. In spite of the tensions between the Eudist and Saint Croix fathers, though, members of the male congregations were more often present during the discussions and decision making than the sisters.

In Isabelle McKee's study of women's religious congregations and their colleges in New Brunswick, she stated that, in addition to unequal power relations and regional rivalries, there were tensions between men's congregations and also between men's and women's congregations.[67] Nonetheless, there were also very effective alliances between men and women, as seen in Father Cormier's co-operation with MacLaggan and between the Hospitallers and the Eudist fathers, who collaborated for the protection of their own programs.

Reflecting on the early years of higher education for francophone women in New Brunswick, Father Cormier wrote that "those who have observed the profound transformations which have occurred during the past decades and who have experienced the *ancient regime* may be nostalgic when recalling these old convents whose customs have disappeared ... [along with] their charm and advantages." However, he also recognized the nuns' role in small communities and their importance in the survival of the French language in the Maritimes.[68] The termination of the nursing program at the Collège Maillet was a substantial loss for Sister Larose, the founder of the college, and for the Hospitallers and the region. One of the principal motivations of the Hospitallers and their supporters was to preserve the programs that had been established in northwestern New Brunswick and not lose them to the new university in Moncton. Bishop Gagnon of Edmundston had written in a letter to Father Cormier in 1964 that the Collège Maillet "is fixed in Saint-Basile and must remain there."[69] As historian Sioban Nelson suggested, nuns had to be "innovative and entrepreneurial ... [and] understand the politics and economics of [their] domain." Successful communities had to develop the skills of "commercialism and business acumen."[70] American scholar Barbra Mann Wall pointed out that nuns, in their role as health care administrators, contributed to local economies by purchasing goods and supplies, developing medical and hospital services, and training many young women through their nursing schools.[71] The Religious Hospitallers of Saint Joseph had been in the northeastern part of the province since the middle of the nineteenth century, and this region, in which the college was situated, also appreciated and depended on the educational institution's contribution to the local economy. As Mann Wall noted, however, nuns who administered hospitals gradually lost much of their autonomy during the twentieth century because of professionalization, the increased regimentation of their religious lives, and government regulations.[72] In the case of the Hospitallers, gender, too, played a part. As directors of the women's colleges, they lost status and voice once the Université de Moncton was established, since they were barred from membership in both the Conseil des regents and the Senate, which were both important decision-making bodies.[73]

## Conclusion

If certain events in the establishment of the nursing school at the Université de Moncton are undoubtedly unique, many of the events reflect similar social and political influences that were present in many nursing schools in the 1960s. Historian Geertje Boschma has written that the history of a faculty of nursing is a story of accommodation, resistance, and creativity in responding to larger social trends.[74] Her argument illustrates the need to examine the wider context surrounding the founding of a school of nursing. Such an investigation will expose the multiple forces that are at play: individual, religious, professional, and regional values as well as politics, gender roles, and economic considerations. Persons not traditionally identified as promoters of nursing education, in this case, Father Cormier, for example, can have a substantial impact on the profession.[75] MacLaggan had first noted his interest in nursing education, and their continued collaboration contributed to the development of university nursing education for francophones through the creation of the school at the Université de Moncton.

The contributions of the Religious Hospitallers of Saint Joseph and other women's congregations to the education of francophone women in New Brunswick are an essential part of the province's history that have not yet been fully acknowledged.[76] The sisters identified needs in education and health care services and founded institutions with their own resources when public institutions did not exist. Years of experience and expertise in their own institutions were no match, however, for the changing social and political environment in New Brunswick during the latter half of the twentieth century, and it became much more difficult for religious congregations to maintain their institutions and programs.

# Notes

## Introduction

1 The second conference was organized by the Canadian Association for the History of Nursing.

2 For just one example of the debates surrounding the meaning and identities in nursing, see Amélie Perron and Dave Holmes, "Advanced Practice: A Clinical or Political Issue?" *Canadian Nurse* 102 (September 2006): 26-29; and the responses to this article in "Readers Speak," *Canadian Nurse* 102 (November 2006): 4-7.

3 Patricia D'Antonio, "Revisiting and Rethinking the Rewriting of Nursing History," *Bulletin of the History of Medicine* 73 (1999): 272.

4 Patricia D'Antonio, "History for a Practice Profession," *Nursing Inquiry* 13 (2006): 243.

5 For writing on Black nurses in Canada, see Karen Flynn, "Race, the State, and Caribbean Immigrant Nurses, 1950-1962," in *Women, Health and Nation: Canada and the United States since 1945,* ed. Georgina Feldberg, Molly Ladd-Taylor, Alison Li, and Kathryn McPherson (Montreal and Kingston: McGill-Queen's University Press, 2003), 247-63; and Karen Flynn, "Experience and Identity: Black Immigrant Nurses to Canada, 1950-1980," in *Sisters or Strangers: Immigrant, Ethnic, and Racialized Women in Canadian History,* ed. Marlene Epp, Franca Iacovetta, and Frances Swyripa (Toronto: University of Toronto Press, 2004), 381-97. See also Agnes Calliste, "Women of 'Exceptional Merit': Immigration of Caribbean Nurses to Canada," *Canadian Journal of Women and the Law* 6 (1992): 85-103; and Tania Das Gupta, *Racism and Paid Work* (Toronto: Garamond Press, 1996). For nursing and the construction of whiteness, see Diana L. Gustafson, "White on Whiteness: Becoming Radicalized About Race," *Nursing Inquiry* 14 (2007): 153-61.

6 Celia Davies, "Rewriting Nursing History – Again?" *Nursing History Review* 15 (2007): 20-21.

7 Sioban Nelson, "The Fork in the Road: Nursing History versus the History of Nursing?" *Nursing History Review* 10 (2002): 175-88.

8 Christina Bates, Dianne Dodd, and Nicole Rousseau, eds., *On All Frontiers: Four Centuries of Canadian Nursing* (Ottawa: University of Ottawa Press and the Canadian Museum of Civilization, 2005). Also published in French under the title *Sans frontières: Quatre siècles de soins infirmiers canadiens* (Ottawa: University of Ottawa Press and the Canadian Museum of Civilization, 2005).

9 Kathryn McPherson and Meryn Stuart, "Writing Nursing History in Canada: Issues and Approaches," *Canadian Bulletin of Medical History* 11 (1994): 3-22; and Cynthia Toman and Meryn Stuart, "Emerging Scholarship in Nursing History," *Canadian Bulletin of Medical History* 21 (2004): 223-27.

10 "Making Nursing Relevant to a New Generation of Practitioners," Plenary Session, Annual Meeting of the Canadian Association for the History of Nursing, Toronto, 2004.

11 Although we are aware of the developing theoretical literature on the geography of nursing that examines the relationship between space, place, and nursing, it was not our intention to situate this collection in it. Future research in this direction would, however, be a useful

path to follow. For two summaries of the rich relationship between cultural geography and nursing, see Gavin J. Andrews, "Locating a Geography of Nursing: Space, Place and the Progress of Geographical Thought," *Nursing Philosophy* 4 (2003): 231-48; and Gavin J. Andrews, "Geographies of Health in Nursing," *Health and Place* 12 (2006): 110-18.

12  Kathryn McPherson, *Bedside Matters: The Transformation of Canadian Nursing, 1900-1990* (Toronto: Oxford University Press, 1996), 17-18.

13  Marion McKay, "Region, Faith, and Health: The Development of Winnipeg's Visiting Nursing Agencies, 1897-1926," this volume, p. 75.

14  Susan Riddell, "'Curing Society's Ills': Public Health Nurses and Public Health Nursing in Rural British Columbia, 1919-1946," MA thesis, Simon Fraser University, Vancouver, 1991; Sharon Richardson, "Frontier Health Care: Alberta's District and Municipal Nursing Services, 1919 to 1976," *Alberta History* 46 (Winter 1998): 2-9; Laurie Meijer Drees and Lesley McBain, "Nursing and Native Peoples in Northern Saskatchewan: 1930s-1950s," *Canadian Bulletin of Medical History* 18 (2001): 43-65; Merle Massie, "Ruth Dulmage Shewchuk: A Saskatchewan Red Cross Outpost Nurse," *Saskatchewan History* 56 (Fall 2004): 35-44; Jayne Elliott, "Blurring the Boundaries of Space: Shaping Nursing Lives at the Red Cross Outposts in Ontario, 1922-1945," *Canadian Bulletin of Medical History* 21 (2004): 303-25.

15  In particular, see David A. Gerber, *Authors of Their Lives: The Personal Correspondence of British Immigrants to North America in the Nineteenth Century* (New York: New York University Press, 2006).

### Chapter 1: "A Loyal Body of Empire Citizens"

1  Margaret Macdonald, "No. 1 Canadian General Hospital on Salisbury Plain and Early Days in France," MG30, E45, Aii, Margaret Macdonald Papers [hereafter Macdonald Papers], Library and Archives Canada (LAC).

2  Ibid.; and "More Nurses Needed," *Mail and Empire,* 6 July 1917, 7. So great was the distinction between home and overseas service that it carried over into the post-war formation of the Overseas Nursing Sisters Association, in which membership was limited to those who had served overseas. Not until early in the Second World War was this restriction lifted. See Jessie Morrison, "Address to Royal Alexandra Hospital Nurses Alumnae – Edmonton, December 9, 1974," Jessie Morrison Fonds, records 87.4, 91.30, and 92.10, Alberta Association of Registered Nurses Museum and Archives.

3  Mabel Clint, *Our Bit: Memories of War Service by a Canadian Nurse* (Montreal: Barwick Limited, 1934), 50.

4  May Bastedo, "My Trip Abroad," letter of 20 October 1915, May Bastedo Papers, Canadian War Museum (CWM), 58A 1 2.1 [hereafter Bastedo letters].

5  See Susan R. Grayzel, *Women's Identities at War: Gender, Motherhood, and Politics in Britain and France during the First World War* (Chapel Hill, NC: University of North Carolina Press, 1999); Angela K. Smith, *The Second Battlefield: Women, Modernism and the First World War* (Manchester: Manchester University Press, 2000); Angela Woollacott, "From Moral to Professional Authority: Secularism, Social Work, and Middle-Class Women's Self-Construction in World War I Britain," *Journal of Women's History* 10 (Summer 1998): 85-111; Miriam Cooke and Angela Woollacott, eds., *Gendering War Talk* (Princeton: Princeton University Press, 1993); Cynthia Enloe, *Does Khaki Become You? The Militarisation of Women's Lives* (Boston: South End Press, 1983); Cynthia Enloe, *Maneuvers: The International Politics of Militarizing Women's Lives* (Berkeley: University of California Press, 2000); Margaret Randolph Higonnet, Jane Jenson, Sonya Michel, and Margaret Collins Weitz, eds., *Behind the Lines: Gender and the Two World Wars* (New Haven, CT: Yale University Press, 1987); Margaret R. Higonnet, *Nurses at the Front: Writing the Wounds of the Great War* (Boston: Northeastern University Press, 2001); Henriette Donner, "Under the Cross – Why V.A.D.s Performed the Filthiest Task in the Dirtiest War: Red Cross Women Volunteers, 1914-1918," *Journal of Social History* 30 (Spring 1997): 687-704; Jean Bethke Elshtain, *Women and War* (New York: Basic Books, 1987); Ruth Roach Pierson, *"They're Still Women after All": The Second World War and Canadian Womanhood* (Toronto: McClelland and Stewart, 1986).

6  Gail Braybon, "Winners or Losers: Women's Symbolic Role in the War Story," in *Evidence, History and the Great War: Historians and the Impact of 1914-1918,* ed. Gail Braybon (New

York and Oxford: Berghahn Books, 2003), 88 and 104-5. As Braybon further elaborated, "the most popular stereotypes are VAD (volunteer aid nurses) and munitions worker ... The VAD, of course, was performing 'standard women's work': her dedication is seen as admirable, but unsurprising – while her sisters who were professional nurses arouse very little attention at all" (at 88).

7 Waltraud Ernst and Bernard Harris, eds., *Race, Science and Medicine, 1700-1960* (London and New York: Routledge, 1999).

8 Gail Braybon, "Introduction," in *Evidence, History and the Great War: Historians and the Impact of 1914-1918*, ed. Gail Braybon, 5 and 21.

9 Clint, *Our Bit*, 50.

10 Historians R.G. Moyles and Doug Owram analyzed the disconnect between the expectations created through literature regarding the "dreams of imperialists – and the reality of actual experience – of colonial life" in Canada at the turn of the century as consisting of nine dominant discourses. Two of these discourses involved a country in need of refinement and an evolving society that was primitive in manner, insular in outlook, lacking artistry, but offering hope and an escape from British problems. See R.G. Moyles and Doug Owram, *Imperial Dreams and Colonial Realities: British Views of Canada, 1880-1914* (Toronto: University of Toronto Press, 1988), 7 and 8-9.

11 Mildred Forbes, letter to Cairine Wilson, 1 October 1915, Carine Reay Wilson Fonds, MG27, III-C6 (R5278-0-4-E), LAC [hereafter Forbes letters].

12 Edward W. Said, *Orientalism* (NY: Vintage Books, 1979), 157 and 206.

13 Said, *Orientalism*, xviii, 1-4, and 206. A growing historiography related to imperialism has relevance for analyses of military nursing. See, for example, Adele Perry, "Whose Sisters and What Eyes? White Women, Race, and Immigration to British Columbia, 1849-1871," in *Sisters or Strangers? Immigrant, Ethnic, and Racialized Women in Canadian History*, ed. Marlene Epp, Franca Iacovetta and Frances Swyripa (Toronto: University of Toronto Press, 2004), 49-70; and Mary Louise Pratt, *Imperial Eyes: Travel Writing and Transculturation* (London and New York: Routledge, 1992), 28 and 33.

14 Said, *Orientalism*, 156 [emphasis in original].

15 Kathleen Wilson, "Empire, Gender, and Modernity in the Eighteenth Century," in *Gender and Empire*, ed. Philippa Levine (Oxford: Oxford University Press, 2004), 18.

16 Catherine Hall, "Of Gender and Empire: Reflections on the Nineteenth Century," in *Gender and Empire*, ed. Philippa Levine, 52.

17 Anne McClintock, *Imperial Leather: Race, Gender and Sexuality in the Colonial Context* (London and New York: Routledge, 1995), 5-6.

18 Katie Pickles, *Female Imperialism and National Identity: Imperial Order Daughters of the Empire* (Manchester: Manchester University Press, 2002), 5 and 9.

19 Carl Berger, *The Sense of Power: Studies in the Ideas of Canadian Imperialism, 1867-1914* (Toronto: University of Toronto Press, 1970).

20 Benedict Anderson, *Imagined Communities: Reflections on the Origin and Spread of Nationalism*, revised edition (New York: Verso, 1991); A.P. Cohen, *The Symbolic Construction of Community* (New York: Tavistock Publications, 1985); Charles Wetherell, Andrejs Plakans, and Barry Wellman, "Social Networks, Kinship, and Community in Eastern Europe," *Journal of Interdisciplinary History* 24 (1994): 639-63; Barry Wellman and Barry Leighton, "Networks, Neighborhoods, and Communities: Approaches to the Study of the Community Question," *Urban Affairs Quarterly* 14 (March 1979): 363-90; and Veronica Strong-Boag, Sherrill Grace, Avigail Eisenberg, and Joan Anderson, eds., *Painting the Maple: Essays on Race, Gender, and the Construction of Canada* (Vancouver: UBC Press, 1998).

21 Barbara Lorenzkowski and Steven High, "Culture, Canada, and the Nation," *Histoire sociale/ Social History* 39 (May 2006): 5.

22 Cecilia Morgan, "'A Choke of Emotion, a Great Heart-Leap': English-Canadian Tourists in Britain, 1880s-1914," *Histoire sociale/Social History* 39 (May 2006): 12-13 and 15.

23 Pratt referred to this particular type of travel writing as "survival literature." See Pratt, *Imperial Eyes*, 20.

24 Nursing Sister Mabel Clint was a member of the Imperial Order Daughters of the Empire (IODE) who published in the organizational literature at least as early as 1904. The mandate

of this elite Anglo-Canadian society of women was to promote and defend Britain. Indeed, there are strong IODE links to wartime nursing through the funding of an entire hospital ship, nineteen ambulances, twenty-two sterilizing units, twelve operating tables, three huts for convalescent soldiers, 942 cots, equipment for thirty-six wards, and a home or "haven of rest" in London for the use of military nurses. See Pickles, *Female Imperialism,* 36 and 43-44.

25 First-hand accounts of experiences on Lemnos and Salonika are included in the published memoirs of Constance Bruce, *Humour in Tragedy: Hospital Life behind Three Fronts by a Canadian Nursing Sister* (London: Skeffington and Son, 1918); Clint, *Our Bit;* and Katherine M. Wilson-Simmie, *Lights Out! A Canadian Nursing Sister's Tale* (Belleville, ON: Mika Publishing, 1981). Maude Wilkinson included sections from the Mediterranean settings as part of three brief autobiographical accounts published in *Canadian Nurse* during her lifetime: "Four Score and Ten," part 1, *Canadian Nurse* 73, no. 10 (1977): 26-29; part 2, *Canadian Nurse* 73, no. 11 (1977): 14-23; and part 3, *Canadian Nurse* 73, no. 12 (1977): 16-23. Posthumously, her family added further material and published *Four Score and Ten: Memoirs of a Canadian Nurse* (Brampton, ON: Margaret M. Armstrong, 2003). Unpublished accounts and oral interviews based wholly or partially on the Mediterranean experience include: Elsie D. Collis, "A Nursing Sister of No. 5: Diary of E.D. Collis, June 1915-March 1919" [in possession of the author with thanks to Glennis Zilm of the British Columbia History of Nursing Professional Practice Group who salvaged and preserved this diary]; Helen Fowlds diaries and letters, boxes 1-2, file 69-001/1/1, Helen Marryat (nee Fowlds) Fonds, Trent University Archives [hereafter Fowlds letter and Fowlds diary]; Forbes letters; Bastedo letters; and the oral history of Mabel Lucas Rutherford, audio-taped interview with Margaret M. Allemang in Oakville, Ontario, 1978, Oral History Collection, Margaret M. Allemang Centre for the History of Nursing. This interview has been partially reprinted in John Gardam, *Seventy Years After: 1914-1984* (Stittsville, ON: published by author, 1983), 46-49. There are several other first-hand accounts by Canadian military nurses who served only on the Western front, of which the most substantial ones are the diaries of Alice Isaacson at the LAC, and the diary of Clare Gass that Susan Mann painstakingly recovered, edited, and published in 2000. Susan Mann, ed., *The War Diary of Clare Gass, 1915-1918* (Montreal and Kingston: McGill-Queen's University Press, 2000).

26 Fowlds letters, 27 February 1916 [emphasis in the original].
27 Ibid., 4 March 1915.
28 William Bridgeman, "Report of an Advisory Committee Appointed by the Army Council to Enquire into the Supply of Nurses," 14 November 1916, in folder XV, MG30 E45, Macdonald Papers, LAC.
29 Maude Abbott, "Lectures on the History of Nursing," *Canadian Nurse* 18 (March 1922): 141.
30 Clint, *Our Bit,* 11.
31 See Andrew Macphail, *The Medical Services: Official History of the Canadian Forces in the Great War, 1914-1919* (Ottawa: King's Printer, 1925); and Carlotta Hacker, "The Bluebirds Who Went Over," *Canadian Nurse* 65 (November 1960): 32-33.
32 Mabel Clint, "Our Bit," *Canadian Nurse* 35 (August 1939): 58 and 460.
33 Fowlds diaries, "Diaries and Autograph Book – World War I."
34 Clint, *Our Bit,* 59-60.
35 Quoted in Hacker, "The Bluebirds Who Went Over," 31-34.
36 Wilson-Simmie, *Lights Out!* 61.
37 For some examples, see the Canadian Expeditionary Force fonds for the personnel files of Nursing Sisters Mabel Clint, Helen Fowlds, Beatrice Mack, Mabel Lucus, and Katharine Wilson contained in RG 150, series 166, files 1803-57, 3245-6, 5828-11, 5779-46, and 10465-46 respectively, LAC.
38 Bastedo letters.
39 Ibid., letter, 26 November 1915.
40 Ibid., letter, 12 December 1915.
41 Wilson-Simmie, *Lights Out!* 94; and Wilkinson, "Four Score and Ten," part 2 (November 1977): 18.

42 Luella Lees, diary 1916-17, copy in possession of author.
43 Collis, "A Nursing Sister of No. 5: Diary of E.D. Collis, June 1915-March 1919," 9 [in possession of the author].
44 Wilson-Simmie, *Lights Out!* 64.
45 Geneva Conventions, 12 August 1949, 1125 U.N.T.S. 3.
46 Margaret Macdonald, "No. 1 Canadian Stationary Hospital," War Diaries of Matrons, folder XII, MG30 E45, Margaret Macdonald Papers, LAC.
47 Clint, *Our Bit,* 62-63.
48 J. Cameron-Smith, "The Story of Moore Barracks," in War Diaries of Matrons, folder XII, MG30 E45, Margaret Macdonald Papers, LAC [emphasis in original].
49 Clint, *Our Bit,* 63.
50 Fowlds diary, 15 September 1915.
51 Myra Goodene, quoted in ibid., 16 January 1916.
52 Fowlds letter, 19 September 1915 [emphasis in original].
53 Fowlds diary, 23 November 1916.
54 Forbes letter, 29 March 1916.
55 Ibid., 6 August 1916.
56 Clint, *Our Bit,* 65.
57 Forbes letters, 29 March 1916, 29 May 1916, and 6 August 1916.
58 Herbert A. Bruce, *Politics and the Canadian Army Medical Corps: A History of Intrigue, Containing Many Facts Omitted from the Official Records, Showing How Efforts at Rehabilitation were Balked* (Toronto: William Briggs, 1919). See also R.C. Fetherstonhaugh, *History of No. 3 CGH (McGill), 1914-1919* (Montreal: Gazette Printing Company, 1928), 69; and Kenneth Cameron, *No. 1 Canadian General Hospital, 1914-1919: History of No. 1 General Hospital Canadian Expeditionary Force* (Sackville, NB: Tribune Press, 1938), 290, for the impact of this commission on two medical units.
59 During the same period, the Australian Army Nursing Service was requested to staff the British general hospitals there. See Jan Bassett, *Guns and Brooches: Australian Army Nursing from the Boer War to the Gulf War* (Oxford: Oxford University Press, 1992), 74-85.
60 Perry, "Whose Sisters and What Eyes?" 60-61.
61 Dea Birkett, "The 'White Woman's Burden' in the 'White Man's Grave': The Introduction of British Nurses in Colonial West Africa," in *Western Women and Imperialism: Complicity and Resistance,* ed. Nupur Chaudhuri and Margaret Strobel (Indianapolis: Indiana University Press, 1992): 180.
62 Clint, *Our Bit,* 59.
63 Ibid., 85.
64 Pratt, *Imperial Eyes,* 28 and 33. There is a very small body of literature on the diverse roles that nurses have played in colonialist or imperialist endeavours. Two examples include Margaret Jones, "Heroines of Lonely Outposts or Tools of the Empire? British Nurses in Britain's Model Colony: Celon, 1878-1948," *Nursing Inquiry* 11 (2004): 148-60; and Helen Sweet, "'Wanted: Sixteen Nurses of the Better Educated Type': Provision of Nurses to South Africa in the Late Nineteenth and Early Twentieth Centuries," *Nursing Inquiry* 11 (2004): 176-84.
65 Margaret M. Allemang Centre for the History of Nursing, Oral History Collection, Mabel Lucas Rutherford, audio-taped interview with Margaret M. Allemang at Oakville, Ontario, 1978.
66 Clint, *Our Bit,* 86.
67 Anonymous Canadian Army Medical Corps Nursing Sister, "Military Nursing," *Canadian Nurse* 13 (August 1917): 485.
68 These accounts are similar to the discourse missionaries used to portray local inhabitants as uncivilized, wherein both narratives and photos represent the "other" through a focus on the unkempt, frequently unclothed, unruly appearance of the "other," and on "divergence from European standards of neatness, cleanliness, and order." See Kim Greenwell, "Picturing 'Civilization': Missionary Narratives and the Margins of Mimicry," *BC Studies* 135 (Autumn 2002): 12.
69 Fowlds diary, 5 March 1916.

70 Wilson-Simmie, *Lights Out!* 57.
71 Lorenzkowski and High, "Culture, Canada, and the Nation," 6.
72 Clint, *Our Bit,* 41.
73 Bassett, *Guns and Brooches,* 74-85.
74 Fowlds letter, 27 February 1916.
75 Fowlds diary, 26 January 1916 [emphasis in original].
76 Fowlds letter, 3 June 1915.
77 Ibid., 28 April 1915.
78 Anonymous reporter quoting Miss Emily B. Forster in "Impressions of a Canadian Nurse," Montreal *Gazette,* 24 November 1915, 2.
79 Fowlds letter, 3 June 1915.

**Chapter 2: Social Sisters**

1 Joan Scott, "The Evidence of Experience," *Critical Inquiry* 17 (Summer 1991): 777.
2 For a discussion of the issues around self-fulfillment and the desire for equality with men in the war context, see Sharon Ouditt, *Fighting Forces, Writing Women: Identity and Ideology in the First World War* (London and New York: Routledge, 1994), 5.
3 Helen Fowlds was typical of graduated nurses. Forty-two percent of working nurses were ages twenty-five to thirty-four, according to the 1931 census. See Kathryn McPherson, *Bedside Matters: The Transformation of Canadian Nursing, 1900-1990* (Toronto: Oxford University Press, 1996), 116.
4 Trent University Archives, Helen Marryat Fonds (née Fowlds) [hereafter Fowlds letter, or Fowlds diary], letter to mother, 18 March 1915, file 69-001/1/1, boxes 1-2.
5 Ibid., letter, 5 April 1915.
6 Margaret Conrad, *Recording Angels: The Private Chronicles of Women from the Maritime Provinces of Canada, 1750-1950* (Ottawa: Canadian Institute for the Advancement of Women, 1982), 1. On the destabilization of the old binaric private/public spheres, see Alison Piepmeier, *Out in Public: Configurations of Women's Bodies in Nineteenth Century America* (Chapel Hill: University of North Carolina Press, 2004), 1-12.
7 Re soldiers' mail, see Desmond Morton, *When Your Number's Up: The Canadian Soldier in the First World War* (Toronto: Random House, 1993), 238. Letters home from First World War Canadian nursing sisters on active service are uncommon in archival or private collections as it seems that families or the nurses themselves threw them away or destroyed them. For example, Vie, the younger sister of Matron-in-Chief Margaret Macdonald, burned all of Macdonald's letters in 1974 after the nurse herself had saved them carefully all her life (Macdonald died in 1948 at the age of seventy-five). Intense family privacy may have accounted for this act. Susan Mann, *Margaret Macdonald: Imperial Daughter* (Montreal and Kingston: McGill-Queen's University Press, 2005), 189. A few other letter collections do exist in Canada, including that of Nursing Sister Mildred Forbes, available at Library and Archives Canada (LAC) in the Cairine Reay Wilson Fonds, MG27, III-C6 (R5278-0-4-E), vol. 1, file 7, microfilm no. 2299. Letters from British and Australian First World War nurses are found in their respective war museums. Published war letters of American nurses, especially the volunteer nurses, for example, can be found in Judith S. Graham, ed., *"Out Here at the Front": The World War One Letters of Nora Saltonstall* (Boston: Northeastern University Press, 2004).
8 Maude Wilkinson, *Four Score and Ten: Memoirs of a Canadian Nurse* (Brampton, ON: Margaret M. Armstrong, 2003). Parts of this memoir were published in the *Canadian Nurse* journal in 1977.
9 Karen Duder, "Public Acts and Private Languages: Bisexuality and the Multiple Discourses of Constance Grey Swartz," *BC Studies* 136 (Winter 2002-03): 5.
10 See Carroll Smith-Rosenberg, *Disorderly Conduct: Visions of Gender in Victorian America* (New York: Alfred A. Kopf, 1985), 245-96.
11 Sir Andrew Macphail, *Official History of the Canadian Forces in the Great War, 1914-1919: The Medical Services* (Ottawa: King's Printer, 1925), 228. These numbers do not include Canadian nurses who volunteered with the American Red Cross Army Nursing Service nor those who enlisted with the British nursing service, Queen Alexandra's Imperial Military Nursing

Service. It is unclear exactly how Macphail came up with the number of nurses and matrons, since numbers vary. The first popular published history of nurses was G.W.L. Nicholson's *Canada's Nursing Sisters*, Canadian War Museum Historical publication no. 13 (Toronto: Samuel Stevens Hakkert and Company, 1975). He wrote that 2,504 nurses went overseas at some time in the war (at 98) and quoted the records in LAC, Margaret Macdonald Papers, MG30, E45.

12  Susan Mann, ed., *The War Diary of Clare Gass, 1915-1918* (Montreal and Kingston: McGill-Queen's University Press, 2000), xxi-xxii. For patriotism and duty, see also two memoirs published after the war and written by nursing sisters themselves: Mabel Clint, *Our Bit, Memories of War Service by a Canadian Nursing Sister* (Montreal: Barwick, 1934) and Maude Wilkinson, *Four Score and Ten*.

13  Susan Mann, "Where Have All the Bluebirds Gone? On the Trail of Canada's Military Nurses, 1914-18," *Atlantis* 26 (Fall/Winter 2001): 38.

14  In his book on the Canadian forces, Macphail devoted three pages to the formation of the nursing service and occasionally inserted nurses' roles into the narrative of the four hundred-dred-page history. He wrote that "the nursing service being an integral part of the medical services, no attempt has been made to segregate its history." Macphail, *Official History of the Canadian Forces*, 229.

15  Tim Cook, *Clio's Warriors: Canadian Historians and the Writing of the World Wars* (Vancouver: UBC Press, 2006), 258. Some exceptions are Bill Rawling, who intermittently discussed nursing in his book *Death Their Enemy: Canadian Medical Practitioners and War* (Québec: AGMV Marquis, 2001); Michel Litalien, who described the nurses who volunteered for the two Québec hospital units (No. 6 General and No. 4 Stationary) in *Dans la tourmente: Deux hôpitaux militaires canadiens-français dans la France en guerre, 1915-1919* (Outremont, QC: Athéna Éditions, 2003). However, a recent official history of the Canadian Forces Medical Service contains only a mention of nurses, who are subsumed under the rubric of "military medicine." See *Canadian Forces Medical Service: Introduction to its History and Heritage* (Ottawa: Director General Health Services, Department of National Defence, 2003), 19.

16  Jan Bassett, *Guns and Brooches: Australian Army Nursing from the Boer War to the Gulf War* (Oxford: Oxford University Press, 1992); and Mary Sarnecky, *A History of the U.S. Army Nurse Corps* (Philadelphia: University of Pennsylvania Press, 1999).

17  G.W.L. Nicholson, *Canada's Nursing Sisters* and *Seventy Years of Service: A History of the R.C.A.M.C.* (Ottawa: Borealis Press, 1977); Carlotta Hacker, "The Bluebirds Who Went Over," *Canadian Nurse* 65 (November 1969): 31-34; Marjorie Barron Norris, *Sister Heroines: The Rose-ate Glow of Wartime Nursing 1914-1918* (Calgary, AB: Bunker to Bunker Publishing, 2002); and Edith Landells, *The Military Nurses of Canada: Recollections of Canadian Military Nurses* (White Rock, BC: Co-Publishing, 1995).

18  Linda Quiney, "Assistant Angels: Canadian Voluntary Aid Detachment Nurses in the Great War," *Canadian Bulletin of Medical History* 15 (1998): 189-206.

19  The published master's thesis is by Mélanie Morin-Pelletier, *Briser les ailes de l'ange: Les infirmières militaires canadiennes, 1914-1918* (Montreal: Athéna Éditions, 2006). Mann, ed., *The War Diary of Clare Gass;* Mann, *Margaret Macdonald, Imperial Daughter.*

20  Concerning sexuality, Mary Sarnecky wrote that among 10,000 nurses in the First World War, forty-four pregnancies were recorded in the official records of army nursing. Military officials considered pregnancies as "major misconducts." Since the American nurses were not officers, more opportunity existed for socializing with enlisted men, causing much consternation about nurses' "social relations." See Sarnecky, *A History of the U.S. Army Nurse Corps*, 116. No official record of any pregnancies has been found for Canadian nursing sisters.

21  On Macdonald's friendships with men and women and on her rumoured "romance" with and potential future marriage to the well-known physician and poet Colonel John MacCrae (who died in 1918), see Mann, *Margaret Macdonald: Imperial Daughter*, 122-23, 133, and 135-38.

22  Katie Holmes, "Day Mothers and Night Sisters: World War I Nurses and Sexuality," in *Gender and War: Australians at War in the Twentieth Century*, ed. Joy Damousi and Marilyn Lake (Cambridge: Cambridge University Press, 1995), 46-53.

23  See Cynthia Toman's chapter in this volume.
24  Fowlds letter, 22 October 1918.
25  Holmes, "Day Mothers and Night Sisters," 45.
26  Fowlds letter, 20 May 1915.
27  Ibid., letter, 11 March 1916
28  Conrad, *Recording Angels*, 1.
29  Thanks to Crystal O'Connell, former Master of Science of Nursing student at the University of Ottawa, for the information regarding the missing pages.
30  Susan Reverby, *Ordered to Care: The Dilemma of American Nursing, 1850-1945* (Cambridge: Cambridge University Press, 1987), 41.
31  Clara S. Weeks, *A Textbook of Nursing: For the Use of Training Schools, Families and Private Students* (New York: D. Appleton and Company, 1885), 16-17.
32  Reverby, *Ordered to Care*, 39-75; and McPherson, *Bedside Matters*, 164-204.
33  On the sexual division of labour in training schools, see McPherson, *Bedside Matters*, 39. As much as the military gendered nursing work female, it gendered medical work male, and typically granted it the male attributes of primary decision making and higher military rank and pay. In fact, it required all medical officers to be male. Despite being a physician, Dr. Margaret Parks was commissioned as a nursing sister and wore the same veil and blue uniform as the nurses. She gave anaesthetics at the Canadian Stationary Hospitals No. 1 and No. 3, and probably did not perform nursing work.
34  Mann, "War Diary of Clare Gass," 88 and 152.
35  LAC, *Instructions for Members of Canadian Army Medical Corps Nursing Service (When Mobilized)*, File: "History of the Nursing Service," MG30, E45, folder 15, chapter 4: 2 and 3. These were a copy of the British instructions.
36  Ibid.
37  See Mann, *Margaret Macdonald: Imperial Daughter*, 138-39, for a discussion of Macdonald's expectations with regard to nurses being "ladies" and her efforts to track down any reported indiscretions.
38  LAC, *Instructions for Members of Canadian Army Medical Corps Nursing Service*, 4: 3 and 6.
39  Ibid., 4: 4 and 6.
40  See, for example, Fowlds letter, 11 March 1916, where Fowlds adds a note to the end of the letter asking for coffee, a book, and writing paper.
41  Ibid., 15 July 1915.
42  Ibid., 10 June 1917.
43  Ibid., 13 December 1915.
44  Erika Rappaport, "The Bombay Debt: Letter Writing, Domestic Economies and Family Conflict in Colonial India," *Gender and History* 16 (August 2004): 233. Rappaport also stated that personal family letters as a source are "under-theorised."
45  Fowlds letter, 9 April 1915.
46  Ibid., 13 February 1916. See also her diary entry from Alexandria on 3 February 1916 regarding shopping through the city.
47  Fowlds letter, 1 October 1916.
48  Victoria de Grazia with Ellen Furlough, eds., *The Sex of Things: Gender and Consumption in Historical Perspective* (Berkeley: University of California Press, 1996), 9 and 10.
49  Rudi Laermans, "Learning to Consume: Early Department Stores and the Shaping of Modern Consumer Culture, 1860-1914," *Theory, Culture and Society* 10 (November 1993): 82.
50  Erika Rappaport, *Shopping for Pleasure: Women in the Making of London's West End* (Princeton, NJ: Princeton University Press, 2000), 142-43.
51  Fowlds letter, 18 April 1918.
52  Mann, *Margaret Macdonald: Imperial Daughter*, 126. See also LAC, *Instructions for Members of Canadian Army Medical Corps Nursing Service*, 4: 6.
53  LAC, *Instructions for Members of Canadian Army Medical Corps Nursing Service*, Appendix A: "Patterns and Materials of Uniforms, 4: 7. The quote about not wearing civilian clothes in France "at any time" is on the same page.
54  Fowlds letter, 13 February 1916.

55  Ibid., 23 September 1915.
56  Kathryn McPherson, "Carving Out a Past: The Canadian Nurses Association War Memorial," *Histoire sociale/Social History* 29 (November 1996): 420. McPherson's article is a critical analysis and "deconstruction" of the bas-relief memorial for Canadian military nurses.
57  For a discussion of Gerald Moira's painting, see Dean Oliver and Laura Brandon, *The Canvas of War: Painting the Canadian War Experience, 1914-1945* (Vancouver: Douglas and McIntryre and Ottawa: Canadian War Museum, 2000), 44. See also the large war painting *Sacrifice* prominently exhibited in the new Canadian War Museum, in which the veiled nursing sister in bright blue is central to helping wounded and despairing European refugees after the war. A crucified Jesus is in the foreground.
58  Sharon Ouditt, *Fighting Forces*, 17 and 18. In the first decades of the twentieth century, Canadian nurses travelling in cities and rural areas to patients' homes were required to wear their uniforms and caps, in part because of the belief that the uniform protected them from sexual assaults.
59  See the comprehensive discussion of the new woman who came of age in the early twentieth century in Smith-Rosenberg, *Disorderly Conduct*, 292-96.
60  Fowlds letter, 15 May 1915.
61  Ibid., 11 August 1915.
62  Ibid., 13 September 1915.
63  Ibid., 19 September 1915.
64  Mann, *War Diary of Clare Gass*, xxv. Mann described Macdonald's intense interest in the romances and overseas marriages of her nurses to the point that she was accused of running a "matrimonial agency." See Mann, *Margaret Macdonald: Imperial Daughter*, 132-33.
65  For example, see Fowlds letter, 28 October 1919.
66  Fowlds diary, 15 September 1915 [emphasis is added].
67  Ibid., 19 November 1915.
68  Surprisingly, she also noted at the end of this entry that two of her patients had died of pneumonia, something never mentioned in the letters to her mother on those dates.
69  Fowlds diary, 3 January 1916; and 8 January 1916.
70  Fowlds letter, 19 September 1915.
71  Fowlds diary, 23 November 1915; and 30 December 1915.
72  Ibid., 9 January 1916.
73  Fowlds letter, 16 February 1916.
74  Peter Bailey, "Parasexuality and Glamour: The Victorian Barmaid as Cultural Prototype," *Gender and History* 2 (Summer 1990): 148.
75  Angela Woollacott, *To Try Her Fortune in London: Australian Women, Colonialism and Modernity* (London: Oxford University Press, 2001), 7.

### Chapter 3: The Healing Work of Aboriginal Women in Indigenous and Newcomer Communities

1  Anne Woywitka, "Pioneers in Sickness and in Health," *Alberta History* 49 (Winter 2001): 16.
2  According to Mary Louise Pratt, contact zones are "social spaces where disparate cultures meet, clash, and grapple with each other, often in highly asymmetrical relations of domination and subordination." Mary Louise Pratt, *Imperial Eyes: Travel Writing and Transculturation* (London and New York: Routledge, 1992), 4.
3  Irene Stewart, ed., *These Were Our Yesterdays: A History of District Nursing in Alberta* (Altona, MB: D.W. Friesen and Sons, 1979), 10.
4  George Bird Grinnell, *Blackfoot Lodge Tales: The Story of a Prairie People* (Lincoln: University of Nebraska Press, 1962), 196-207. See also Sandra Leslie Peacock, "Piikani Ethnobotany: Traditional Plant Knowledge of the Piikani Peoples of the Northwestern Plains," MA thesis, University of Calgary, Calgary, 1992, 22-23.
5  Patricia Jasen, "Race, Culture, and the Colonization of Childbirth in Northern Canada," *Social History of Medicine* 10 (1997): 383-400.
6  Ibid., 392.

7   Maureen Lux, *Medicine That Walks: Disease, Medicine, and Canadian Plains Native People, 1880-1940* (Toronto: University of Toronto Press, 2001), 91-95.
8   For an example of contemporary discussions of childbirth in northern Native communities, see Betty-Anne Daviss, "Heeding Warnings from the Canary, the Whale and the Inuit: A Framework for Analyzing Competing Types of Knowledge about Childbirth," in *Childbirth and Authoritative Knowledge: Cross-Cultural Perspectives*, ed. Robbie Davis-Floyd and Carolyn Sargent (Berkeley: University of California Press, 1997), 441-73; and John O'Neil and Patricia Kaufert, "*Irniktakpunga!* Sex Determination and the Inuit Struggle for Birthing Rights in Northern Canada," in *Conceiving the New World Order: The Global Politics of Reproduction*, ed. Faye Ginsburg and Rayna Rapp (Berkeley: University of California Press, 1995), 59-73.
9   *An Act to Amend and Consolidate the Laws Respecting Indians, S.C., 1876.*
10  Sarah Carter, *Aboriginal People and Colonizers of Western Canada to 1900* (Toronto: University of Toronto Press, 1999), 162-64.
11  Katherine Pettipas, *Severing the Ties That Bind: Government Repression of Indigenous Religious Ceremonies on the Prairies* (Winnipeg: University of Manitoba Press, 1994), 3-7.
12  P.B. Waite, *Canada, 1874-1896: Arduous Destiny* (Toronto: McClelland and Stewart, 1971), 149.
13  Sheila McManus, *The Line Which Separates: Race, Gender, and the Making of the Alberta-Montana Borderlands* (Edmonton: University of Alberta Press, 2005), 142-43.
14  W.H. Long, ed., *Fort Pelly Journal of Daily Occurrences, 1863* (Regina: Regina Archaeological Society, 1987), 128. Fort Pelly was located at the northeast elbow of the Assiniboine River, eight miles west of the present-day village of Pelly, Saskatchewan. It was built in 1824, burned down in 1842, rebuilt, and then moved to another location in 1856-57, and eventually closed in 1912.
15  For information about the accident, see John Julius Martin, *The Prairie Hub: An Outline of Early Western Events from the Hand Hills to the Buffalo Hills* (Rosebud: Strathmore Standard, 1967), 179. For further information about Rundle's career, see Frits Pannekoek, "Robert T. Rundle," *Dictionary of Canadian Biography Online*, http://www.biographi.ca/EN/ShowBio. asp?BioId=40534&query=pannekoek.
16  United Church of Canada/Victoria College Archives, John Maclean Papers, Diaries and Notebooks, February-April 1888, entry dated 29 February 1888, box 11, file 5.
17  John Webster Grant, *Moon of Wintertime: Missionaries and the Indians of Canada in Encounter since 1534* (Toronto: University of Toronto Press, 1984), 105; and S.A. Archer, ed., *A Heroine of the North: Memoirs of Charlotte Selina Bompas, 1830-1917* (London: Society for Promoting Christian Knowledge, 1929), 74-76.
18  Kristin Burnett, "Aboriginal and White Women in the Publications of John Maclean, Egerton Ryerson Young, and John McDougall," in *Unsettled Pasts: Reconceiving the West through Women's History*, ed. Sarah Carter et al. (Calgary: University of Calgary Press, 2005), 115-16.
19  Myra Rutherdale, *Women and the White Man's God: Gender and Race in the Canadian Mission Field* (Vancouver: UBC Press, 2002), 45.
20  Ibid., 4.
21  François Adam, "Duhamel," *Alberta Folklore Quarterly* 1 (1945): 14-15.
22  Saskatchewan Archives Board (SAB), Regina Women's Canadian Club Conventions, 1924: Essays on Pioneer Days, Mrs. J.A. Reid, "The Neighbourhood of Battleford," R-176II, 15.
23  SAB, Effie Storer Papers, "The Story of My Life, 1868-1940," unpublished manuscript, box 4, file 9, 24.
24  Martin, *The Prairie Hub*, 179.
25  Elaine Silverman, *The Last Best West: Women on the Alberta Frontier, 1880-1930* (Calgary: Fifth House, 1998), 84-85.
26  SAB, Charles Cantlon Bray, 1883, Wolseley, Saskatchewan, pioneer questionnaire, X2, file 8, Health.
27  SAB, Regina Women's Canadian Club Conventions, 1924: Essays on Pioneer Days, Mrs. J.A. Reid, "The Neighbourhood of Battleford."
28  Grant MacEwan, *... And Mighty Women Too: Stories of Notable Western Canadian Women* (Saskatoon: Western Producer Books, 1975), 1-6 and 8. Written as an addendum to an earlier

work by MacEwan, *Fifty Mighty Men* (Saskatoon: Western Producer Books, 1982), this work writes women, especially white women, into the story of settlement. The moss bag was made of leather or fabric with lace and attached to a cradleboard. Moss was placed inside the bag as a diaper.

29  Elizabeth Bailey Price, "Pioneers of the Foothills," *Maclean's Magazine*, 1 July 1927, 85; and Annie McDougall, "Pioneer Life in the 1870s," *Alberta History* 46 (Summer 1998): 26.
30  Price, "Pioneers of the Foothills," 85.
31  Glenbow Museum and Archives (GMA), F.C. Cornish Papers, Recollections and Papers as a Pioneer Indian Agent, M266, 13.
32  Ibid.
33  Stephen Hume, *Lilies and Fireweed: Frontier Women of British Columbia* (Madeira Park: Harbour Publishing, 2004), 73-76.
34  Margaret Ormsby, ed., *A Pioneer Gentlewoman in British Columbia: The Recollections of Susan Allison* (Vancouver: UBC Press, 1976), 28.
35  Ibid.
36  Ibid., 60.
37  Emmy Preston, ed., *Pioneers of Grandview District* (Steinbach, MB: Carillon Press, 1976), 103.
38  Ibid., 102-3.
39  Nanci Langford, "Childbirth on the Canadian Prairies,1880-1939," in *Telling Tales in Western Women's History,* ed. Catherine Cavanaugh and Randi Warne (Vancouver: UBC Press, 2000), 156.
40  Helen MacMurchy, *Maternal Mortality in Canada* (Ottawa: Department of Health, 1928), 23.
41  Jacalyn Duffin, *Langstaff: A Nineteenth Century Medical Life* (Toronto: University of Toronto Press, 1993).
42  GMA, Gooderham Family Papers, "Treaty Indians and Doctors," M4738, box 2, file 12, 2.
43  SAB, Effie Storer Papers, "The Story of My Life," box 4 file 9, 10 and 11.
44  Frog Lake Community Club, *Land of Red and White* (Heinsburg: Frog Lake Community Club, 1977), 98.
45  M.K. Lux, Assiniboine Field Notes, interview with Kay Thompson, January 1998, cited in Lux, *Medicine That Walks*, 95-96.
46  Regina Flannery, *Ellen Smallboy: Glimpses of a Cree Woman's Life* (Montreal and Kingston: McGill-Queen's University Press, 1995), 51.
47  MacMurchy, *Maternal Mortality in Canada,* 12.
48  SAB, Mrs. Maggie Whyte, 1883, Indian Head, Saskatchewan, pioneer questionnaire; and Mrs. Ellen W. Hubbard, 1894, Grenfell, Saskatchewan, pioneer questionnaire, X2, file 8, Health.
49  GMA, McDougall Family Papers, address delivered by Mrs. (Rev.) John McDougall at the evening service of the Pincher Creek United Church, 16 June 1935, M729, file 21.
50  GMA, F.C. Cornish Papers, Recollections and Papers as a Pioneer Indian Agent, 13.
51  J. Maclean, *Canadian Savage Folk: The Native Tribes of Canada* (Toronto: William Briggs, 1896), 201. Maclean did not include in his numerous publications, which catalogued the cultures of North American First Nations people, the effectiveness of certain treatments used by Aboriginal healers.
52  For examples of Maclean's writing, see *The Indians: Their Manners and Customs* (Toronto: William Briggs, 1907); *H.B. Steinhauer: His Work among the Cree Indians of the Western Canadian Plains* (Toronto: William Briggs, n.d.); *McDougall of Alberta* (Toronto: Ryerson Press, 1927); and *Vanguards of Canada* (Toronto: Missionary Society of the Methodist Church, 1918).
53  Sarah Carter, *Capturing Women: The Manipulation of Cultural Imagery in Canada's Prairie West* (Montreal: McGill-Queen's University Press, 1997), 5.
54  Jennifer S.H. Brown, "A Cree Nurse in a Cradle of Methodism: Little Mary and the Egerton R. Young Family at Norway House and Berens River," in *Canadian Family History: Selected Readings,* ed. Bettina Bradbury (Toronto: Copp Clark Pitman, 1992), 90-110. Similarly, the wife of Methodist missionary Egerton Ryerson Young relied on the help of a Cree woman

named Little Mary to care for her children during the family's tenure in the West. Little Mary does not appear in any of Young's writings. It was not until shortly before his death that Eddie, one of the children Little Mary had cared for, wrote about his affection for her.

55  Andrea Smith, *Conquest: Sexual Violence and American Indian Genocide* (Cambridge, MA: South End Press, 2005), 9.
56  Pettipas, *Severing the Ties That Bind,* 87-125.
57  Library and Archives Canada, RG10/1009: file 628, 596-635, L. Vankoughnet to Macdonald, 15 November 1883. See also Carter, *Capturing Women,* 187-88.
58  Sarah Carter, "Categories and Terrains of Exclusion: Constructing the 'Indian Woman' in the Early Settlement Era in Western Canada," in *Out of the Background: Readings on Canadian Native History,* ed. Ken Coates and Robin Fisher (Toronto: Copp Clark, 1996), 177-95.
59  Constance Backhouse, "Nineteenth Century Canadian Prostitution Law: Reflection of a Discriminatory Society," *Histoire sociale/Social History* 18 (1985), 420-22.
60  Carter, "Categories and Terrains of Exclusion," 181-84.
61  Backhouse, "Nineteenth Century Canadian Prostitution Law," 422. Carter, *Capturing Women,* 169-81.
62  Carter, "Categories and Terrains of Exclusion," 188.
63  Langford, "Childbirth on the Canadian Prairies," 147-73.

**Chapter 4: Cleansers, Cautious Caregivers, and Optimistic Adventurers**
1  Eugenie Louise Myles, *Remember Nurse* (Toronto: Ryerson, 1960), 5.
2  For a description of her workspace, see ibid., 26. I use the original place names out of respect for the original people who occupied these communities.
3  Ibid., 79.
4  Ibid., 78.
5  Betty Lee, *Lutiapik* (Toronto: McClelland Stewart, 1975), 54.
6  Ibid., 58.
7  "Lucy Wilson" is a pseudonym. Glenbow Museum and Archives (GMA), Frontier Nursing Project, letter from Lucy Wilson to her family, 12 November 1962, M4745/7.
8  This chapter is part of a larger study that analyzes the experiences of nurses and doctors who worked in northern Canada in the years between 1945 and 1970. There is a rich biographical and autobiographical collection of sources on this topic, as well as a good set of government records that include details about the establishment and maintenance of the various nursing stations and information on the personnel who worked in the medical field in the north. A few examples of the medical life writing genre include: Amy V. Wilson, R.N., *No Man Stands Alone* (Sidney: Gray Publishing, 1965); Joseph P. Moody with W. de Groot van Embden, *Arctic Doctor* (New York: Dodd, Mead and Company, 1955); and Gareth Howerd, *Dew Line Doctor* (London: Robert Hale, 1960). See also J. Karen Scott with Joan E. Kieser, *Northern Nurses: True Nursing Adventures from Northern Canada* (Oakville: Kokum Publications, 2002). Popular histories tend also to be very useful in our attempts to put together the story of northern medical services. See, for example, Bob Burrows, *Healing in the Wilderness: A History of the United Church Mission Hospitals* (Madeira Park: Harbour Publishing, 2004).
9  Eugenie Louise Myles graduated from the University of Alberta in 1927. She worked as an editorial staff member on the *Edmonton Journal* for a number of years and also published non-fiction accounts of life in western and northern Canada.
10  The following is contained in a letter from Knight to P.E. Moore, director of Indian Health Services 1945-65. While it is not overly critical, it suggests some cynicism: "The proposed new communication system, whereby the Eskimos are supplied with radios to report illnesses to the post, sounds too good to be true. If put into effect it will be a great step forward and will be really tangible evidence of our interest in the health of the Eskimos." See Library and Archives Canada (LAC), Department of National Health and Welfare, letter from Knight to Moore, August 1958, RG29, vol. 3433, file 800-1-X861.
11  The history of newcomer health care workers in northern and/or Aboriginal communities has received much scholarly attention recently. See especially, Laurie Meijer Drees and Lesley McBain, "Nursing and Native Peoples in Northern Saskatchewan, 1930s-1950s,"

*Canadian Bulletin of Medical History* 18 (2001), 43-65; Kathryn McPherson, "Nursing and Colonization: The Work of Indian Health Services Nurses in Manitoba, 1945-1970," in *Women, Health and Nation: Canada and the United States since 1945,* ed. Georgina Feldberg et al. (Montreal and Kingston: McGill-Queen's University Press, 2003), 223-46; Nicole Rousseau and Johanne Daigle, "Medical Service to Settlers: The Gestation and Establishment of a Nursing Service in Quebec, 1932-1943," *Nursing History Review* 8 (2000): 95-116; Patricia Jasen, "Race, Culture, and the Colonization of Childbirth in Northern Canada," in *Rethinking Canada: The Promise of Women's History,* ed. Veronica Strong-Boag et al. (Toronto: Oxford University Press, 2002), 353-66. On northern nursing, see Judith Bender Zelmanovits, "'Midwife Preferred': Maternity Care in Outpost Nursing Stations in Northern Canada, 1945-1988," in *Women, Health and Nation,* ed. Feldberg et al., 161-88. For first-hand experiences, see Scott and Kieser, eds., *Northern Nurses: True Nursing Adventures from Canada's North.* For an American comparison, see Effie Graham et al., eds., *With a Dauntless Spirit: Alaska Nursing in Dog-Team Days – Six Personal Accounts* (Fairbanks: University of Alaska Press, 2003).

12 Alice K. Smith, "Nursing with Indian and Northern Health Services," *Canadian Nurse* 59 (February 1963): 130.

13 Ibid.

14 John D. O'Neil, "Self-Determination, Medical Ideology and Health Services in Inuit Communities," in *Northern Communities: The Prospects for Empowerment,* ed. Gurston Dacks and Kenneth C. Coates (Edmonton: University of Alberta Press, 1988), 34.

15 Walter J. Vanast, "Hastening the Day of Extinction: Canada, Quebec, and the Medical Care of Ungava's Inuit, 1867-1967," *Études/Inuit Studies* 15 (1991): 76.

16 Mary-Ellen Kelm, *Colonizing Bodies: Aboriginal Health and Healing in British Columbia* (Vancouver: UBC Press, 1998), 57. See also Maureen Lux, *Medicine That Walks: Disease, Medicine and Canadian Plains Native People, 1880-1940* (Toronto: University of Toronto Press, 2001), 226. For an international perspective on medicine and colonization, see David Arnold, *Colonizing the Body: State Medicine and Epidemic Disease in Nineteenth-Century India* (Berkeley: University of California Press, 1993); Alison Bashford, *Imperial Hygiene: A Critical History of Colonialism, Nationalism and Public Health* (London and New York: Palgrave, 2004). For interesting discussions on the nexus between the body and colonization, see Tony Ballantyne and Antoinette Burton, eds., *Bodies in Contact: Rethinking Colonial Encounters in World History* (Durham and London: Duke University Press, 2005); Katie Pickles and Myra Rutherdale, eds., *Contact Zones: Aboriginal and Settler Women in Canada's Colonial Past* (Vancouver: UBC Press, 2005); Myra Rutherdale, "Ordering the Bath: Children, Health and Hygiene in Northern Canadian Communities, 1900-1970," in *Children's Health Issues in Historical Perspective,* ed. Cheryl Krasnick Warsh and Veronica Strong-Boag (Waterloo, ON: Wilfrid Laurier University Press, 2005), 305-27; Warwick Anderson, "States of Hygiene: Race Improvement and Biomedical Citizenship in Australia and the Colonial Philippines," in *Haunted By Empire: Geographies of Intimacy in North American History,* ed. Ann Laura Stoler (Durham and London: Duke University Press, 2006), 94-115.

17 Cited in Kathryn McPherson, *Bedside Matters: The Transformation of Canadian Nursing, 1900-1990* (Toronto: Oxford University Press, 1996), 86. See also Wendy Mitchinson, *The Nature of Their Bodies: Women and Their Doctors in Victorian Canada* (Toronto: University of Toronto Press, 1991), 41.

18 Myles, *Remember Nurse,* 3.

19 Ibid., 7.

20 Ibid.

21 Ibid., 185.

22 Ibid., 55.

23 Ibid.

24 Ibid., 231.

25 For a full discussion of the connection between citizenship and health care provision, see Dorothy Porter, *Health, Citizenship and the State: A History of Public Health from Ancient to Modern Times* (London and New York: Routledge, 1999). See particularly her chapter on conditional citizenship (at 231-77).

26   Myles, *Remember Nurse,* 74.
27   Ibid.
28   Ibid., 75.
29   Ibid., 76.
30   Ibid.
31   Ibid., 197.
32   Ibid., 223.
33   Lee, *Lutiapik,* 17-18.
34   Ibid., 45.
35   Ibid., 98. Emphasis in the original.
36   Ibid., 31.
37   Ibid., 235.
38   Ibid., 213.
39   Ibid.
40   Ibid., 175.
41   Ibid., 218.
42   Sheryl Nestel, "(Ad)ministering Angels: Colonial Nursing and the Extension of Empire in Africa," *Journal of Medical Humanities* 19 (1998): 257-77; and Margaret Jones, "Heroine of Lonely Outposts or Tools of Empire? British Nurses in Britain's Model Colony: Ceylon, 1878-1948," *Nursing Inquiry* 11 (2004): 1-17.
43   Christina Bates, Dianne Dodd, and Nicole Rousseau, eds., *On All Frontiers: Four Centuries of Canadian Nursing* (Ottawa: University of Ottawa Press and the Canadian Museum of Civilization, 2005), 149. The entire chapter on outpost nursing in Canada beautifully exemplifies the experiences of many northern nurses.
44   Helen Gilbert, "Great Adventures in Nursing: Colonial Discourse and Health Care Delivery in Canada's North," *Jouvert* 7 (2003): 4.
45   Ibid. 3.
46   GMA, Frontier Nursing Project, letter from Lucy Wilson to her family, 27 October 1960.
47   Ibid., 12 February 1961.
48   Ibid., 19 April 1962.
49   Ibid., 4 August 1962.
50   Ibid., 3 December 1960.
51   Ibid., 12 February 1961.
52   See Joan Sangster, "The *Beaver* as Ideology: Constructing Images of Inuit and Native Life in Post-World War Two Canada," forthcoming in *Anthropologia,* Fall 2007.
53   GMA, Frontier Nursing Project, letter from Lucy Wilson to her family, 18 January 1963.

### Chapter 5: Region, Faith, and Health

 1   Karen Buhler-Wilkerson, *No Place Like Home: A History of Nursing and Home Care in the United States* (Baltimore: Johns Hopkins University Press, 2001).
 2   Jennifer Koslow, "Eden's Underbelly: Female Reformers and Public Health in Los Angeles 1889-1932," PhD dissertation, University of California, Los Angeles, 2001.
 3   Beverly Boutilier, "Helpers or Heroines? The National Council of Women, Nursing, and 'Women's Work' in Late Victorian Canada," in *Caring and Curing: Historical Perspectives on Women and Healing in Canada,* ed. Dianne Dodd and Deborah Gorham (Ottawa: University of Ottawa Press, 1991), 17-47; John Gibbon, *The Victorian Order of Nurses for Canada: Fiftieth Anniversary 1897-1947* (Montreal: Southam Press, 1947); and Sheila Penney, *A Century of Caring: The History of the Victorian Order of Nurses for Canada* (Ottawa: Victorian Order of Nurses Canada, 1996).
 4   Sharon Richardson, "Women's Enterprise: Establishing the Lethbridge Nursing Mission, 1909-1919," *Nursing History Review* 5 (1997): 105-30; Sharon Richardson, "Political Women, Professional Nurses, and the Creation of Alberta's District Nursing Service, 1919-1925," *Nursing History Review* 6 (1998): 25-50; and Dianne Dodd, Jayne Elliott, and Nicole Rousseau, "Outpost Nursing in Canada," in *On All Frontiers: Four Centuries of Canadian Nursing,* ed. Christina Bates, Dianne Dodd, and Nicole Rousseau (Ottawa: University of Ottawa Press and the Canadian Museum of Civilization, 2005), 142-43.

5   Karen Buhler-Wilkerson, *False Dawn: The Rise and Decline of Public Health Nursing, 1900-1930* (New York: Garland Publishing, 1989), 112-15.
6   Megan J. Davies, "Competent Professionals and Modern Methods: State Medicine in British Columbia during the 1930s," *Bulletin of the History of Medicine* 76 (2002): 58.
7   Meryn Stuart, "'Half a Loaf Is Better Than No Bread:' Public Health Nurses and Physicians in Ontario, 1920-1925," *Nursing Research* 41 (1992): 21-27; Meryn Stuart, "'Let Not the People Perish for Lack of Knowledge:' Public Health Nursing and the Ontario Rural Child Welfare Project, 1916-1930," PhD dissertation, University of Pennsylvania, Philadelphia, 1987.
8   See, for example, Sara Burke, *Seeking the Highest Good: Social Service and Gender at the University of Toronto, 1888-1937* (Toronto: University of Toronto Press, 1996); Ruth Crocker, *Social Work and Social Order: The Settlement Movement in Two Industrial Cities, 1880-1930* (Madison: University of Wisconsin Press, 1989); Wendy J. Deichmann Edwards and Carolyn De Swart Gifford, eds., *Gender and the Social Gospel* (Chicago: University of Chicago Press, 2003); Linda Gordon, *Pitied but Not Entitled: Single Mothers and the History of Welfare, 1890-1935* (Cambridge, MA: Harvard University Press, 1994); Regina Kunzel, *Fallen Women, Problem Girls: Unmarried Mothers and the Professionalization of Social Work* (New Haven, CT: Yale University Press, 1993); and Margaret Little, *No Car, No Radio, No Liquor Permit: The Moral Regulation of Single Mothers in Ontario, 1920-1997* (Toronto: Oxford University Press, 1998).
9   Mary Taylor Huber and Nancy C. Lutkehaus, "Introduction: Gendered Missions at Home and Abroad," in *Gendered Missions: Women and Men in Missionary Discourse and Practice,* ed. Mary Taylor Huber and Nancy C. Lutkehaus (Ann Arbor, MI: University of Michigan Press, 1999), 1-28; Dana L. Robert, *American Women in Mission: A Social History of Their Thought and Practice* (Macon: Mercer University Press, 1996); Myra Rutherdale, *Women and the White Man's God: Gender and Race in the Canadian Mission Field* (Vancouver: UBC Press, 2002); and Susan Thorne, "Missionary-Imperial Feminism," in *Gendered Missions,* ed. Huber and Lutkehaus, 39-66.
10  Kunzel, *Fallen Women,* 3. See also Linda Gordon, *Heroes of Their Own Lives: The Politics and History of Family Violence* (New York: Viking, 1988); Gordon, *Pitied but Not Entitled;* Susan Kent, *Sex and Suffrage in Britain: 1860-1914* (Princeton: Princeton University Press, 1987); Andrée Lévesque, "Deviants Anonymous: Single Mothers at the Hôpital de la Miséricorde in Montreal, 1929-1939," in *Delivering Motherhood: Maternal Ideologies and Practices in the Nineteenth and Twentieth Centuries,* ed. Katherine Arnup, Andrée Lévesque, and Ruth Roach Pierson (London and New York: Routledge, 1990), 108-25; Linda Mahood, *Policing Gender, Class and Family: Britain 1850-1940* (London: University College London Press, 1995); Linda Mahood, *The Magdalenes: Prostitution in the Nineteenth Century* (London and New York: Routledge, 1990); Frank Mort, *Dangerous Sexualities: Medico-moral Politics in England since 1830,* 2nd edition (London and New York: Routledge, 2000); Caroline Strange, *Toronto's Girl Problem: The Perils and Pleasures of the City, 1880-1929* (Toronto: University of Toronto Press, 1995); and Judith Walkowitz, *Prostitution and Victorian Society: Women, Class and the State* (New York: Cambridge University Press, 1980).
11  Considerable debate ensued regarding the proper use of the terms "visiting nursing" and "public health nursing." In the early years of both the Margaret Scott Nursing Mission (MSNM) and the Victorian Order of Nursing (VON), many members referred to bedside nursing care in the home as visiting or district nursing and described health promotion and health education programs as public health nursing. At the VON's 18 November 1915 annual meeting, Miss Mackenzie, the dominion superintendent, "expressed regret" that city council did not employ the VON nurses as public health nurses, "as they were specially trained for such work." Similarly, at a meeting on 21 January 1920, Miss Hall, the western superintendent, urged the local branch to "emphasize public health nursing." This chapter will maintain the above distinction between these two terms. See VON, Manitoba Branch. The Winnipeg Branch of the VON's archives are held by VON Manitoba. Sources are listed by date and event.
12  Alan F.J. Artibise, *Gateway City: Documents on the City of Winnipeg 1873-1913* (Winnipeg: University of Manitoba Press, 1979); Alan F.J. Artibise, "Boosterism and the Development of Prairie Cities," in *The Prairie West: Historical Readings,* 2nd edition, ed. R. Douglas Francis and Howard Palmer (Edmonton: Pica Pica Press, 1995), 515-43; Alan F.J. Artibise, *Winnipeg:*

*A Social History of Urban Growth 1874-1914* (Montreal and Kingston: McGill-Queen's University Press, 1975); and William Morton, *Manitoba: A History* (Toronto: University of Toronto Press, 1967), 215 and 223.

13  "Editorial," *Winnipeg Telegram*, 13 May 1901. These remarks have been attributed to W. Sanford Evans, who became editor of the *Winnipeg Telegram* in 1901. See Stella M. Hyrniuk and Neil G. McDonald, "The Schooling Experience of Ukrainians in Manitoba," in *The Prairie West: Historical Readings*, 293. Evans served as Winnipeg's mayor from 1905-11. J.M. Bumsted, *Dictionary of Manitoba Biography* (Winnipeg: University of Manitoba Press, 1999), 78.

14  Historians and contemporary observers have extensively documented the anti-Semitic and anti-Slavic attitudes held by some members of Winnipeg's social elite during the early twentieth century. Contemporary accounts, both biographical and fictional, include Douglas Durkin, *The Magpie* (Toronto: Hodder and Stoughton, 1923); James Gray, *The Boy from Winnipeg* (Toronto: McMillan Canada, 1970); and John Marlyn, *Under the Ribs of Death* (Toronto: McClelland and Stewart, 1957; reprinted 1993). Historians writing on the same topic include Alan F.J. Artibise, "Divided City: The Immigrant in Winnipeg Society, 1874-1921," in *The Canadian City: Essays in Urban and Social History*, ed. Gilbert A. Stelter and Alan F.J. Artibise (Ottawa: Carleton University Press, 1984), 300-36; Gerald Friesen, *The Canadian Prairies: A History* (Toronto: University of Toronto Press, 1887), 242-73; Gerald Friesen, *The West: Regional Ambitions, National Debates, Global Age* (Toronto: Penguin Books, 1999), 57-59; and Daniel Hiebert, "Class, Ethnicity and Residential Structure: The Social Geography of Winnipeg, 1901-1921," *Journal of Historical Geography* 17 (1991): 56-86.

15  All population figures reported are from the federal census. More inflated population estimates were reported by the city's assessment office. All data are found in Artibise, *Winnipeg*, 130-33 and 142; and Artibise, "Divided City," 312.

16  Artibise, *Winnipeg*, 169 and 163.

17  Hiebert, "Class, Ethnicity and Residential Structure," 73 and 57; and Esyllt Jones, "Contact across a Diseased Boundary: Urban Space and Social Interaction during Winnipeg's Influenza Epidemic, 1918-1919," *Journal of the Canadian Historical Association* 13 (2002): 119.

18  "Editorial," *Winnipeg Telegram*, 13 May 1901.

19  Several historians have used the term "charter group" to characterize the Anglo-Canadian middle-class residents of Winnipeg who dominated the city's business and political institutions. See, for example, Artibise, "Divided City," 308.

20  James Shaver Woodsworth (1874-1942), ordained Methodist minister, labour supporter, pacifist, and founder of the Cooperative Commonwealth Federation party, served as superintendent of the All People's Mission in Winnipeg's North End from 1907 to 1913. Increasingly dissatisfied with Methodist doctrine, he resigned from the church in 1918. He was arrested on charges of seditious libel in the aftermath of the 1919 Winnipeg general strike but was later released. First elected to Parliament in 1921, he served the same riding in Winnipeg North Centre until his death in 1942. A social democrat, Woodsworth had a significant impact on Canadian social policy. He was directly involved in the establishment of federal old-age pension legislation and advocated for many other social welfare programs, including medicare. Bumsted, *Dictionary of Manitoba Biography*, 268; and Kenneth McNaught, *A Prophet in Politics: A Biography of J.S. Woodsworth* (Toronto: University of Toronto Press, 1971).

21  James S. Woodsworth, *Strangers within Our Gates or Coming Canadians*, edited by Michael Bliss (Toronto: University of Toronto Press, 1972; originally published 1909), 9 and 46-47

22  Artibise, "Divided City," 312; Artibise, *Winnipeg*, 160; Hiebert, "Class, Ethnicity and Residential Structure," 61; and Jones, "Contact across a Diseased Boundary," 119.

23  Ralph Connor, *The Foreigner: A Tale of Saskatchewan* (Toronto: Westminster Company, 1909), 253.

24  For further analysis of the complexities of Canadian attitudes to immigrants, see, for example, Robert Adamoski, Dorothy E. Chunn, and Robert Menzies, eds., *Contesting Canadian Citizenship: Historical Readings* (Peterborough: Broadview Press, 1994); Gerald Friesen, *The Canadian Prairies: A History* (Toronto: University of Toronto Press, 1987); Howard Palmer, ed., *Immigration and the Rise of Multiculturalism* (Vancouver: Copp Clark, 1975); Patricia Roy,

*A White Man's Province: British Columbia Politicians and Chinese and Japanese Immigrants 1858-1914* (Vancouver: UBC Press, 1989); and Patricia Roy, *The Oriental Question: Consolidating a White Man's Province, 1914-1941* (Vancouver: UBC Press, 2003)

25  Ross Mitchell, *Medicine in Manitoba: The Story of Its Beginnings* (Winnipeg: Stovel-Advocate Press, 1954), 77-79.

26  Artibise, *Winnipeg*, 187-88 and 192-94.

27  The National Council of Women (NCW) had discussed the issue of providing skilled "nursing" assistance to Canadian women as early as 1894. In February 1897, Lady Aberdeen, president of the NCW, proposed that the organization mark Queen Victoria's diamond jubilee by establishing the Victorian Order of Home Helpers to assist child-bearing women in the Northwest Territories. In the initial version of this plan, the helpers were not trained nurses. Instead, Lady Aberdeen recommended that they be drawn from the ranks of well-respected local women who could live with the family for several weeks, providing domestic assistance during the mother's lying-in period. Physicians and nurses vigorously opposed this proposal. By March 1897, just prior to the meetings in Winnipeg, it was changed to the Victorian Order of Nurses (VON), which would employ only trained hospital nurses with additional preparation in visiting nursing. As well, the focus of the order shifted from rural prairie women to the urban poor. For a more extended discussion of the early debates about district nursing in Canada and the formation of the VON, see Boutilier, "Helpers or Heroines?" 17-47.

28  "The Woman's Council," *Manitoba Free Press*, 3 May 1897, 3; "The Home Helpers," *Manitoba Free Press*, 22 May 1897, 5.

29  Dr. H.H. Chown, professor of surgery and future dean of the Manitoba Medical School, spearheaded medical opposition to the plan. Ian Carr and Robert Beamish, *Manitoba Medicine: A Brief History* (Winnipeg: University of Manitoba Press, 1999), 27-29, 40-43, 48, and 52; "The Home Helpers," 5; "Order Approved," *Manitoba Free Press*, 8 June 1897, 1; "Victorian Order," *Manitoba Free Press*, 5 June 1897, 5.

30  "Order Approved," 4.

31  Ibid.

32  "Not in Sympathy," *Manitoba Free Press*, 28 May 1897, 6.

33  Ibid.

34  "The Home Helpers," 5; "Victorian Order," 4.

35  Carr and Beamish, *Manitoba Medicine*, 35; "Hospital Jubilee Ward," *Manitoba Free Press*, 12 June 1897, 4.

36  "The Home Helpers," 5.

37  "Hospital Jubilee Ward," 4; "The General Hospital," *Manitoba Free Press*, 15 June 1897, 4. The subscription form for the appeal appeared in the *Manitoba Free Press* on 26 June 1897, 7.

38  "The General Hospital," *Manitoba Free Press*, 1 June 1897, 4; "The General Hospital," 15 June 1897, 4.

39  Gibbon, *Victorian Order of Nurses for Canada*, 116-19; Penney, *A Century of Caring*, 33 and 36-40; VON, Manitoba Branch, minutes of 9 April 1901 to 12 April 1905.

40  Archives of Manitoba (AM), Margaret Scott Nursing Mission Papers, *Annual Report*, 1935, MG10, B9, box VI, 4.

41  Nurses Alumni Association Winnipeg General Hospital/Health Sciences Centre Archives, Winnipeg General Hospital, *Annual Report*, 1900, 46.

42  "Margaret Scott Nursing Mission," *Manitoba Free Press*, 17 May 1904, 8.

43  Artibise, *Winnipeg*, 190-91; Bumsted, *Dictionary of Manitoba Biography*, 224; Diane DeGraves, "Margaret Scott, 1856-1931: Health and Social Service Innovator," in *Extraordinary Women: Manitoba Women and Their Stories*, ed. Colleen Armstrong (Winnipeg: Canadian Federation of University Women, 2000), 66; Helena Macvicar, *Margaret Scott: A Tribute: The Margaret Scott Nursing Mission* (Winnipeg: Margaret Scott Nursing Missing, c. 1948), 10; Edith Paterson, "It Happened Here: Margaret Scott Devotes Life to Winnipeg's Needy," *Winnipeg Free Press*, 18 January 1975, 5; "The Florence Nightingale of Winnipeg: The Story of Mrs. Margaret Scott and Her Labor of Great Love," *Canadian Nurse* 10 (1915): 139-42; Lillian Benyon

Thomas, "Some Manitoba Women Who Did First Things," *Manitoba Historical Society Transaction Series* 3, no. 4 (1947-48). Available online at http://www.mhs.mb.ca/docs/transactions/3/firstwomen.shtml.

44   "Florence Nightingale of Winnipeg," 143.

45   Macvicar, *Margaret Scott,* 8-10; City of Winnipeg Archives (CWA), Market, Licence and Health Committee Minutes, 21 January 1902, item 325.

46   A budget line for a district nurse first appears in the 1903-04 estimates for the City of Winnipeg Health Department.

47   "Devoted Work of the District Nurse," *Manitoba Free Press,* 16 May 1904.

48   "Nursing Mission for Winnipeg Poor," *Manitoba Free Press,* 10 June 1904, 10.

49   AM, Margaret Scott Nursing Mission Papers, box IV, undated letter from Mrs. A.M. Fraser. A copy of this letter is attached to the front of the 8 November 1909 to 10 October 1920 minute book.

50   "A Home for the District Nurses," *Manitoba Free Press,* 13 May 1904, 4.

51   A. Richard Allen, *The Social Passion: Religion and Reform in Canada* (Toronto: University of Toronto Press, 1973); Paul Merkley, "The Vision of the Good Society in the Social Gospel: What, Where and When in the Kingdom of God?" *Historical Papers: Canadian Historical Association* (1987): 138-56.

52   Bumsted, *Dictionary of Manitoba Biography,* 95.

53   "Nursing at Home Society," *Manitoba Free Press,* 26 May 1904, 10.

54   "Margaret Scott Nursing Mission," 8; and "Nursing at Home Society," 10.

55   A.J. Douglas, "Chairman's Address, Section of Municipal Health Officers, American Public Health Association," *American Journal of Public Health* 2, no. 2 (1912): 85-86.

56   AM, Margaret Scott Nursing Mission Papers, minutes of 12 May 1904, box IV; "Devoted Work of the District Nurse," 8; "Margaret Scott Nursing Mission," 8; and "A Work of Noble Philanthropy," *Manitoba Free Press,* 31 October 1905, 7.

57   AM, Margaret Scott Nursing Mission Papers, *First Annual Report,* 1905, box VI, 6 and 8. Lamont's tenure at the mission was quite short, and Beveridge was serving as the superintendent by November 1905.

58   AM, Margaret Scott Nursing Mission Papers, *First Annual Report,* 1905, box VI; *Twenty-fourth Annual Report,* 1928, box VI; minutes of 13 May 1907, box IV; minutes of 2 August 1931, box V.

59   Ibid., Applications for Nursing Attendance and Relief, boxes VII-1X. Approximately 11,000 case files, covering the period from August 1908 to December 1921, are contained in the mission's papers.

60   Connor, *The Foreigner,* 13 and 87.

61   AM, Margaret Scott Nursing Mission Papers, minutes of 11 November 1905, box IV.

62   Ibid., Applications for Nursing Attendance and Relief, boxes VII-X.

63   Artibise, *Winnipeg,* Table 11, 169.

64   Artibise, *Winnipeg,* 117-80; University of Manitoba Archives (UMA), Gerald Friesen Fonds, MSS 154, PC 171, Winnipeg Elite Files, boxes 17-19.

65   AM, Margaret Scott Nursing Mission Papers, Applications for Nursing Attendance and Relief, boxes VII-X; Terry Copp, *The Anatomy of Poverty: The Condition of the Working Class in Montreal 1897-1929* (Toronto: University of Toronto Press, 1974), 31-32; Michael Piva, *The Condition of the Working Class in Toronto, 1900-1921* (Ottawa: University of Ottawa Press, 1979), 171; Joseph Harry Sutcliffe, "Economic Background of the Winnipeg General Strike: Wages and Working Conditions," PhD dissertation, University of Manitoba, 1972, 9-17 and 139-41.

66   AM, Margaret Scott Nursing Mission Papers, minutes of 9 December 1907, box IV.

67   No single factor shaped the practice for referring patients to the Board of Director's visitors' committee. In part, the physical, social, and language differences between the board members and the patients that the mission served may have created the board's dependence on Beveridge to supply names of suitable patients. As well, board members may have consciously or unconsciously depended on Margaret Scott's ongoing lay missionary work to generate referrals for home nursing care. However, by the early twentieth century, the increased complexity and size of visiting nursing associations made it less likely that board members

were directly involved in the day-to-day operations of the organization. Instead, they employed head nurses or matrons to supervise staff and make decisions about which individuals and families were eligible to be placed on the agency's caseload. See, for example, Karen Buhler-Wilkerson, *No Place Like Home*, 29-34.

68 AM, Margaret Scott Nursing Mission Papers, minutes of 13 January 1908, box IV; minutes of 12 November 1917, box IV; minutes of 10 December 1934, box V.

69 "Annual Meeting of the Margaret Scott Mission," *Winnipeg Free Press*, 29 October 1906, 9.

70 E.M. Wood's undated (c. January 1920) letter is in the possession of the author.

71 "Obituary," *Winnipeg Telegram*, 16 April 1918.

72 Huber and Lutkehaus, eds., *Gendered Missions*, 1-28; Dana L. Robert, *American Women in Mission: A Social History of Their Thought and Practice* (Macon: Mercer University Press, 1996); Rutherdale, *Women and the White Man's God;* and Thorne, "Missionary-Imperial Feminism," 39-66.

73 Leonore Davidoff and Catherine Hall, *Family Fortunes: Men and Women of the English Middle Class, 1780-1930* (London: Hutchinson, 1987); Geoff Eley, "Culture, Nation and Gender," in *Gendered Nations: Nationalism and Gender Order in the Long Nineteenth Century,* ed. Ida Blom, Karen Hagemann, and Catherine Hall (Oxford: Berg, 2000), 32-33; Seth Koven and Sonya Michel, "Womanly Duties: Maternalist Politics and the Origins of the Welfare States in France, Germany, Great Britain, and the United States, 1880-1920," *Radical History Review* 43 (1989): 1088; Alan Hunt, *Governing Morals: A Social History of Moral Regulation* (Cambridge: Cambridge University Press 1999), 1-3; Anne McClintock, *Imperial Leather: Race, Gender and Sexuality in the Colonial Conquest* (London and New York: Routledge, 1995); and Joan Wallach Scott, *Gender and the Politics of History* (New York: Columbia University Press, 1988), 42.

74 Nancy Lutkehaus, "Missionary Maternalism: Gendered Images of the Holy Spirit Sisters in Colonial New Guinea," in *Gendered Missions,* ed. Huber and Lutkehaus, 208-9.

75 For further reading about moral regulation and its theoretical difference from social control theory, see Mary Louise Adams, "In Sickness and in Health: State Formation, Moral Regulation and Early VD Initiatives in Ontario," *Journal of Canadian Studies* 28 (April 1993): 117-30; Linda Gordon, "Family Violence, Feminism and Social Control," in *Women, The State, and Welfare,* ed. Linda Gordon (Madison: University of Wisconsin Press, 1990), 178-98; Nikolas Rose, *Governing the Soul: The Shaping of the Private Self* (London and New York: Routledge, 1991); Carolyn Strange and Tina Loo, *Making Good: Law and Moral Regulation in Canada, 1867-1939* (Toronto: McClelland and Stewart, 1997); Mariana Valverde, *The Age of Light, Soap, and Water: Moral Reform in English Canada, 1885-1925* (Toronto: McClelland and Stewart, 1991). Of particular interest is the debate between Linda Gordon and Joan Wallach Scott. See Linda Gordon, "Response to Scott," *Signs* 15 (1990): 852-53; and Joan Wallach Scott, "Book Review: Heroes of Their Own Lives: The Politics and History of Family Violence," *Signs* 15 (1990): 848-52. For a haunting fictional analysis of the impact that internalizing the cultural norms of the Anglo-Canadian majority might have had on Winnipeg's immigrant community, see John Marlyn, *Under the Ribs of Death.*

76 Artibise, *Winnipeg,* 158-62, 186-89, and 207-45.

77 CWA, Health Department, *Annual Report,* 1911, 7.

78 AM, Margaret Scott Nursing Mission Papers, "Annual Meeting of the Margaret Scott Nursing Mission," box IV. This 1906 newspaper article is pasted in the 1906 minute book.

79 For an extended discussion of the moral reform movement in Canada, which was at its height at the time that the Margaret Scott Nursing Mission was founded in 1904, see Valverde, *The Age of Light, Soap, and Water.*

80 "A Work of Noble Philanthropy," *Winnipeg Free Press*, 30 October 1905. This remark was made by the Very Reverend George Coombs, dean of the Anglican Diocese of Rupertsland, which was headquartered at St. John's Cathedral in Winnipeg.

81 AM, Margaret Scott Nursing Mission Papers, "Annual Meeting of the Margaret Scott Nursing Mission," box IV, pasted in the 1906 minute book.

82 Ibid., *First Annual Report,* 1905, box VI, 4-5.

83 "A Work of Noble Philanthropy," 7.

84 "Devoted Work of the District Nurse," 8.

85  AM, Margaret Scott Nursing Mission Papers, C. DeNully Frazer, "A Peep into the Day's Routine of a District Nurse at the Margaret Scott Nursing Mission," *Third Annual Report,* 1907, 9-10, box VI.

86  Ibid., Applications for Nursing Attendance and Relief, Application 6127, boxes VII-X.

87  This information was drawn from the Mission Board of Management Minutes and Annual Reports, correspondence, newspaper clippings and information documented in the Applications for Nursing Attendance and Relief.

88  Adams, "In Sickness and in Health," n. 13; Strange and Loo, *Making Good,* 140; and Patrick Brantlinger, *Crusoe's Footprints: Cultural Studies in Britain and America* (London and New York: Routledge, 1990), 97.

89  AM, Margaret Scott Nursing Mission Papers, Applications for Nursing Attendance and Relief, Application 6057, boxes VII-X.

90  Ibid., Applications for Nursing Attendance and Relief, Application 7649; Application 10192, boxes VII-X.

91  Ibid., minutes of 11 September and 13 November 1911; 10 June, 13 June, 9 September, and 26 October 1912, box IV.

92· Brantlinger, *Crusoe's Footprints,* 92; Dina Copelman, *London's Women Teachers: Gender, Class, and Feminism 1870-1930* (London and New York: Routledge, 1996); Anna Davin, *Growing Up Poor: Home, Street and School in London 1897-1914* (London: Hutchinson, 1987); Neil Sutherland, "To Create a Strong and Healthy Race: School Children in the Public Health Movement, 1880-1914," in *Medicine in Canadian Society: Historical Perspectives,* ed. S.E.D. Shortt (Montreal and Kingston: McGill-Queen's University Press, 1981), 361-93. Similar strategies were described in Connor, *The Foreigner.*

93  AM, Margaret Scott Nursing Mission Papers, minutes of 9 September 1912, box IV.

94  VON, Winnipeg Branch, minutes of 31 October 1904.

95  Ibid., minutes of 12 April 1905.

96  Ibid., minutes of 11 October 1905.

97  Ibid., minutes of 10 January 1906.

98  "Winnipeg News," *Canadian Nurse* 2 (January 1906): 56; "Victorian Nurse's Work," *Manitoba Free Press,* 15 November 1906, 15.

99  VON, Winnipeg Branch, minutes of 10 January 1906.

100  "Winnipeg News," *Canadian Nurse* 2 (June 1906): 54; VON, Winnipeg Branch, minutes of 11 April 1906; minutes of 10 October 1906.

101  VON, Winnipeg Branch, minutes of 11 December 1907.

102  VON, Winnipeg Branch, *Twenty-First Annual Report,* 6; and minutes of 15 October 1924; 23 April 1923; 17 March 1936; 16 March 1927; and 18 September 1929.

103  AM, Margaret Scott Nursing Mission Papers, minutes of Special Board Meeting, 7 July 1919, box IV.

104  VON, Winnipeg Branch, minutes of the Special Meeting of Executive and Medical Advisory Committee, 27 March 1923.

105  Ibid., minutes of 27 March 1923.

106  Ibid. See also the minutes of 18 April 1923; 24 September, 15 October, and 17 December 1924; 15 April and 18 November 1925; and 16 April 1926.

107  Ibid., minutes of 21 March and 27 March 1923.

108  Ibid., *Twentieth Annual Report,* 1921, 14; *Twenty-first Annual Report,* 1922, 6 and 15; and *Twenty-second Annual Report,* 1923, 7.

109  Ibid., minutes of 27 March and 18 April 1923.

110  Ibid., minutes of 15 April and 25 April 1925; and 15 September 1926.

### Chapter 6: "Suitable Young Women"

1  Provincial Archives of Manitoba (PAM), Canadian Red Cross Society (CRCS), Manitoba Division, "Nursing Stations, c. 1920s-1935," Kinosota, 30 September 1921, P4478, file 12, 16.

2  PAM, CRCS, Manitoba Division, Minute Books and Reports, "Report: Provincial Nursing Committee," 28 November 1922, MG10, B29, box 8.

3  PAM, P4478, CRCS, Manitoba Division, "Fisher Branch, July 1921," 16; and PAM, CRCS, Manitoba Division, Minute Books and Reports, "Report: Provincial Nursing Committee," September 1922, MG10, B29.

4 PAM, CRCS, Manitoba Division, Minute Books and Reports, "Minutes of a Meeting of Policy Committee," 8 February 1920, MG10, B29, box 8, 13-14.

5 CRCS, *Crusade for Good Health* (Toronto: CRCS, 1921).

6 CRCS Library and Archives, Box CRCS History, "Canadian Red Cross Society: National Peace Policy," file 1919-1939.

7 Cynthia R. Comacchio, *"Nations Are Built of Babies": Saving Ontario's Mothers and Children, 1900-1940* (Montreal and Kingston: McGill-Queen's University Press, 1993), 13-14. See also Mona Gleason, "Race, Class and Health: School Medical Inspection and 'Healthy' Children in British Columbia, 1890-1930," *Canadian Bulletin of Medical History* 19 (2002): 95-112; Cynthia Comacchio, "The Rising Generation: Laying Claim to the Health of Adolescents in English Canada, 1920-1970," *Canadian Bulletin of Medical History* 19 (2002): 139-79; and Kari Delhi, "'Health Scouts for the State?': School and Public Health Nurses in Early Twentieth Century Ontario," *Historical Studies in Education* 2 (1990): 247-64.

8 Mary H. Conquest, "Sunny Alberta," *Canadian Red Cross* 1, no. 8 (November 1922): 6-7.

9 Suzann Buckley, "Ladies or Midwives? Efforts to Reduce Infant and Maternal Mortality in Canada between the Two World Wars," *Atlantis* 2, no. 2 (Spring 1977): 76-84; Desmond Morton and Glenn Wright, *Winning the Second Battle: Canadian Veterans and the Return to Civilian Life, 1915-1930* (Toronto: University of Toronto Press, 1987), 25; Desmond Morton, *When Your Number's Up: The Canadian Soldier in the First World War* (Toronto: Random House, 1993), 257; and CRCS, *Crusade for Good Health*, 54.

10 CRCS, *Crusade for Good Health*, 54; League of Red Cross Societies, *Proceedings of the Medical Conference*, Cannes, France, April 1919 (Geneva: League of Red Cross Societies, 1919), 135-36. See also Jayne Elliott, "'Keep the Flag Flying': Medical Outposts and the Red Cross in Northern Ontario, 1922-1984," PhD dissertation, Queen's University, Kingston, 2004, 7; Cynthia Comacchio Abeele, "'The Infant Soldier': The Great War and the Medical Campaign for Child Welfare," *Canadian Bulletin of Medical History* 5 (1988): 99-119.

11 Helen Randal, "CNATN Conference 1918," *Canadian Nurse* 14, no. 8 (August 1918): 1237; CRCS, *Annual Report*, 1921, 30; PAM, CRCS, Executive Committee Minute Book, "Twenty-First Meeting of the Central Council," 9-10 September 1919; and Ian Carr and Robert F. Beamish, *Manitoba Medicine: A Brief History* (Winnipeg: University of Manitoba Press, 1999).

12 CRCS, *Divisional Annual Report: Manitoba, 1921*, 14-23; and CRCS, *Annual Report*, 1920, 40-43.

13 CRCS, Executive Committee Minute Book, "Twenty-First Meeting of the Central Council," 9-10 September 1919.

14 The Duke of Devonshire was governor general at the time of the address, 5 February 1920. CRCS, *Annual Report*, 1920, 16.

15 CRCS, "Report of Special Committee on Future Policy," 29 January 1920.

16 Meryn Stuart, "War and Peace: Professional Identities and Nurses' Training, 1914-1930," in *Challenging Professions: Historical and Contemporary Perspectives on Women's Professional Work*, ed. Elizabeth Smyth, Sandra Acker, Paula Bourne, and Alison Prentice (Toronto: University of Toronto Press, 1999), 184-85.

17 Lee Stewart, *"It's Up to You": Women at UBC in the Early Years* (Vancouver: UBC Press, 1990), 37; and Mackenzie Porter, *To All Men: The Story of the Canadian Red Cross* (Toronto: McClelland and Stewart, 1960), 58. The five programs were at the University of British Columbia, Dalhousie University, University of Toronto, University of Western Ontario, and McGill University. See also Rondalyn Kirkwood, "Blending Vigorous Leadership and Womanly Virtues: Edith Kathleen Russell at the University of Toronto, 1920-1952," *Canadian Bulletin of Medical History* 11 (1994): 175-205.

18 CRCS, "Manitoba Division," *Canadian Red Cross* 1, no. 3 (April 1922): 10.

19 Kathryn McPherson, *Bedside Matters: The Transformation of Canadian Nursing, 1900-1990* (Toronto: Oxford University Press, 1996), 62-63.

20 Marian McKay, "The Role of Winnipeg's Voluntary Agencies in the Development of Visiting and Public Health Nursing in Winnipeg, 1904-1945," unpublished paper presented at the Hannah Nursing History Conference, Ottawa, June 2005 [on file with the author].

21 CRCS, "Manitoba Division," *Canadian Red Cross* 1, no. 3 (April 1922): 10; and CRCS, "Report of Special Committee on Future Policy," 5-6.

22  CRCS, "Report of Special Committee on Future Policy," 5. The districts cited at the time were listed as Fort Nelson, Amaranth, Ashen, and the Greater Winnipeg Water Works Railway.

23  G.J. Seale, commissioner, "Nursing Outposts," *Canadian Red Cross* 1, no. 3 (April 1922): 2.

24  PAM, CRCS, Manitoba Division, Minute Book, "Provincial Nursing Committee," 28 November 1922, MG10 B29, box 8, 1.

25  By April 1922, the Reynolds station was relocated to East Braintree as the fourth nursing station. See PAM, CRCS, Manitoba Division, "Memoirs Fisher Branch Nursing Station, c. 1922," P4478, File 11, 1.

26  PAM, CRCS, Manitoba Division, Executive Committee Minute Book, September 1919-20, "Minutes," 8 March 1920, MG10b B29, box 8.

27  CRCS, "Provincial Nursing Committee," 15 April 1920, 28 May 1920, June 1920, and 6 July 1920.

28  CRCS, Manitoba Division, Executive Committee Minute Book, "Report of Nursing Committee," September 1920.

29  Ibid., October 1920.

30  PAM, CRCS, Manitoba Division, Minute Books and Reports 1923, "Nursing Service: Reynolds," May-June 1923, MG10 B29, box 8; and "Nursing Service: Grahamdale," June-August 1923, MG10, B29.

31  McPherson, *Bedside Matters,* 62.

32  CRCS, "Nursing Stations c. 1920s-1935," minutes of Provincial Executive, 23 May 1923, P4478, file 12, 8.

33  "Provincial Nursing Committee," 28 November 1922, 1.

34  Elliott, "Keep the Flag Flying," 51; and CRCS, *Annual Report,* 1923, 64.

35  PAM, CRCS, Manitoba Division, "East Braintree Nursing Station and Nursing Service Report," P4478, file 8, 1931.

36  Elliott, "Keep the Flag Flying," 58.

37  PAM, CRCS, Minute Books and Reports, "Policy Committee," 8 February 1920, P4478, 13-14.

38  Jean Gunn, "President's Address, CNATN Convention," *Canadian Nurse* 15 (August 1919): 1922; and Jean Gunn, "The Services of Canadian Nurses and Voluntary Aids during the War," *Canadian Nurse* 15 (September 1919): 1978.

39  Elliott, "Keep the Flag Flying," 51.

40  Linda J. Quiney, "'Assistant Angels': Canadian Women as Voluntary Aid Detachment Nurses During and After the Great War, 1914-1930," PhD dissertation, University of Ottawa, Ottawa, 2002, chapter 2.

41  Jean Gunn was an Ontario native, but Elva Gunn was from the Maritimes. No apparent familial connection exists between the two nurses.

42  The reluctance of middle-class families to have a daughter enter a nursing career is a common theme in Canadian nursing histories. See Natalie Riegler, *Jean I. Gunn: Nursing Leader* (Toronto: Associated Medical Services and Fitzhenry and Whiteside, 1997), 13 and 15-28. It was not unusual for a nurse of this era to earn a teaching certificate, frequently financing her subsequent nursing studies with her teacher's earnings.

43  Stuart, "War and Peace," 178-79; PAM, CRCS, Manitoba Division, Executive Committee Minutes, "Provincial Nursing Committee," 1 October 1920.

44  CRCS, Manitoba Division Executive Committee Minutes, "Provincial Nursing Committee," October 1920.

45  CRCS, "Nursing Stations, c. 1920s-1935," minutes of Provincial Executive, 10 November 1920, 5.

46  Rondolyn Kirkwood, "The Development of University Nursing Education in Canada, 1920-1975: Two Case Studies," PhD dissertation, University of Toronto, Toronto, 1988; CRCS, *The Story of the Red Cross* (Toronto: CRCS, 1927), 9-10. The CRCS initially funded the earliest university-based public health nursing programs in Canada, promoting them by offering scholarships for qualified nursing graduates.

47  McPherson, *Bedside Matters,* 115-63.

48 PAM, CRCS, Manitoba Division, "Flora Hill Correspondence, 1930s," letter, 27 April 1938, P4478, file 3; and letter from chairman, Nursing Stations Committee, n.d.
49 PAM, CRCS, Manitoba Division, "Flora Hill Correspondence, 1930s," P4478, file 3.
50 The Kinosota station opened on 21 July 1921 with Nurse Edith Macey. The Reynolds station opened 27 July 1921 with Elva Gunn. Nurse Macey was transferred to the Fisher Branch when it opened on 1 December 1921. Grahamdale followed in 1922, and Rorketon in 1924. Later, Kinosota was relocated to Alonsa, and Reynolds to East Braintree, each with the same nurse in charge. See also Dianne Dodd, Jayne Elliott, and Nicole Rousseau, "Outpost Nursing in Canada," in *On All Frontiers: Four Centuries of Canadian Nursing,* ed. Christina Bates, Dianne Dodd, and Nicole Rousseau (Ottawa: University of Ottawa Press and the Canadian Museum of Civilization, 2005), 148.
51 Jayne Elliott, "Blurring the Boundaries of Space: Shaping Nursing Lives at the Red Cross Outposts in Ontario, 1922-1945," *Canadian Bulletin of Medical History* 21 (2004): 306. An overview of outpost nursing can be found in Dodd, Elliott, and Rousseau, "Outpost Nursing in Canada," 139-52.
52 Seale, "Nursing Outposts," 2.
53 Elliott, "Blurring the Boundaries of Space," 305.
54 PAM, CRCS, Manitoba Division, "Memoirs, Fisher Branch Nursing Station," c. 1922, P4478, file 11, 2.
55 Elliott, "Blurring the Boundaries of Space," 310.
56 PAM, CRCS, Manitoba Division, "Memoirs, Fisher Branch Nursing Station," 2.
57 Ibid., 22.
58 Ibid., 29; and CRCS, "Manitoba Nursing Stations," *Canadian Red Cross* 4, no. 5 (May 1925): 16.
59 Elliott, "Blurring the Boundaries of Space," 310; Sharon Richardson, "Frontier Health Care: Alberta's District Nursing Service," *Alberta History* 46 (Winter 1998): 5; Laurie Meijer Drees and Lesley McBain, "Nursing and Native Peoples in Northern Saskatchewan, 1930s-1950s," *Canadian Bulletin of Medical History* 18 (2001): 43-65.
60 The literature on wartime military nursing is extensive. Some examples include "Halifax Disaster and Relief Work Performed," *Canadian Nurse* 14 (November 1918): 1404-6; V.A. Macdonald, R.N., "Nursing in Disasters," *Canadian Nurse* 18 (January 1922): 9-10; Linda J. Quiney, "'Sharing the Halo': Social and Professional Tensions in the Work of World War One Canadian Volunteer Nurses," *Journal of the Canadian Historical Association* 9 (1998): 105-24; Eileen Crofton, *The Women of Royaumont: A Scottish Woman's Hospital on the Western Front* (East Lothian: Tuckwell, 1997); Lyn Macdonald, *The Roses of No Man's Land* (London: Penguin, 1993; originally published c. 1980); Susan Mann, ed., *The War Diary of Clare Gass, 1915-1918* (Montreal and Kingston: McGill-Queen's University Press, 2000); and Constance Bruce, R.N., *Humour in Tragedy: Hospital Life behind Three Fronts, by a Canadian Nursing Sister* (London: Skeffington and Son, c. 1918).
61 Stuart, "War and Peace," 178-79.
62 Seale, "Nursing Outposts," 10.
63 PAM, CRCS, Manitoba Division, "Flora Hill Correspondence, 1930s," letter from Mrs. H.C. Bonnett to Mrs. Speechley, 22 July 1931, P4478, file 3; PAM, CRCS, Manitoba Division, letter from A. Perks Cameron to Mrs. A.C. Bonnett, 24 July 1931 [2 letters], P4478; and PAM, CRCS, Manitoba Division, memo from Rorketon, n.d., P4478.
64 PAM, CRCS, Manitoba Division, letter from Flora Hill to Mrs. Speechley, 15 July 1931, P4478; and PAM, CRCS, Manitoba Division, note from Mrs. Speechley, 19 July 1931 [not addressed], P4478.
65 Margaret Andrews, "Medical Attendance in Vancouver, 1886-1920," *BC Studies* 40 (Winter 1978-79): 32-56. See also S.E.D. Shortt, "Before the Age of Miracles: The Rise, Fall and Rebirth of General Practice in Canada, 1890-1940," in *Health, Disease and Medicine: Essays in Canadian Medical History,* ed. Charles Roland (Toronto: Clarke, Irwin, 1984), 123-52.
66 PAM, CRCS, Manitoba Division, letter from Nursing Stations' Committee to Flora Hill, n.d., P4478, file 3; and PAM, CRCS, Manitoba Division, letter from A. Purkis Cameron, commissioner to Flora Hill, 12 March 1938, P4478, file 3.

67  PAM, CRCS, "Nursing Stations c. 1920s-1935," minutes of Provincial Executive, November 1920, P4478, file 12, 23.
68  PAM, CRCS, Manitoba Division, "Flora Hill Correspondence, 1930s," letter from A. Purkis Cameron to Mrs. Bonnett, 24 July 1931, P4478, file 3.
69  PAM, CRCS, Manitoba Division, *Minute Book 1929-1930*, "Interim Report – Nursing Outpost," 30 December 1930, MG10, B29, box 9.
70  Ibid., 12-13.
71  Ibid., 14 and 19.
72  J.M. Bumsted, *The Peoples of Canada: A Post-Confederation History* (Don Mills, ON: Oxford University Press, 2003), 96 and 100-2; and CRCS, Manitoba Division, *Canadian Red Cross* 1, no. 3 (April 1922): 10.
73  Bumsted, *The Peoples of Canada*, 203-6; and Ken Coats and Fred McGuinness, *Manitoba: The Province and the People* (Edmonton: Hurtig Publishing, 1987), 98-99.
74  Morton and Wright, *Winning the Second Battle*, 22 and 45. In western Canada, nearly one-quarter of returned soldiers in 1918-19 applied for loans to buy farmland. Desmond Morton and J.L. Granatstein, *Marching to Armageddon: Canadians and the Great War, 1914-1919* (Toronto: Lester and Orpen Dennys, 1989), 6-9.
75  W.L. Morton, *Manitoba: A History* (Toronto: University of Toronto Press, 1967), 363-71.
76  PAM, CRCS, Manitoba Division, "Nursing Stations c. 1920s-1935," minutes of Provincial Executive, 28 November 1922, P4478, file 12, 18.
77  Seale, "Nursing Outposts," 12.
78  PAM, CRCS, Manitoba Division, "Nursing Stations c. 1920s-1935," minutes of Provincial Executive, 28 November 1922, P4478, file 12, 18.
79  Tom Mitchell and James Naylor, "The Prairies in the Eye of the Storm," in *The Worker's Revolt in Canada, 1917-1925*, ed. Craig Heron (Toronto: University of Toronto Press, 1998), 183-84.
80  Seale, "Nursing Outposts," 12.
81  Mrs. C.B. Waagen, "New Canadian Citizens," *Canadian Red Cross* 1, no. 2 (March 1922): 12.
82  Ibid., 1-2; and PAM, CRCS, Manitoba Division, "Nursing Stations c. 1920s-1935," Minutes of Provincial Executive, 28 November 1922, P4478, file 12, 18-19.
83  PAM, CRCS, Minute Books and Reports, "Provincial Nursing Committee," 28 November 1922, MG10, B29, box 8, 2.
84  PAM, CRCS Manitoba Division, "Nursing Stations, c. 1920-1935," Minutes of Provincial Executive, 28 November 1922, P4478, file 12, 7. The cost of a station was estimated at an average of $2,500 per annum.
85  Gleason, "Race, Class and Health," 95-112.
86  PAM, CRCS, Executive Committee Minute Book, September 1919-20, 8 March 1920, MG10, B29, box 8.
87  PAM, CRCS, Manitoba Division, Minute Books and Reports, "Provincial Nursing Committee," 28 November 1922, MG10, B29, box 8, 1-2; and PAM, CRCS Manitoba Division, "Nursing Stations, c. 1920s-1935," Minutes of Provincial Executive, 28 November 1922, P4478, file 12, 18-19.
88  PAM, CRCS, Manitoba Division, "Nursing Stations, c. 1920s-1935," Minutes of Provincial Executive, 28 November 1922, P4478, file 12, 27 and 31.
89  PAM, CRCS, "Memoirs of a Red Cross Outpost," Margaret Litton Hodgins, c. 1922-30, P4478, file 12.
90  Ina J. Bramadat and Marion Saydak, "Nursing on the Canadian Prairies, 1900-1930: Effects of Immigration," *Nursing History Review* 1 (1993): 107.
91  PAM, CRCS, Manitoba Division, "Nursing Stations, c. 1920s-1935," Minutes of Provincial Executive, 28 November 1922, P4478, file 12, 10 and 16.
92  For a broader perspective on outpost nursing, see Bramadat and Saydak, "Nursing on the Canadian Prairies," 105-18; Johanne Daigle and Nicole Rousseau, "Medical Service to Settlers: The Gestation and Establishment of a Nursing Service in Quebec, 1932-1943," *Nursing History Review* 8 (2000): 95-116; Drees and McBain, "Nursing and Native Peoples in Northern Saskatchewan"; Gertrude LeRoy Miller, *Mustard Plasters and Hand Cars: Through the Eyes of a Red Cross Outpost Nurse* (Toronto: Natural Heritage Books, 2000); Sharon Richardson, "Alberta's Provincial Travelling Clinic, 1924-1942," *Canadian Bulletin of Medical History* 9

(2002): 245-63; Meryn Stuart, "Ideology and Experience: Public Health Nursing and the Ontario Rural Child Welfare Project, 1920-1925," *Canadian Bulletin of Medical History* 6 (1989): 111-31; and J. Karen Scott and Joan E. Kieser, eds., *Northern Nurses: True Nursing Adventures from Canada's North* (Oakville: Kokum Publications, 2002).

93 Note that the late John Hutchinson was extremely skeptical of the post-war ambitions of the International Council of the Red Cross, citing a lack of explicit direction as to how they could be achieved. See John F. Hutchinson, *Champions of Charity: War and the Rise of the Red Cross* (Boulder: Westview Press, 1996), 343.

**Chapter 7: The Call of the North**

1 The Medical Service to Settlers (MSS) was quietly created in 1936 and placed under the authority of the department of the provincial secretary, under the heading "medical help for settlers." It was then placed under the provincial Ministry of Health, which produced the first annual reports for the service in 1944. Johanne Daigle and Nicole Rousseau, "Le Service médical aux colons: gestation et implantation d'un service infirmier au Québec (1932-1943)," *Revue d'histoire de l'Amérique française* 52 (1998): 47-72; and Nicole Rousseau and Johanne Daigle, "Medical Service to Settlers: The Gestation and Establishment of a Nursing Service in Quebec, 1932-1943," *Nursing History Review* 8 (2000): 95-116.

2 Dianne Dodd, Jayne Elliott, and Nicole Rousseau, "Le nursing en régions éloignées au Canada," in *Sans frontières: Quatre siècles de soins infirmiers canadiens,* ed. Christina Bates, Dianne Dodd, and Nicole Rousseau, translated by Marie-Claude Rochon with Marielle Gaudreault and Renée Thivierge (Ottawa: University of Ottawa Press and the Canadian Museum of Civilization, 2005), 139-52. Among the nursing services mentioned are the Alberta District Nursing Services, the philanthropic Grenfell Mission for Newfoundland and Labrador, the Newfoundland Outpost Nursing and Industrial Association (NONIA) for Newfoundland, the MSS for Québec, the Canadian Red Cross Society, and nursing stations under the aegis of the federal government. Other health care organizations eventually absorbed or closed down all but the federal services, as was the case with the MSS, with the creation of public sector health care and social services systems in Canada.

3 Alberta farmers' associations and particularly farmwomen had pushed to obtain maternity services for settler women for many years. However, it was not until 1919, when 25,000 soldiers, demobilized after the First World War, moved to the settlement lands in the western provinces that the Alberta government established the District Nursing Service. Sharon Richardson, "Political Women, Professional Nurses and the Creation of Alberta's District Nursing Service, 1919-1925," *Nursing History Review* 6 (1998): 25-50. Testimonials by nurses who worked in this service in the most recent periods have been collected, notably in Irene Stewart, ed., *These Were Our Yesterdays: A History of District Nursing in Alberta* (Altona, MB: D.W. Friesen and Sons, 1979).

4 Meryn Stuart, "War and Peace: Professional Identities and Nurses' Training, 1914-1930," in *Challenging Professions: Historical and Contemporary Perspectives on Women's Professional Work,* ed. Elizabeth Smyth, Sandra Acker, Paula Bourne, and Alison Prentice (Toronto: University of Toronto Press, 1999), 171-93.

5 See Janet C. Ross-Kerr, *Prepared to Care: Nurses and Nursing in Alberta, 1859 to 1996* (Edmonton: University of Alberta Press, 1998), xxii. For information on the United States, see Esther Lucile Brown, *Nursing for the Future* (New York: Russell Sage Foundation, 1948), in which she explained that people were habituated to the presence of nurses.

6 Notably for maternity care, "nursing educators provided students with thorough instructions pertaining to prenatal and postnatal care of mother and child, preparing a sterile area in which the delivery could occur safely and recognizing the various pathologies and difficulties that might occur during labour." Kathryn McPherson, *Bedside Matters: The Transformation of Canadian Nursing, 1900-1990* (Toronto: Oxford University Press, 1996), 96.

7 Johanne Daigle, "Devenir infirmière: le système d'apprentissage et la formation professionnelle à l'Hôtel-Dieu de Montréal, 1920-1970," PhD dissertation, Université du Québec, Montreal, 1990.

8 Denyse Baillargeon, *Un Québec en mal d'enfants: La médicalisation de la maternité, 1910-1970* (Montreal: Éditions du Remue-ménage, 2004). François Guérard argued that the

professionalization of nurses and the rapid increase in their numbers "was part of a broader process of medicalization in Quebec society." François Guérard, *Histoire de la santé au Québec,* collection Boréal Express (Montreal: Boréal, 1996), 59.

9   Sara Mills, "'Gender and Colonial Space,'" in *Feminist Postcolonial Theory: A Reader,* ed. Reina Lewis and Sara Mills (London and New York: Routledge, 2003), 692-719.

10  McCallum analyzed *Canadian Nurse, Canadian Medical Association Journal,* and *Canadian Journal of Public Health.* Mary Jane McCallum, "This Last Frontier: Isolation and Aboriginal Health," *Canadian Bulletin of Medical History* 22 (2005): 103-20. Marita E. Bardenhagen, "Professional Isolation and Independence of Bush Nurses in Tasmania 1910-1957: 'We Were Very Much Individuals on Our Own,'" PhD dissertation, School of History and Classics, University of Tasmania, Launceston, 2003.

11  Jayne Elliott, "Blurring the Boundaries of Space: Shaping Nursing Lives at the Red Cross Outposts in Ontario, 1922-1945," *Canadian Bulletin of Medical History* 21 (2004): 303-25.

12  The definition that they use is taken from Mary Louise Pratt, *Imperial Eyes: Travel Writing and Transculturation* (London and New York: Routledge, 1992), 6: "The space in which peoples geographically and historically separated come into contact with each other and establish ongoing relations, usually involving conditions of coercion, radical inequality, and intractable conflict." Katie Pickles and Myra Rutherdale, eds., "Introduction," *Contact Zones: Aboriginal and Settler Women in Canada's Colonial Past* (Vancouver: UBC Press, 2005), 4.

13  Judith Bender Zelmanovits, "'Midwife Preferred': Maternity Care in Outpost Nursing Stations in Northern Canada, 1945-1988," in *Women, Health, and Nation: Canada and the United States since 1945,* ed. Georgina Feldberg, Molly Ladd-Taylor, Alison Li, and Kathryn McPherson (Montreal and Kingston: McGill-Queen's University Press, 2003), 161-88.

14  Laurie Meijer Drees and Lesley McBain, "Nursing and Native Peoples in Northern Saskatchewan: 1930s-1950s," *Canadian Bulletin of Medical History* 18 (2001): 43-65.

15  Nicole Rousseau and professional researcher Clara Benezara conducted most of the interviews.

16  See, in particular, Philippe Joutard, ed., *Ces voix qui nous viennent du passé* (Paris: Hachette, 1983), 217-44.

17  Most of the interviews took place between forty and sixty years after the "settlement" experiences, and most of the nurses were over seventy years of age. Following a review of the historiography on oral studies, which is too long to be presented here, we have also observed in our group a "saturation point" beyond which the recurrence of themes collected won out over new data.

18  Recalling the history of district nurses in Alberta, the province's minister of public health, Dr. Malcolm R. Bow, wrote that nurses "were stationed in frontier communities in which neither medical nor hospital facilities of any kind are available. Some of these nurses [were] located in districts sixty miles from the nearest doctor or hospital. A district nurse [was] often required in the course of her duties to assume the role of doctor, dispenser, bedside nurse and any other role the occasion may require. Her duties [were], however, chiefly in maternity and first-aid work." Malcolm R. Bow and F.T. Cook, "The History of the Department of Public Health of Alberta," *Canadian Journal of Public Health* 26 (1935): 390. Reproduced in Ross-Kerr, *Prepared to Care,* 88-89. Dr. Peter H. Bryce, who in 1904 became the first person at the federal level responsible for health care for people with Indian status, promoted nursing support on the local community level. The first nursing station operated by the Bureau of Indian Affairs was inaugurated only in 1930, in the Fisher River reservation in Manitoba.

19  Newfoundland recognized the status of midwives. However, Alberta was the only province to legally allow nurses to act as midwives and to give emergency care under certain conditions. See the *Public Health Nurses Act,* S.A. 1919, c. 7, s. 49. Reproduced in Ross-Kerr, *Prepared to Care,* 87-88. François Guérard emphasizes the importance of the role that nurses played in applying public health policies in Québec in Guérard, *Histoire de la santé au Québec,* 45-59.

20  Dr. Helen MacMurchy, director of the Division of Childhood for the federal Department of Health, produced a detailed guide for women settlers in the West and isolated regions on how to attend an emergency childbirth without professional care, which was distributed

in 1923 as a supplement to the *Canadian Mother's Book*. Dianne Dodd, "Helen MacMurchy: Popular Midwifery and Maternity Services for Canadian Pioneer Women," in *Caring and Curing: Historical Perspectives on Women and Healing in Canada*, ed. Dianne Dodd and Deborah Gorham (Ottawa: University of Ottawa Press, 1994), 135-81.

21  Dr. Alphonse Lessard, "De l'amélioration des conditions hygiéniques constatées dans les familles," *Bulletin sanitaire* 18 (1918): 103, reproduced in Baillargeon, *Un Québec en mal d'enfants*, 73.

22  Denyse Baillargeon, "Entre la 'Revanche' et la 'Veillée' des berceaux: Les médecins québécois francophones, la mortalité infantile et la question nationale, 1910-1940," *Canadian Bulletin of Medical History* 19 (2002): 113-37.

23  Susan Mann Trofimenkoff presents a good analysis of the debates surrounding this question within the clerico-nationalist elite in *The Dream of Nation: A Social and Intellectual History of Quebec* (Toronto: Macmillan, 1982).

24  Antoine Labelle, "Lettre du 10 juin 1888 à O. Reclus, RLC-BM 1 Fol. 55-66; 60s," reproduced in Gilles Dusseault, *Le curé Labelle: Messianisme, utopie et colonisation au Québec, 1850-1900* (Montreal: Éditions Hurtubise HMH, 1983), 90.

25  This subject is discussed in a number of analyses of the history of the Roman Catholic Church in Québec. According to father Jacques Cousineau, s.j., this program, conceived as a way to get rid of the Depression, was inspired by the papal encyclical letter, *Quadragesimo Anno* (1931). In fact, an ambitious action plan for French Canadians (Catholic unions, co-operatives, social welfare initiatives, etc.) was viewed as an alternative to the "economic dictatorship" of the Liberal government of the province. Jacques Cousineau, s.j., *L'Église d'ici et le social, 1940-1960* (Montreal: Bellarmin, 1982), 132-42.

26  Esdras Minville, *L'oeuvre de la colonisation* (Montreal: École sociale populaire/Imprimerie du Messager, 1933), 32.

27  Robert H. Wiebe provides an enlightening definition of nationalist ideology in *Who We Are: A History of Popular Nationalism* (Princeton: Princeton University Press, 2002). He wrote: "Nationalism is the desire among people who believe that they share a common ancestry and a common destiny to live under their own government on land sacred to their history." It is reproduced in Johan Agnew, "Nationalism," in *A Companion to Cultural Geography*, ed. J. Duncan, N. Johnson, and R. Schein (London: Blackwell, 2004), 223. See also Christian Morissonneau, *La Terre promise: Le mythe du Nord québécois*, collection Ethnologie (Quebec City: Cahiers du Québec/Hurtubise HMH, 1978); and Serge Courville, *Introduction à la géographie historique* (Quebec City: Presses de l'Université Laval, 1995), 237.

28  Morissonneau, *La Terre promise*, 60-61.

29  Arthur Buies, *La province de Québec* (Province du Québec: Département de l'Agriculture, 1900), 80-81.

30  Serge Courville, *Immigration et colonisation: Du rêve américain au rêve colonial* (Quebec City: Éditions MultiMondes, 2002), 616-21.

31  See Morissonneau, *La Terre promise*, 175.

32  Dusseault, *Le curé Labelle*, and Courville, *Immigration et colonisation*, give detailed assessments of the main literature on this issue.

33  Courville, *Immigration et colonisation*, 635.

34  Normand Séguin, *La conquête du sol au 19e siècle* (Montreal: Éditions du Boréal Express, 1977), has shown how the agroforestry system worked in the second half of the nineteenth century using the example of the Notre-Dame d'Hébertville parish in Lac-Saint-Jean.

35  "Being a settler meant very explicitly to acquire public farmland, according to determined and resolutory conditions for settlement. The granting by the state of property titles meant that all of these conditions had been satisfactorily met. And this put an end to the status of settler, a status whose duration was a function of the time spent satisfying the settlement requirements set by the state." Séguin, *La conquête du sol*, 26.

36  The most detailed study on Labelle is by Dusseault, *Le curé Labelle*. The quote is reported in A. Chintre, "St-Jérôme et l'abbé Labelle," *La Minerve* (September 1881), reproduced in Dusseault, *Le curé Labelle*, 187. Dusseault mentioned that Curé Labelle had made a plan for a chapel school, estimating the construction costs at $500. Missionary nuns often quickly agreed to work in isolated communities, especially among Aboriginal populations

and pioneers in the western territories. See, in particular, Mary George Edmond, s.s.a., *North to Share: The Sisters of Saint Ann in Alaska and the Yukon Territory* (Victoria: Sisters of St. Ann, 1992); and Pauline Paul, "Les congrégations religieuses soignantes: une présence remarquable dans l'Ouest canadien," in Bates, Dodd, and Rousseau, eds., *Sans frontières,* 125-38.

37  M.C. Marquis, *Rapport du comité permanent sur l'agriculture, l'immigration et la colonisation* (Quebec City: A. Côté, 1868), 77, reproduced in Dusseault, *Le curé Labelle,* 9.

38  Yves Frenette, *Brève histoire des Canadiens français* (Montreal: Éditions Boréal, 1998), 103.

39  Of the almost six thousand people affected, 5,440 went to settle in the Abitibi-Témiscamingue region alone. Courville, *Introduction à la géographie historique,* 276.

40  This was explained by Dr. A. Lessard to some three hundred delegates in a discussion on the Vautrin Plan. A. Lessard, *Actes du Congrès de la colonisation tenu à Québec les 17 et 18 octobre 1934 sous la présidence de l'honorable Irénée Vautrin, ministre de la Colonisation* (Province du Québec, 1935), 215-16. Lessard added: "We are suffering a crisis, and in extraordinary times we must take extraordinary measures."

41  Léo-Pierre Bernier, "Genèse d'une colonie québécoise (1931-1935) Saint-Émile d'Auclair et LeJeune, comté de Témiscouata," in *Naissance et vie d'une "colonie" québécoise: Saint-Émile d'Auclair, 1931-1971,* Rodier Voisine, ed., parish souvenir book (n.p., 1971), 4.

42  Gérard Ouellet (the name was added in ballpoint pen on the cover page), *Sainte-Monique de Rollet ou La Rivière Solitaire,* souvenir book (Province du Québec: Ministère de la colonisation, 1958), 3.

43  The abandonment rate was estimated at 28 percent for the Abitibi-Témiscamingue region alone, even before the expiration of the Gordon Plan. Odette Vincent, ed., *Histoire de L'Abitibi-Témiscamingue,* collection "Les regions du Québec" (Quebec City: Institut québécois de recherche sur la culture, 1995), 241.

44  A number of authors described the Vautrin Plan, among them Courville, *Introduction à la géographie historique,* 277-78. With regard to its application in the Abitibi-Témiscamingue region, see Roger Barette, "Le plan Vautrin et l'Abitibi-Témiscamingue," in *L'Abitibi et le Témiscamingue: Hier et aujourd'hui,* ed. Maurice Asselin and Benoît Beaudry-Gourd (Rouyn, QC: Université du Québec à Rouyn, Département d'histoire et de géographie, 1975), 105-10; and Odette Vincent, ed., *Histoire de L'Abitibi-Témiscamingue,* collection Histoires régionales (Quebec City: Institut québécois de recherche sur la culture, 1995), particularly chapter 7.

45  Speech by Dr. Alphonse Lessard, in *Actes du Congrès de la colonisation de 1934,* 215-16.

46  There were many such attempts, all unfruitful. See the articles cited in note 1.

47  Courville, *Introduction à la géographie historique,* 280-81, presents an enlightening analysis.

48  AEG, drawer *Brébeuf,* "François de Casey à Mgr Ross," 29 November 1938, quoted in Bélanger et al., *Histoire de la Gaspésie* (Montreal: Boréal Express, 1981), 556.

49  Accounts reported in Bélanger et al., *Histoire de la Gaspésie,* 559-60.

50  Paul Claval, *Géographie culturelle: Une nouvelle approche des sociétés et des milieux* (Paris: Armand Colin, 2003), 110.

51  Antoine Labelle, *Projet d'une société de colonisation du diocèse de Montréal pour Coloniser la Vallée de l'Outaouais et le Nord de ce diocèse* (Montreal: Cie d'imprimerie canadienne, 1879), 10, reproduced in Dusseault, *Le curé Labelle,* 184.

52  Accounts reported in Vincent, ed., *Histoire de l'Abitibi-Témiscamingue,* 375 [emphasis in original].

53  Comité du cinquantenaire, Antoine Lacasse, manager, *1933-Roquemaure-1983, Cinquante ans de coopération, ça se fête,* souvenir album (Province du Québec, 1983), 171.

54  This experience is described in Père Louis Garnier, *Du cométique à l'avion: Les Pères Eudistes sur la Côte Nord (1903-1946)* (Province du Québec: A. D'Amours, C.J.M., 1947), 179-212.

55  The first health units were created in 1926. They became permanent in 1933 to monitor health in all counties of Québec. The *Social Assistance Act* passed in 1921 and, in fact, served to provide state support for the private initiative. The Department of Social Assistance, which was formed in 1922 to apply the act, became operational only in 1925, over the protests of clerico-nationalist organizations, which feared state mismanagement. See Guérard, *Histoire de la santé,* particularly chapter 4.

56 Vincent, *Histoire de l'Abitibi-Témiscamingue*. A number of authors mention the persistence of a high birth rate in the peripheral regions of Québec.
57 Archives Nationales du Québec (ANQ), Service medical aux colons (SMC), letter from Émile Nadeau, assistant director of Service provincial d'hygiène (SPH), to Nurse Blais, nurse in Auclair, Quebec City, 14 January 1933, B4-D1.
58 See note 1 for works discussing this issue.
59 ANQ, SMC, "Rapport concernant le dispensaire de Rollet," by Dr. Émile Martel, 14 October 1936, B4-D5; and ANQ, SMC, "Rapport anonyme et non daté du Ministère de la Santé," B4-D5.
60 A nurse in Abitibi received the following directive: "Until you receive further orders, in the case of certain people who are in a position to pay something for your care, you must require a reasonable amount for remedies in order to make a necessary distinction between indigents and others. These moneys must be handed over to Dr. Émile Martel, at the end of each month ... and he will forward them to us." ANQ-Rouyn (Abitibi-Témiscamingue), contract from Dr. Émile Nadeau, interim director, Ministère de la Santé, to nurse Marcelle Gingras, for the Canton Castagnier dispensary, 30 December 1936.
61 In Canada, for example, Alberta's District and Municipal Nursing program involved three nurses' stations in 1919, eight in 1934, twenty-five in 1939, and thirty-seven in 1951, while only twelve remained in operation in 1965. See Sharon Richardson, "Frontier Health Care: Alberta's District and Municipal Nursing Services, 1919 to 1976," *Alberta History* 46 (Winter 1998): 2-9. NONIA in Newfoundland involved twenty-seven outposts between 1920 and 1934. See Edgar House, *The Way Out: The Story of NONIA, 1920-40* (St. John's, NF: Creative Publishers, 1990); the Canadian Red Cross Society outposts in Ontario comprised forty-four stations between 1922 and 1984, with a peak in 1940 when the society had thirty-one stations in operation simultaneously. Elliott, "Blurring the Boundaries of Space," 303-25. In 1948, the federal government operated eighteen nursing stations for the Aboriginal populations of Canada, although it also had recourse to services implemented by the provinces. Meijer Drees and McBain, "Nursing and Native People." In Australia, the Bush Nursing Order of Australia had fifty bush nursing centres between 1911 and 1956. Bardenhagen, "Professional Isolation and Independence."
62 Nurse Anna Forest-Poirier, *Souvenir d'une infirmière en pays de colonisation* (Mont-Brun, Abitibi: Comité de recherche sur le 50e de la paroisse, May 1986), 3.
63 Interview with Monique Lachance, stationed at Rochebaucourt, Abitibi, 1972 (15 October 1992).
64 Interview with Georgette Boutin-Turgeon, stationed at Saint-Dominique, Abitibi, 1948-49 (18 January 1993). Another nurse who had lived in several dispensaries in the same region in the 1950s went so far as to say: "I had good memories of people there. They were charitable, and it was like a big family in the end." Interview with Nicole Dionne-De-La-Chevrotière, stationed at Saint-Janvier-de-Chazel, Rollet, and Cadillac, Abitibi, 1950-74 (9 December 1992).
65 Interview with Anita Dionne-Ott, stationed at L'Anse-Saint-Jean, 1932-38 (26 February 1993). The nurse stationed at Saint-Charles-Garnier in Bas-Saint-Laurent in the 1950s also said: "There was a group of very nice parishioners, you know ... it was very united." Interview with Marguerite Pelletier-Martin, stationed at Saint-Charles-Garnier, Bas-Saint-Laurent, 1952-58 (18 November 1993).
66 Interview with Edna Lachance, stationed at La Tabatière, Côte-Nord, 1972-74 (9 February 1993).
67 Marguerite Turgeon, *Mémoires d'une infirmière de colonies en Abitibi: Un récit* (Terrebonne, QC: Les Éditions Berthiaume, 1997), 15.
68 Interview with Juliette Jourdain-Dumont, stationed at Saint-Dominique-du-Rosaire, Abitibi, 1949-52 (12 November 1992).
69 Interview with Louisette Beaudoin-Mercier, stationed in Abitibi, 1942-78 (7 December 1992).
70 Interview with Annette Bélanger-Beaupré, stationed at Les Étroits (Saint-Marc-du-lac-long), Bas-Saint-Laurent, 1950-53 (20 January 1993).

71  Interview with Nurse No. 4, stationed at Abitibi-Témiscamingue, 1936-43 (16 February 1993).
72  Interview with Louisette Beaudoin-Mercier, stationed at Beaucanton, Abitibi, 1942-78 (7 December 1992).
73  Interview with Jeannette Coulombe-Morneau, stationed at Saint-Janvier-de-Chazal, 1944-48 and 1954-79 (19 October 1992).
74  Interview with Nurse No. 8, stationed in the Saguenay–Lac-Saint-Jean region, 1952-57 (13 May 1993).
75  Interview with Nurse No. 39, stationed in Bas-Saint-Laurent, 1960-75, and in the Mauricie–Bois-Francs region, 1980-83. She also spent time in Côte-Nord, 1983-87 (10 November 1992).
76  Ibid.
77  Interview with Louisette Beaudoin-Mercier, stationed at Beaucanton, Abitibi, 1942-78 (7 December 1992).
78  Interview with Nurse No. 43, stationed in a health unit in Bas-Saint-Laurent, 1936-76 (19 March 1993).
79  Interview with Bérangère Martel-Méthot, stationed at Sainte-Paule, Gaspé, 1960-69 (4 February 1993).
80  Interview with Angéline Hudon-Langlois, stationed at Bégin, Saguenay–Lac-Saint-Jean, 1966-73 (8 February 1993).
81  Interview with Nurse No. 1, stationed in Bas-Saint-Laurent–Gaspésie, 1936-76 (24 November 1992).
82  Interview with Nurse No. 36, stationed in Bas-Saint-Laurent–Gaspésie, 1950-74 (18 November 1992).
83  Interview with Thérèse Mercier, stationed at Île-aux-Grues, Chaudière-Appalaches region, 1955-78 (27 February 1993).
84  Interview with Louisette Beaudoin-Mercier, stationed at Beaucanton, Abitibi, 1942-78 (7 December 1992).
85  Interview with Jeanne Lussier-Gosselin, Saint-Mathias-de-Bonneterre, Estrie region, 1948-51 (12 April 1993).
86  Interview with Marguerite Turgeon, stationed in Abitibi, 1936-42 (20 July 1992).
87  Interview with Nurse No. 12, stationed in Abitibi, 1958-62 (6 October 1992).
88  Interview with Juliette Jourdain-Dumont, stationed at Saint-Dominique-du-Rosaire, Abitibi, 1949-52 (12 November 1992).
89  Interview with Marguerite Pelletier-Martin, stationed at Saint-Charles-Garnier, Bas-Saint-Laurent, 1952-58 (18 November 1993).
90  Interview with Nurse No. 36, stationed in Bas-Saint-Laurent–Gaspésie, 1950-74 (18 November 1992).
91  Interview with Alberte Labrie, Sainte-Marthe, Bas-Saint-Laurent–Gaspésie, 1965-67 (11 February 1993).
92  Turgeon, *Mémoires d'une infirmière*, 12.
93  Interview with Marcelle Laliberté-Saint-Aubin, stationed in Abitibi-Témiscamingue, 1950-60 and 1971-88 (22 October 1992).
94  Interview with Nurse No. 1, stationed in Bas-Saint-Laurent–Gaspé, 1936-76 (24 November 1992).
95  Interview with Hénédine Gendron-Beaupré, stationed at Sacré-Cœur, Gaspésie, 1953-65 (21 January 1993).
96  Interview with Bibiane Trottier-Dumont, stationed at Manneville, Abitibi, 1940-43 (27 January 1993).
97  Interview with Mary Leblanc, stationed at Saint-Jogues, Gaspé, 1941-46 (27 November 1992).
98  Interview with Jeanne Lussier-Gosselin, Saint-Mathias-de-Bonneterre, Estrie region, 1948-51 (12 April 1993).
99  Interview with Anita Dionne-Ott, stationed at L'Anse-Saint-Jean, 1932-38 (26 February 1993).
100 Interview with Nurse No. 11, stationed in Côte-Nord, 1978-79 (10 March 1992).
101 Interview with Nurse No. 3, stationed in Côte-Nord starting in 1988 (26 February 1993).

102 Interview with Edna Lachance, stationed at La Tabatière, Côte-Nord, 1972-74 (9 February 1993).
103 Interview with Nicole Dionne-De-La-Chevrotière, stationed at Saint-Janvier-de-Chazel, Rollet, and Cadillac, Abitibi, 1950-74 (9 December 1992).
104 Interview with Marie-Hélène Gagné-Roy, stationed at Saint-Jogues, Gaspésie, 1940 (8 July 1992).
105 Interview with Nurse No. 39, stationed in Bas-Saint-Laurent, 1960-75, and in the Mauricie–Bois-Francs region, 1980-83. She also spent time in Côte-Nord, 1983-87 (10 November 1992).
106 Interview with Alberte Labrie, Sainte-Marthe, Bas-Saint-Laurent–Gaspésie, 1965-67 (11 February 1993).
107 Interview with Nurse No. 39, stationed in Bas-Saint-Laurent, 1960-75, and in the Mauricie–Bois-Francs region, 1980-83. She also spent time in Côte-Nord, 1983-87 (10 November 1992).
108 Interview with Nurse Irène Bergeron-Dupont, stationed at Parent, Mauricie, 1965-77 (3 October 1991).
109 Interview with Georgette Boutin-Turgeon, stationed at Saint-Dominique, Abitibi, 1948-49 (18 January 1993).
110 Interview with Georgette Soumis, stationed in Abitibi, 1956-78 (20 January 1993).
111 Morissonneau, *La Terre promise,* 114.
112 Interview with Alberte Labrie, Sainte-Marthe, Bas-Saint-Laurent–Gaspésie, 1965-67 (11 February 1993).

## Chapter 8: (Re)constructing the Identity of a Red Cross Outpost Nurse

1 "Lauds Nurses' Work at Dionne Births, Madame de Kirilene [sic], Red Cross Nurse, Interviewed When Off Duty," *The Nugget,* June 1934.
2 Louise de Kiriline, *The Quintuplets' First Year: The Survival of the Famous Five Dionne Babies and Its Significance for All Mothers* (Toronto: MacMillan, 1936), xiii.
3 Pierre Berton, *The Dionne Years: A Thirties Melodrama* (Toronto: McClelland and Stewart, 1977); and Katherine Arnup, "Raising the Dionne Quintuplets: Lessons for Modern Mothers," *Journal of Canadian Studies* 29 (Winter 1994-95): 65-85.
4 Linda Quiney, "'Suitable Young Women': Red Cross Nursing Pioneers and the Crusade for Healthy Living in Manitoba, 1920-," in this volume; and Merle Massie, "Ruth Dulmage Shewchuk: A Saskatchewan Red Cross Outpost Nurse," *Saskatchewan History* 52, no. 2 (2004): 35-44.
5 Jayne Elliott, "'Keep the Flag Flying': Medical Outposts and the Red Cross in Northern Ontario, 1922-1984," PhD dissertation, Queen's University, Kingston, 2004, 228.
6 Joy Parr, *The Gender of Breadwinners: Women, Men, and Change in Two Industrial Towns, 1880-1950* (Toronto: University of Toronto Press, 1990), 9.
7 The last letter in this collection is dated 28 February 1937. Included in the overall de Kiriline collection but not consulted for this article are letters by de Kiriline's mother, which make this already rich resource even more valuable as a two-sided conversation. All translations are by the author.
8 Library and Archives Canada (LAC), Louise de Kiriline Lawrence Papers, 31 May 1934, MG31, J18, vol. 12, file 1.1. Apart from her book on the Dionne quintuplets, de Kiriline never did write about her Bonfield years "among the French-Canadians."
9 Wendy Cameron, Sheila Haines, and Mary McDougall Maude, eds., *English Immigrant Voices: Labourers' Letters from Upper Canada in the 1830s* (Montreal and Kingston: McGill-Queen's University Press, 2000), xi.
10 Rebecca Earle, ed., *Epistolary Selves: Letters and Letter-Writers, 1600-1945* (Aldershot, UK: Ashgate, 1999), 2.
11 James How, *Epistolary Spaces: English Letter Writing from the Foundation of the Post Office to Richardson's Clarissa* (Aldershot, UK: Ashgate, 2003), 2.
12 David Fitzpatrick, ed., *Oceans of Consolation: Personal Accounts of Irish Migration to Australia* (Ithaca, NY: Cornell University Press, 1994), 23-24.
13 David A. Gerber, *Authors of Their Lives: The Personal Correspondence of British Immigrants to North America in the Nineteenth Century* (New York: New York University Press, 2006), 73.

14  Ibid., 113.
15  Biographical information in this section is taken from Louise de Kiriline Lawrence, *Another Winter, Another Spring: A Love Remembered* (Toronto: Natural Heritage, 1987, previously published by McGraw-Hill Book Company, 1977). The name Lawrence comes from her marriage to Len Lawrence in the mid-1930s.
16  LAC, Louise de Kiriline Lawrence Papers, scrapbook of newspaper clippings, vol. 10, file 4.
17  Sharon Ouditt, *Fighting Forces, Writing Women: Identity and Ideology in the First World War* (London and New York: Routledge, 1994), 40.
18  Ontario Medical Association (OMA), Corporate Records Department, oral interview with Louise de Kiriline Lawrence conducted by Barry Penhale, 26-27 September 1978, OHR001417.
19  "Why Did You Come to Canada?" *Chatelaine* (October 1937): 53.
20  Georgina Gladbach Rawn, quoted in Merilyn Mohr, "To Whom the Wilderness Speaks: The Remarkable Life of Louise de Kiriline Lawrence," *Harrowsmith* 13 (1989): 75.
21  H. Arnold Barton, *Letters from the Promised Land: Swedes in America, 1840-1941* (Minneapolis: University of Minnesota Press, 1975), 204-7; 305-7. Barton's figures and analysis are focused on the United States. The raw Canadian census data demonstrates that the total resident population of people born in Sweden more than doubled from 28,246 in 1911 to 61,503 in 1921 and then grew more slowly by 1931 to 81,576. A. Ernest Epp, *Nordic People in Canada: A Study in Demography 1861-2001* (Thunder Bay: Lakehead Social History Institute, 2004), 20d, 21e, and 24e.
22  Frank Thistlethwaite, "Migration from Europe Overseas in the Nineteenth and Twentieth Centuries," in *A Century of European Migrations, 1830-1930,* ed. Rudolph J. Vecoli and Suzanne M. Sinke (Urbana and Chicago: University of Illinois Press, 1991), 22. See also Joy K. Lintelman, "'America Is the Woman's Promised Land': Swedish Immigrant Women and Domestic Service," *Journal of American Ethnic History* 8 (Spring 1989): 9-23.
23  "Why Did You Come to Canada?" *Chatelaine* (October 1937): 53.
24  Meryn Stuart, "War and Peace: Professional Identities and Nurses' Training, 1914-1930," in *Challenging Professions: Historical and Contemporary Perspectives on Women's Professional Work,* ed. Elizabeth Smyth, Sandar Acker, Paula Bourne, and Alison Prentice (Toronto: University of Toronto Press, 1999), 178.
25  Ibid., 178-79.
26  "In Romantic Woodland Home Louise de Kiriline is Writing the Story of Her Remarkable Life," *North Bay News,* 2 January 1936.
27  De Kiriline Lawrence, *Another Winter,* 32.
28  LAC, Louise de Kiriline Lawrence Papers, letters, 20 August and 19 November 1927, vol. 11, file 1.9.
29  Ibid., 19 November and 31 July 1927, vol. 11, file 1.9. For some examples of nursing anxiety around midwifery requirements, see Gertrude Leroy Miller, *Mustard Plasters and Handcars: Through the Eyes of a Red Cross Outpost Nurse* (Toronto: Natural Heritage Books, 2000), 32; Judith Bender Zelmanovits, "'Midwife Preferred': Maternity Care in Outpost Nursing Stations in Northern Canada, 1945-1988," in *Women, Health and Nation: Canada and the United States Since 1945,* ed. Georgina Feldberg, Molly Ladd-Taylor, Alison Li, and Kathryn McPherson (Montreal and Kingston: McGill-Queen's University Press, 2003), 161.
30  LAC, Louise de Kiriline Lawrence Papers, letters, 24 June 1928, vol. 12, file 2.1.
31  Rondalyn Kirkwood, "Blending Vigorous Leadership and Womanly Virtues: Edith Kathleen Russell at the University of Toronto, 1920-52," *Canadian Bulletin of Medical History* 11 (1994): 178-79.
32  LAC, Louise de Kiriline Lawrence Papers, letters, 17 June 1928, vol. 12, file 2.1.
33  Ibid., 10 May 1928, vol. 12, file 2.1; and 20 November 1928, vol. 12, file 2.2.
34  Ibid., 8 March 1928, vol. 12, file 2.1.
35  Ibid., 15 June 1927, vol. 11, file 1.8.
36  Ibid., 20 August 1927, vol. 11, file 1.9.
37  Ibid., 8 March 1928, vol. 12, file 2.1.
38  Ibid.

39  De Kiriline Lawrence, *Another Winter,* 32.
40  LAC, Louise de Kiriline Lawrence Papers, letters, 14 August 1928, vol. 12, file 2.2; and 9 June 1934, vol. 12, file 2.11.
41  OMA, Corporate Records Department, interview conducted by Barry Penhale, 26-27 September 1978, 35.
42  LAC, Louise de Kiriline Lawrence Papers, letters, 23 September 1928, 1 October 1928, and 12 December 1928, vol. 12, file 2.2; and 12 January 1929, vol. 12, file 2.3.
43  Barton, *Letters from the Promised Land,* 5.
44  In another, smaller set of letters, Canadian Red Cross Society nurse Maude Weaver corresponded with both her mother and her sister from her outpost in Atikokan in 1933-34. Weaver's letters to her own mother were similar to those de Kiriline sent in that they contained more social than medical content. Weaver, however, eagerly relayed in great detail the medical treatment she had provided for her patients to her sister Gwen, who was at that time a medical intern at the Moose Jaw Hospital. Letters from Maude Weaver to her mother and to her sister Gwen, 21 and 24 July (likely 1933) [copies in possession of author].
45  Gerber, *Authors of their Lives,* 55; and David A. Gerber, "Epistolary Ethics: Personal Correspondence and the Culture of Emigration in the Nineteenth Century," *Journal of American Ethnic History* 19 (Summer 2000): especially 11-16.
46  De Kiriline hinted in her autobiography that her mother was initially less than happy with her decision to marry a Russian soldier who had little means of financial support, but she went ahead anyway, in spite of family misgivings. See de Kiriline Lawrence, *Another Winter,* 56.
47  Bettina Bradbury and Tamara Myers, eds., *Negotiating Identities in Nineteenth and Twentieth-Century Montreal* (Vancouver and Toronto: UBC Press, 2005), 4.
48  LAC, Louise de Kiriline Lawrence Papers, letters, 10 May 1928 and 3 June 1928, vol. 12, file 2.1.
49  Ibid., 3 June 1928, vol. 12, file 2.1.
50  Brigitte Violette, "Gertrude Duchemin," in *On All Frontiers: Four Centuries of Canadian Nursing,* ed. Christina Bates, Dianne Dodd, and Nicole Rousseau (Ottawa: University of Ottawa Press and the Canadian Museum of Civilization, 2005), 145; Marita Bardenhagen and Jayne Elliott, "Uniform as Costume in the Performance of Rural Nursing: Tasmanian Bush Nursing and Red Cross Outpost Nursing in Ontario, Canada," unpublished paper presented to the Biennial Conference of the Australia New Zealand American Studies Association, University of Tasmania, Launceston, July 2006.
51  Marita Bardenhagen, "Professional Isolation and Independence of Bush Nurses in Tasmania 1910-1957, 'We're Very Much Individuals on Our Own,'" PhD dissertation, School of History and Classics, University of Tasmania, Launceston, 2003, 120-36.
52  Elliott, "Keep the Flag Flying," 247.
53  LAC, Louise de Kiriline Lawrence Papers, letters, 15 July 1928, vol. 12, file 2.2. Oral interview conducted by Jayne Elliott with Jean Birch Williamson, 9 May 2000, and Margaret Maclachlan, 10 February 2000 [transcripts in possession of author].
54  LAC, Louise de Kiriline Lawrence Papers, letters, 1 November 1928, vol. 11, file 2.2.
55  A.D. Kean, "Swedish Girl Ministering Angel to Ontario French-Canadians," *Toronto Star Weekly,* 21 March 1931, 43.
56  "Bonfield's Nurse Has Had Thrilling Life Experience," *The Nugget,* October 1929.
57  *North Bay News,* 2 January 1936.
58  LAC, Louise de Kiriline Lawrence Papers, letters, 20 January 1929, vol. 12, file 2.3.
59  Ibid., 23 October 1927, vol. 11, file 1.9.
60  Ibid., 1 November 1928, vol. 12, file 2.2.
61  Epp, *Nordic People in Canada,* 24 and 28.
62  Quoted in Orm Øverland, *Immigrant Minds, American Identities: Making the United States Home, 1870-1930* (Urbana and Chicago: University of Illinois Press, 2000), 58.
63  LAC, Louise de Kiriline Lawrence Papers, letters, 9 November 1927, vol. 11, file 1.9.
64  Karen Dubinsky, *Improper Advances: Rape and Heterosexual Conflict in Ontario, 1880-1929* (Chicago and London: Chicago University Press, 1993), 155-56.

65   LAC, Louise de Kiriline Lawrence Papers, letters, 28 October 1927, vol. 11, file 1.9.
66   Ibid., 18 January 1928, vol. 12, file 1. De Kiriline used the Swedish word "pigor," which translates as "maids" or "domestic servants."
67   Ibid., 17 June 1928, vol. 12, file 2.1.
68   Meryn Stuart, "Ideology and Experience: Public Health Nursing and the Ontario Rural Child Welfare Project, 1920-25," *Canadian Bulletin of Medical History* 6 (1989): 111-31.
69   LAC, Louise de Kiriline Lawrence Papers, letters, 29 July 1927, vol. 11, file 1.8; and 12 October 1927, vol. 11, file 1.9.
70   Ibid., 23 September 1928, vol. 12, file 2.2.
71   See, for examples, H.J.G. Geggie, *The Extra Mile: Medicine in Rural Quebec 1885-1965*, edited by Norma and Stuart Geggie (self-published, 1987), 34 and 47; Hugh MacLean, "A Pioneer Prairie Doctor," *Saskatchewan History* 15 (1962): 60-61; and Jacalyn Duffin, *Langstaff: A Nineteenth-Century Medical Life* (Toronto: University of Toronto Press, 1993), 27, 182.
72   LAC, Louise de Kiriline Lawrence Papers, letters, 28 June 1928, vol. 12, file 2.2.
73   Ibid., 20 November 1928, vol. 12, file 2.2.
74   Ibid., 20 March 1929, vol. 12, file 2.3.
75   Kathryn McPherson, *Bedside Matters: The Transformation of Canadian Nursing, 1900-1910* (Toronto: Oxford University Press, 1996), 165.
76   Canadian Red Cross Society Library and Archives, Box CRCS History, *Annual Report*, 1920, 42.
77   OMA, Corporate Records Department, interview conducted by Barry Penhale, 26-27 September 1978, 71.
78   Ibid., 74.
79   Krista Cowman and Louise A. Jackson, "Middle-Class Women and Professional Identity," *Women's History* Review 14 (2005): 165-80. For an example in nursing, see Kathryn McPherson, "'The Country Is a Stern Nurse': Rural Women, Urban Hospitals and the Creation of a Western Canadian Nursing Work Force, 1920-1940," *Prairie Forum* 20 (1995): 198.
80   Since I have not yet translated the letters in Swedish for this period, I am referring here to the letters de Kiriline wrote in English after she retired.
81   Many years later, de Kiriline stated that she continued to help some women at childbirth, but what I mean here is that she never again (in her English letters at least) self-identified herself as a nurse. See OMA, Corporate Records Department, interview conducted by Barry Penhale, 58. Patricia D'Antonio suggests that a nursing identity may have informed women's status and activities in their communities even if they had left the profession. See Patricia D'Antonio, "Revisiting and Rethinking the Rewriting of Nursing History," *Bulletin of the History of Medicine* 73 (1999): 268-90. For one example of nurses in "retirement," see Miller, *Mustard Plasters and Handcars*, 171-82.

### Chapter 9: University Nursing Education for Francophones in New Brunswick in the 1960s

1   Helen K. Mussallem, *Nursing Education in Canada*, Report to the Royal Commission on Health Services (Ottawa: Queen's Printer, 1964), 5.
2   Della M.M. Stanley, *Louis Robichaud: A Decade of Power* (Halifax: Nimbus Publishing, 1984).
3   New Brunswick, *Preface to the Commission royale d'enquête sur l'enseignement supérieur au Nouveau-Brunswick* (Fredericton: Government of New Brunswick, 1962).
4   George W. Weir, *Survey of Nursing Education in Canada* (Toronto: University of Toronto Press, 1932). Edith K. Russell, *Report of a Study of Nursing Education in New Brunswick* (Fredericton: University of New Brunswick, 1956). Helen K. Mussallem, *Spotlight on Nursing Education: The Report of the Pilot Project of the Evaluation of Schools of Nursing in Canada* (Ottawa: Canadian Nurses Association, 1962). This last study was undertaken to see if schools were ready for accreditation, but it identified many serious deficiencies.
5   Canada, *Royal Commission on Health Services* (Ottawa: Queen's Printer, 1964), 64-69. It recommended that nursing education be organized and financed as were other forms of professional education.
6   New Brunswick, *Commission royale d'enquête sur l'enseignement supérieur*.

7 Michel Cormier, "Que reste-t-il de l'héritage de Louis J. Robichaud? In *L'Ère Louis J. Robichaud, 1960-1970,* ed. Institut canadien de recherche sur le développement régional (Université de Moncton: [ICRDR], 2001), 206.

8 *Financing of Higher Education in New Brunswick,* a brief submitted to the provincial cabinet by denominational colleges, 20 December 1960. Financial resources are compared to support provided by other provinces for higher education. See Stanley, *Louis Robichaud,* 64.

9 See Jean Daigle, *Acadians of the Maritimes: Thematic Studies* (Moncton: Centre d'études acadiennes, Université de Moncton, 1982) for a comprehensive history of the Acadians.

10 The two other women's colleges, the Collège Notre-Dame d'Acadie in Moncton under the direction of the Notre-Dame du Sacré-Cœur sisters, and the Collège Jésus-Marie at Shippegan, near Bathurst, directed by the Religieuses Jesus-Marie, were not involved in the founding of the French baccalaureate nursing program.

11 Michel Cormier, *Louis J. Robichaud: Une révolution si peu tranquille* (Moncton: Éditions de la Francophonie, 2004), 135. In an interview, Robichaud admitted that Judge Cormier had been a good friend for many years.

12 Robert Pichette, "Culture et langues officielles," in *L'Ère Louis J. Robichaud,* ICRDR, 71.

13 Stanley, *Louis Robichaud,* 10. For a description of the Quiet Revolution in Québec, see Lucia Ferretti, "La révolution tranquille," *Action nationale* 89 (1999): 59-91. The author states that the specificity of the Quiet Revolution was the conjunction of reform and an "effervescence of nationalism" (at 2).

14 Jacques-Paul Couturier, *Construire un savoir: l'enseignement supérieur au Madawaska 1946-1974* (Moncton: Éditions d'Acadie, 1999), 145.

15 Cormier, *Louis J. Robichaud,* 136.

16 New Brunswick, *Royal Commission on Finances and Municipal Taxation.* See the online summary where it is acknowledged that the commission's recommendations changed the look of the province in a fundamental way. See Government of New Brunswick, www.lib.unb.ca/Texts/NBHistory/Commissions/ES81E/Byrne_1E.html.

17 Robert A. Young, "Le programme de Chances égales pour tous: une vue d'ensemble," in *L'Ère Louis J. Robichaud,* ICRDR, 26.

18 Stanley, *Louis Robichaud,* 131. For example, the 422 school districts were eventually reduced to thirty-three.

19 Young, "Le programme de Chances égales pour tous," 24, 28.

20 A speech by Robichaud, "Un programme d'égalité sociale," 16 November 1965, quoted in Young, "Le programme de Chances égales pour tous," 24 and 28.

21 Canada, *Royal Commission on Health Services,* 68.

22 Committee for the Study of Nursing Education, *Nursing and Nursing Education in the United States* (New York: Macmillan, 1923).

23 Weir, *Survey of Nursing Education,* 116.

24 Mussallem, *Spotlight on Nursing Education.* See also her survey for the Royal Commission on Health Services. Mussallem, *Nursing Education in Canada,* 137-38.

25 Alice Wright, "Report of the Health Survey Committee of New Brunswick for the 1951 Health Survey," in *The Report of a Study of Nursing Education in New Brunswick,* ed. E.K. Russell (Fredericton: UNB Press, 1956), 11. See also Margaret McPhedran, Irene Leckie, and Shirley M. Alcoe, *Reflections: Faculty of Nursing UNB 1958-1983* (Fredericton: UNB Press, no date), 2.

26 Russell, ed., *Report of a Study of Nursing Education,* 48 and 58-60. Mussallem's study four years later found thirteen schools of nursing in the province and 270 graduates per year. See Mussallem, *Spotlight on Nursing Education,* 31.

27 Georgette Desjardins and Corinne LaPlante, "Oeuvre des Hospitalières de Saint-Joseph du Nouveau-Brunswick 1868-1986," *Revue de la Société historique du Madawaska* 14, nos. 1 and 2 (1986): 3 and 47.

28 Sr. Bertille Beaulieu, "Notice biographique de Sœur Marie-Rhéa Larose," http://personal.nbnet.nb.ca/rhsjnda/page38.html (accessed 18 April 2008).

29 Couturier, *Construire un savoir,* 137. See A.L. Laplante, *Le Collège de Bathurst: Chronique des années 1949-1975* (self-published, 1975). He mentioned a little-known post-registered nursing program that existed at the college between 1952 and 1953, "L'École supérieure des sciences hospitalières," the Institut de la Ferre.

30   Centre Universitaire Saint-Louis Maillet, Fonds des services pédagogiques, submission made by the Collège Maillet to the Royal Commission on Higher Education, 12 December 1961, non-classified.

31   New Brunswick, *Commission royale sur l'enseignement supérieur,* 90. Isabelle McKee, in her doctoral dissertation, related the history of the women's colleges and described the impact of the higher-education reforms that led to the closing of these institutions. Isabelle McKee, "Rapports ethniques et rapports de sexe en Acadie: les communautés religieuses de femmes et leurs collèges classiques," Université de Montréal, Montreal, 1995.

32   Couturier, *Construire un savoir,* 143. The author quoted Father Louis Cyr, a professor and later president of the Collège Saint-Louis, in a speech to a local club in 1967. Couturier also stated that Father Clément Cormier wrote the first drafts of the Deutsch Commission report (at 144).

33   Katherine MacLaggan had been a member of the Nursing Education Committee from 1955-56 when E.K. Russell was undertaking her survey of nursing education in New Brunswick. Regarded by the Kellogg Foundation as a "particularly enthusiastic and intelligent leader," MacLaggan later became well known for her published study of nursing in New Brunswick. Her book, *Portrait of Nursing: A Plan for the Education of Nurses in the Province of New Brunswick* (Fredericton: New Brunswick Association of Registered Nurses (NBARN), 1965) was research she had completed for her doctoral dissertation at Columbia University. W.K. Kellogg Foundation, *Annual Report* (Battle Creek, MI: W.K. Kellogg Foundation, 1962), cited in Mussallem, *Nursing Education in Canada,* 127. She was also actively involved in professional activities, assuming the presidency of the Canadian Nurses Association from 1966 until her sudden death in 1967. See also Arlee H. McGee, "Profile of a Leader: Katherine MacLaggan: New Brunswick's Nurse Revolutionist with Evolutionary Strategies," *Canadian Journal of Nursing Leadership* 14, no. 1 (2001): 1-4.

34   McPhedran, Leckie, and Alcoe, *Reflections* 2 and 17. It is clear from his personal archives that Father Cormier had been interested in nursing education for several years. In the late 1940s and during the 1950s, he contacted administrators at several Canadian universities in order to obtain information on their nursing programs. He wrote in his notes that a university nursing program should provide, through a comprehensive education, not only professional knowledge and technical skills but also personal enrichment and religious conviction.

35   Centre d'études acadiennes (CEA), Fonds Clément Cormier, letter from Katherine MacLaggan to Father Cormier, 15 February 1960, file 177-1056.

36   Clément Cormier, *L'Université de Moncton: historique* (Moncton: Centre d'études acadiennes, 1975), 60.

37   Cormier described the letter this way in the first history of the school that he co-wrote with the nursing director at that time, Huberte Richard. See the part written by Cormier in *École des sciences infirmières, Université de Moncton: les dix premières années* (Université de Moncton: École des sciences infirmières, 1975), 8.

38   Nurses Association of New Brunswick (NANB), Nursing History Center, minutes of a meeting of the NBARN Executive Committee, 29 August 1962, Fredericton.

39   Ibid., minutes of a special meeting of the NBARN Executive, 18 September 1962.

40   Letter signed by Sr. Larose to NBARN, 3 January 1963, cited in *Histoire de l'école d'infirmières au Collège Maillet* (Saint-Basile: Archives de l'Hôtel-Dieu Saint-Basile, 1964), 13.

41   Couturier, *Construire un savoir,* 144. In 1962, three lay and three religious students were admitted into the program.

42   Ibid., 157-58.

43   Cormier, *L'Université de Moncton,* 64. The university opened in 1965.

44   CEA, Fonds Université de Moncton, minutes of the Senate of the Université de Moncton, 15 July 1963, file E38-347.

45   Couturier, *Construire un savoir,* 150 and 160.

46   CEA, Fonds Clément Cormier, minutes of the Senate of the Université de Moncton, 21 June 1964, file 171-206.

47   Ibid., letter by Gwendolyn Herman of the NBARN to Mère –, 7 February 1964, file 177-2131.

48 Ibid., letter by Gwendolyn Herman, secretary of the NBARN to Clément Cormier, 7 February 1964, file 177-2131.
49 Ibid., letter from the provincial secretary of the RHSJ to Clément Cormier, 8 September 1964, file 177-1450.
50 Ibid., letter from Clément Cormier to Mère –, 8 October 1964, file 177-1450.
51 Centre Universitaire Saint-Louis Maillet, Fonds des services pédagogiques, letter from Sr. Bouchard to Mère –, 28 February 1965. See also letter of 22 March 1965, Sr. Bouchard to Mère –.
52 Ibid., letter from Mère – to Sr. Bouchard, 2 April 1965.
53 Ibid., letter from Sr. B to Mère –, 22 March 1965, where she presents her analysis of the situation.
54 CEA, Fonds Université de Moncton, letter by Mère – to Sr. Bouchard, 3 June 1964, file ESI 347.
55 Centre Universitaire Saint-Louis Maillet, Fonds des services pédagogiques, letter by Mère – to Sr. Bouchard, 5 April 1965.
56 Cormier and Richard, *École des sciences infirmières*, 10. The author of this chapter was a student in the first class admitted and was quite unaware at the time of the events preceding the opening of the school.
57 CEA, Fonds Clément Cormier, report of the special meeting of the Senate, 21 June 1964 file 171-206; and CEA, Fonds Clément Cormier, letter by Sr. Bouchard to Mère –, 24 March 1965, file 177-1450.
58 Cormier, *L'Université de Moncton*, 126.
59 Cormier and Richard, *École des sciences infirmières*, 11.
60 Aline Charles, "Women's Work in Eclipse: Nuns in Quebec Hospitals, 1940-1980," in *Women, Health and Nation: Canada and the United States since 1945*, ed. Georgina Feldberg, Molly Ladd-Taylor, Alison Li, and Kathryn McPherson (Montreal and Kingston: McGill-Queen's University Press, 2003), 276. During the 1960s, many nuns left their congregation, and recruitment also declined.
61 Cormier, *Louis J. Robichaud*, 135. Cited in an interview on 17 December 1998 in Cormier, "Que reste-t-il de l'héritage," 206, when Robichaud was asked which of his accomplishments gave him the most pride, he replied without hesitation that it was the Université de Moncton. See Robert Pichette, "Culture et langues officielles," in *L'Ère Louis J. Robichaud*, IDRCR, 69, for a description of his other important contributions, including the *Official Languages Act* (New Brunswick Statutes, 1968-69, C14), that made New Brunswick the only bilingual province in Canada.
62 Charles, "Women's Work in Eclipse," 269.
63 Interview with a Hospitaller who was a participant in these events and who confirmed this interpretation.
64 CEA, Fonds Université de Moncton, Report by Sr. Jacqueline Bouchard to the Academic Senate, 25 June 1965, file E38-347.
65 Stanley, *Louis Robichaud*, 64. Barbra Mann Wall, *Unlikely Entrepreneurs: Catholic Sisters and the Hospital Marketplace, 1865-1925* (Columbus, OH: Ohio State University Press, 2005), 191, stated that government regulations limited the nuns' autonomy and described the decreasing influence of the religious congregations on health care institutions.
66 Couturier, *Construire un savoir*, 160.
67 McKee, "Rapports ethniques et rapports de sexe," 175.
68 Cormier, *Université de Moncton*, 24.
69 CEA, Fonds Clément Cormier, letter by Bishop Gagnon to Clément Cormier, 28 February 1964, file 177-474.
70 Sioban Nelson, *Say Little, Do Much: Nurses, Nuns and Hospitals in the Nineteenth Century* (Philadelphia: University of Pennsylvania Press, 2001), 6 and 8.
71 Mann Wall, *Unlikely Entrepreneurs*, 188.
72 Ibid., 191.
73 Cormier, *L'Université de Moncton*, 69-71.
74 Geertje Boschma, *Faculty of Nursing on the Move: Nursing at the University of Calgary 1969-2004* (Calgary: University of Calgary Press, 2005), 2 and 3.

75  Christine Hallett, "The Bachelor of Nursing Degree at the University of Manchester: A His-
    torical Study of an Innovation in Community Nursing Education," paper presented at the
    Annual Conference of the Canadian Association for the History of Nursing, Ottawa, June
    2005. Hallett described the influence of Fraser Brockington, a professor of social and pre-
    ventative medicine, on the development of the Bachelor of Nursing degree, one of the first
    British degrees granted to nurses.
76  See Tracy Schier and Cynthia Russett, eds., *Catholic Women's Colleges in America* (Baltimore:
    Johns Hopkins University Press, 2002); and Charles, "Women's Work in Eclipse," for at-
    tempts to make the work of religious women better known.

# Selected Bibliography

Adams, Mary Louise. "In Sickness and in Health: State Formation, Moral Regulation and Early VD Initiatives in Ontario." *Journal of Canadian Studies* 28 (April 1993): 117-30.

Anderson, Benedict. *Imagined Communities: Reflections on the Origin and Spread of Nationalism*, revised edition. New York: Verso, 1991.

Arnup, Katherine. "Raising the Dionne Quintuplets: Lessons for Modern Mothers." *Journal of Canadian Studies* 29 (Winter 1994-95): 65-85.

Baillargeon, Denyse. "Entre la 'Revanche' et la 'Veillée' des berceaux: Les médecins québécois francophones, la mortalité infantile, et la question nationale, 1910-1940." *Canadian Bulletin of Medical History* 19 (2002): 113-37.

–. *Un Québec en mal d'enfant: La médicalisation de la maternité, 1910-1970*. Montreal: Éditions du Remue-ménage, 2004.

Ballantyne, Tony, and Antoinette Burton, eds. *Bodies in Contact: Rethinking Colonial Encounters in World History*. Durham and London: Duke University Press, 2005.

Barron Norris, Marjorie. *Sister Heroines: The Roseate Glow of Wartime Nursing 1914-1918*. Calgary, AB: Bunker to Bunker Publishing, 2002.

Bashford, Alison. *Imperial Hygiene: A Critical History of Colonialism, Nationalism and Public Health*. London and New York: Palgrave, 2004.

Bassett, Jan. *Guns and Brooches: Australian Army Nursing from the Boer War to the Gulf War*. Oxford: Oxford University Press, 1992.

Bates, Christina, Dianne Dodd, and Nicole Rousseau, eds. *On All Frontiers: Four Centuries of Canadian Nursing*. Ottawa: University of Ottawa Press and the Canadian Museum of Civilization, 2005. Also published in French under the title *Sans frontières: Quatre siècles de soins infirmiers canadiens*. Ottawa: University of Ottawa Press and the Canadian Museum of Civilization, 2005.

Boutilier, Beverly. "Helpers or Heroines? The National Council of Women, Nursing, and 'Women's Work' in Late Victorian Canada." In *Caring and Curing: Historical Perspectives on Women and Healing in Canada*, ed. Dianne Dodd and Deborah Gorham, 17-47. Ottawa: University of Ottawa Press, 1991.

Bradbury, Bettina, and Tamara Myers, eds. *Negotiating Identities in Nineteenth and Twentieth-Century Montreal*. Vancouver and Toronto: UBC Press, 2005.

Bramadat, Ina J., and Marion Saydak. "Nursing on the Canadian Prairies, 1900-1930: Effects of Immigration." *Nursing History Review* 1 (1993): 105-17.

Buckley, Suzann. "Ladies or Midwives? Efforts to Reduce Infant and Maternal Mortality in Canada between the Two World Wars." *Atlantis* 2 (Spring 1977): 76-84.

Buhler-Wilkerson, Karen. *False Dawn: The Rise and Decline of Public Health Nursing, 1900-1930*. New York: Garland Publishing, 1989.

–. *No Place Like Home: A History of Nursing and Home Care in the United States*. Baltimore: Johns Hopkins University Press, 2001.

Burrows, Bob. *Healing in the Wilderness: A History of the United Church Mission Hospitals.* Madeira Park: Harbour Publishing, 2004.

Cameron, Wendy, Sheila Haines, and Mary McDougall Maude, ed. *English Immigrant Voices: Labourers' Letters from Upper Canada in the 1830s.* Montreal and Kingston: McGill-Queen's University Press, 2000.

Carter, Sarah. "Categories and Terrains of Exclusion: Constructing the 'Indian Woman' in the Early Settlement Era in Western Canada." In *Out of the Background: Readings on Canadian Native History,* ed. Ken Coates and Robin Fisher, 177-95. Toronto: Copp Clark, 1996.

Charles, Aline. "Women's Work in Eclipse: Nuns in Quebec Hospitals, 1940-1980." In *Women, Health and Nation: Canada and the United States since 1945,* ed. Georgina Feldberg, Molly Ladd-Taylor, Alison Li, and Kathryn McPherson, 264-91. Montreal and Kingston: McGill-Queen's University Press, 2003.

Comacchio, Cynthia R. *"Nations Are Built of Babies": Saving Ontario's Mothers and Children, 1900-1940.* Montreal and Kingston: McGill-Queen's University Press, 1993.

–. "The Rising Generation: Laying Claim to the Health of Adolescents in English Canada, 1920-1970." *Canadian Bulletin of Medical History* 19 (2002): 139-79.

Cooke, Miriam, and Angela Woollacott, eds. *Gendering War Talk.* Princeton: Princeton University Press, 1993.

Cormier, Michel. *Louis J. Robichaud: Une révolution si peu tranquille.* Moncton: Éditions de la Francophonie, 2004.

D'Antonio, Patricia. "Revisiting and Rethinking the Rewriting of Nursing History." *Bulletin of the History of Medicine* 73 (1999): 268-90.

Davies, Megan J. "Competent Professionals and Modern Methods: State Medicine in British Columbia during the 1930s." *Bulletin of the History of Medicine* 76 (2002): 56-83.

de Kiriline, Louise. *The Quintuplets' First Year: The Survival of the Famous Five Dionne Babies and Its Significance for All Mothers.* Toronto: MacMillan, 1936.

Delhi, Kari. "'Health Scouts for the State?' School and Public Health Nurses in Early Twentieth Century Ontario." *Historical Studies in Education* 2 (1990): 247-64.

Dodd, Dianne. "Helen MacMurchy: Popular Midwifery and Maternity Services for Canadian Pioneer Women." In *Caring and Curing: Historical Perspectives on Women and Healing in Canada,* ed. Dianne Dodd and Deborah Gorham, 135-81. Ottawa: University of Ottawa Press, 1994.

Dusseault, Gilles. *Le curé Labelle: Messianisme, utopie et colonisation au Québec, 1850-1900.* Montreal: Éditions Hurtubise HMH, 1983.

Elliott, Jayne. "Blurring the Boundaries of Space: Shaping Nursing Lives at the Red Cross Outposts in Ontario, 1922-1945." *Canadian Bulletin of Medical History* 21 (2004): 303-25.

Elshtain, Jean Bethke. *Women and War.* New York: Basic Books, 1987.

Enloe, Cynthia. *Does Khaki Become You? The Militarisation of Women's Lives.* Boston: South End Press, 1983.

–. *Maneuvers: The International Politics of Militarizing Women's Lives.* Berkeley, CA: University of California Press, 2000.

Fitzpatrick, David, ed. *Oceans of Consolation: Personal Accounts of Irish Migration to Australia.* Ithaca, NY: Cornell University Press, 1994.

Flynn, Karen. "Experience and Identity: Black Immigrant Nurses to Canada, 1950-1980." In *Sisters or Strangers? Immigrant, Ethnic, and Racialized Women in Canadian History,* ed. Marlene Epp, Franca Iacovetta, and Frances Swyripa, 381-97. Toronto: University of Toronto Press, 2004.

Gerber, David A. *Authors of Their Lives: The Personal Correspondence of British Immigrants to North America in the Nineteenth Century.* New York: New York University Press, 2006.

Gilbert, Helen. "Great Adventures in Nursing: Colonial Discourse and Health Care Delivery in Canada's North." *Jouvert* 7 (2003): 1-15.

Gleason, Mona. "Race, Class and Health: School Medical Inspection and 'Healthy' Children in British Columbia, 1890-1930." *Canadian Bulletin of Medical History* 19 (2002): 95-112.

Graham, Judith S., ed. *"Out Here at the Front": The World War One Letters of Nora Saltonstall.* Boston: Northeastern University Press, 2004.

Grayzel, Susan R. *Women's Identities at War: Gender, Motherhood, and Politics in Britain and France during the First World War*. Chapel Hill, NC: University of North Carolina Press, 1999.

Guérard, François. *Histoire de la santé au Québec*. Montreal: Boréal, 1996.

Higonnet, Margaret Randolph. *Nurses at the Front: Writing the Wounds of the Great War*. Boston: Northeastern University Press, 2001.

Higonnet, Margaret Randolph, Jane Jenson, Sonya Michel, and Margaret Collins Weitz, eds. *Behind the Lines: Gender and the Two World Wars*. New Haven, CT: Yale University Press, 1987.

Holmes, Katie. "Day Mothers and Night Sisters: World War One Nurses and Sexuality." In *Gender and War: Australians at War in the Twentieth Century*, ed. Joy Damousi and Marilyn Lake, 46-53. Cambridge: Cambridge University Press, 1995.

Hutchinson, John F. *Champions of Charity: War and the Rise of the Red Cross*. Boulder, CO: Westview Press, 1996.

Jasen, Patricia. "Race, Culture, and the Colonization of Childbirth in Northern Canada." *Social History of Medicine* 10 (1997): 383-400.

Jones, Esyllt. "Contact across a Diseased Boundary: Urban Space and Social Interaction during Winnipeg's Influenza Epidemic, 1918-1919." *Journal of the Canadian Historical Association* 13 (2002): 119-39.

Jones, Margaret. "Heroines of Lonely Outposts or Tools of Empire? British Nurses in Britain's Model Colony: Ceylon, 1878-1948." *Nursing Inquiry* 11 (2004): 1-17.

Kelm, Mary-Ellen. *Colonizing Bodies: Aboriginal Health and Healing in British Columbia*. Vancouver: UBC Press, 1998.

Kirkwood, Rondalyn. "Blending Vigorous Leadership and Womanly Virtues: Edith Kathleen Russell at the University of Toronto, 1920-1952." *Canadian Bulletin of Medical History* 11 (1994): 175-205.

Landells, Edith. *The Military Nurses of Canada: Recollections of Canadian Military Nurses*. White Rock, BC: Co-Publishing, 1995.

Langford, Nanci. "Childbirth on the Canadian Prairies, 1880-1939." In *Telling Tales: Essays in Western Women's History*, ed. Catherine Cavanaugh and Randi Warne, 147-73. Vancouver: UBC Press, 2000.

Lawrence, Louise de Kiriline. *Another Winter, Another Spring: A Love Remembered* (Toronto: Natural Heritage, 1987, previously published by McGraw-Hill Book Company, 1977).

LeRoy Miller, Gertrude. *Mustard Plasters and Hand Cars: Through the Eyes of a Red Cross Outpost Nurse*. Toronto: Natural Heritage Books, 2000.

Lux, Maureen. *Medicine That Walks: Disease, Medicine, and Canadian Plains Native People, 1880-1940*. Toronto: University of Toronto Press, 2001.

Macphail, Andrew. *The Medical Services: Official History of the Canadian Forces in the Great War, 1914-1919*. Ottawa: King's Printer, 1925.

Mann, Susan. *Margaret Macdonald: Imperial Daughter*. Montreal and Kingston: McGill-Queen's University Press, 2005.

–, ed. *The War Diary of Clare Gass, 1915-1918*. Montreal and Kingston: McGill-Queen's University Press, 2000.

Mann Trofimenkoff, Susan. *The Dream of Nation: A Social and Intellectual History of Quebec*. Toronto: Macmillan, 1982.

Mann Wall, Barbra. *Unlikely Entrepreneurs: Catholic Sisters and the Hospital Marketplace, 1865-1925*. Columbus, OH: Ohio State University Press, 2005.

McCallum, Mary Jane. "This Last Frontier: Isolation and Aboriginal Health." *Canadian Bulletin of Medical History* 22 (2005): 103-20.

McPherson, Kathryn. *Bedside Matters: The Transformation of Canadian Nursing, 1900-1990*. Toronto: Oxford University Press, 1996.

–. "Carving Out a Past: The Canadian Nurses Association War Memorial," *Histoire sociale/Social History* 29 (November 1996): 417-29.

–. "'The Country Is a Stern Nurse': Rural Women, Urban Hospitals and the Creation of a Western Canadian Nursing Work Force, 1920-1940." *Prairie Forum* 20 (1995): 175-206.

–. "Nursing and Colonization: The Work of Indian Health Services Nurses in Manitoba, 1945-1970." In *Women, Health and Nation: Canada and the United States since 1945*, ed.

Georgina Feldberg, Molly Ladd-Taylor, Alison Li, and Kathryn McPherson, 223-46. Montreal and Kingston: McGill-Queen's University Press, 2003.

McPherson, Kathryn, and Meryn Stuart. "Writing Nursing History in Canada: Issues and Approaches. *Canadian Bulletin of Medical History* 11 (1994): 3-22.

Meijer Drees, Laurie, and Lesley McBain. "Nursing and Native Peoples in Northern Saskatchewan: 1930s-1950s." *Canadian Bulletin of Medical History* 18 (2001): 43-65.

Morin-Pelletier, Mélanie. *Briser les ailes de l'ange: Les infirmières militaires canadiennes, 1914-1918*. Montreal: Athena Editions, 2006.

Morton, Desmond. *When Your Number's Up: The Canadian Soldier in the First World War*. Toronto: Random House, 1993.

Morton, Desmond, and Glenn Wright. *Winning the Second Battle: Canadian Veterans and the Return to Civilian Life, 1915-1930*. Toronto: University of Toronto Press, 1987.

Mussallem, Helen K. *Spotlight on Nursing Education: The Report of the Pilot Project of the Evaluation of Schools of Nursing in Canada*. Ottawa: Canadian Nurses Association, 1962.

Myles, Eugenie Louise. *Remember Nurse*. Toronto: Ryerson, 1960.

Nelson, Sioban. "The Fork in the Road: Nursing History versus the History of Nursing?" *Nursing History Review* 10 (2002): 175-88.

–. *Say Little, Do Much: Nurses, Nuns and Hospitals in the Nineteenth Century*. Philadelphia: University of Pennsylvania Press, 2001.

Nestel, Sheryl. "(Ad)ministering Angels: Colonial Nursing and the Extension of Empire in Africa." *Journal of Medical Humanities* 19 (1998): 257-77.

Nicholson, G.W.L. *Canada's Nursing Sisters*. Canadian War Museum Historical publication no. 13. Toronto: Samuel Stevens Hakkert and Company, 1975.

Ouditt, Sharon. *Fighting Forces, Writing Women: Identity and Ideology in the First World War*. London and New York: Routledge, 1994.

Øverland, Orm. *Immigrant Minds, American Identities: Making the United States Home, 1870-1930*. Urbana and Chicago: University of Illinois Press, 2000.

Penney, Sheila. *A Century of Caring: The History of the Victorian Order of Nurses for Canada*. Ottawa: Victorian Order of Nursing Canada, 1996.

Perry, Adele. "Whose Sisters and What Eyes? White Women, Race, and Immigration to British Columbia, 1849-1871." In *Sisters or Strangers? Immigrant, Ethnic, and Racialized Women in Canadian History*, ed. Marlene Epp, Franca Iacovetta, and Frances Swyripa, 49-70. Toronto: University of Toronto Press, 2004.

Pickles, Katie, and Myra Rutherdale, eds. *Contact Zones: Aboriginal and Settler Women in Canada's Colonial Past*. Vancouver: UBC Press, 2005.

Pierson, Ruth Roach. *"They're Still Women after All": The Second World War and Canadian Womanhood*. Toronto: McClelland and Stewart, 1986.

Pratt, Mary Louise. *Imperial Eyes: Travel Writing and Transculturation*. London and New York: Routledge, 1992.

Quiney, Linda. "Assistant Angels: Canadian Voluntary Aid Detachment Nurses in the Great War." *Canadian Bulletin of Medical History* 15 (1998): 189-206.

–. "'Sharing the Halo': Social and Professional Tensions in the Work of World War One Canadian Volunteer Nurses." *Journal of the Canadian Historical Association* 9 (1998): 105-24.

Reverby, Susan. *Ordered to Care: The Dilemma of American Nursing, 1850-1945*. Cambridge: Cambridge University Press, 1987.

Richardson, Sharon. "Frontier Health Care: Alberta's District and Municipal Nursing Services, 1919 to 1976." *Alberta History* 46 (Winter 1998): 2-9.

–. "Political Women, Professional Nurses and the Creation of Alberta's District Nursing Service, 1919-1925." *Nursing History Review* 6 (1998): 25-50.

Riegler, Natalie. *Jean I. Gunn: Nursing Leader*. Toronto: Associated Medical Services and Fitzhenry and Whiteside, 1997.

Ross-Kerr, Janet C. *Prepared to Care: Nurses and Nursing in Alberta, 1859 to 1996*. Edmonton: University of Alberta Press, 1998.

Rousseau, Nicole, and Johanne Daigle, "Medical Service to Settlers: The Gestation and Establishment of a Nursing Service in Quebec, 1932-1943." *Nursing History Review* 8 (2000): 95-116.

Russell, Edith K. *Report of a Study of Nursing Education in New Brunswick.* Fredericton: University of New Brunswick, 1956.

Rutherdale, Myra. "Ordering the Bath: Children, Health and Hygiene in Northern Canadian Communities, 1900-1970." In *Children's Health Issues in Historical Perspective,* ed. Cheryl Krasnick Warsh and Veronica Strong-Boag, 305-27. Waterloo, ON: Wilfrid Laurier University Press, 2005.

–. *Women and the White Man's God: Gender and Race in the Canadian Mission Field.* Vancouver: UBC Press, 2002.

Sarnecky, Mary. *A History of the U.S. Army Nurse Corps.* Philadelphia: University of Pennsylvania Press, 1999.

Scott, J. Karen with Joan E. Kieser. *Northern Nurses: True Nursing Adventures from Northern Canada.* Oakville, ON: Kokum Publications, 2002.

Silverman, Eliane. *The Last Best West: Women on the Alberta Frontier, 1880-1930.* Calgary: Fifth House, 1998.

Stanley, Della M.M. *Louis Robichaud: A Decade of Power.* Halifax: Nimbus Publishing, 1984.

Stewart, Irene, ed. *These Were Our Yesterdays: A History of District Nursing in Alberta.* Altona, MB: D.W. Friesen and Sons, 1979.

Strong-Boag, Veronica, Sherrill Grace, Avigail Eisenberg, and Joan Anderson, eds. *Painting the Maple: Essays on Race, Gender, and the Construction of Canada.* Vancouver: UBC Press, 1998.

Stuart, Meryn. "'Half a Loaf Is Better Than No Bread:' Public Health Nurses and Physicians in Ontario, 1920-1925." *Nursing Research* 41 (1992): 21-27.

–. "Ideology and Experience: Public Health Nursing and the Ontario Rural Child Welfare Project, 1920-1925." *Canadian Bulletin of Medical History* 6 (1989): 111-31.

–. "War and Peace: Professional Identities and Nurses' Training, 1914-1930." In *Challenging Professions: Historical and Contemporary Perspectives on Women's Professional Work,* ed. Elizabeth Smyth, Sandra Acker, Paula Bourne, and Alison Prentice, 171-93. Toronto: University of Toronto Press, 1999.

Toman, Cynthia, and Meryn Stuart. "Emerging Scholarship in Nursing History." *Canadian Bulletin of Medical History* 21 (2004): 223-27.

Weir, George W. *Survey of Nursing Education in Canada.* Toronto: University of Toronto Press, 1932.

Wilkinson, Maude. *Four Score and Ten: Memoirs of a Canadian Nurse.* Brampton, ON: Margaret M. Armstrong, 2003.

Zelmanovits, Judith Bender. "'Midwife Preferred': Maternity Care in Outpost Nursing Stations in Northern Canada, 1945-1988." In *Women, Health and Nation,* ed. Georgina Feldberg, Molly Ladd-Taylor, Alison Li, and Kathryn McPherson, 161-88. Montreal and Kingston: McGill-Queen's University Press, 2003.

# Contributors

**Anne-Marie Arseneault** taught at l'École de science infirmière at the Université de Moncton from 1973 to 2006, primarily in community health nursing, health promotion, professional issues, and nursing ethics. Although a course in nursing history was not part of the curriculum, she strove to include historical aspects in her teaching. Her long-standing interest in nursing history led her to become a founding member of the Canadian Association for the History of Nursing, on which she served on the Executive Committee for several years, including a term as president from 2003 to 2005.

**Kristin Burnett** is an assistant professor in the Department of History at Lakehead University. The article published in this volume is part of a larger body of work that looks at the healing and nursing work of Aboriginal and non-Aboriginal women in indigenous and newcomer communities in western Canada, using health, medicine, and gender as lenses through which to examine Canada's internal colonial project.

**Johanne Daigle**'s primary research interests are in the socio-cultural history of Québec in the nineteenth and twentieth centuries. She and Nicole Rousseau, professor emerita in the nursing science program at Laval University, are preparing to publish a manuscript on the Medical Service to Settlers, which provided nurses for rural colonization projects during the Depression until the 1970s. Daigle is currently the chair of the undergraduate program in the Department of History at Laval University.

**Jayne Elliott** is the research facilitator and administrator of the Associated Medical Services Nursing History Research Unit in the School of Nursing at the University of Ottawa. Her research interests include the history of nursing and medical care in the rural and remote regions of Canada.

**Marion McKay** is a senior instructor and Associate Dean of the Undergraduate Programs in the Faculty of Nursing at the University of Manitoba. She teaches community health nursing in the faculty's undergraduate programs and is currently conducting research on the history of public health nursing in Manitoba. She is a co-investigator on a SSHRC grant with seven other historians of nursing across Canada exploring the relationships of nurses and nursing work to ideas of colonialism, nationalism, and citizenship.

**Linda Quiney**'s doctoral dissertation on Canadian volunteer nurses in the First World War military hospitals at home and overseas was followed by Hannah post-doctoral research into women's roles in the transformation of the Canadian Red Cross Society from wartime military support to peacetime public health and emergency response. She currently teaches Canadian and medical history in the Department of History, University of British Columbia.

**Myra Rutherdale** is an assistant professor in the Department of History at York University. She is the author of *Women and the White Man's God: Gender and Race in the Canadian Mission Field* (UBC Press, 2002) and most recently co-edited with Katie Pickles *Contact Zones: Aboriginal and Settler Women in Canada's Colonial Past* (UBC Press, 2005).

**Meryn Stuart**, a historian of nursing and women, is the founder and Director of the Associated Medical Services Nursing History Research Unit in the School of Nursing at the University of Ottawa. She most recently co-authored *Out of the Ivory Tower: Feminist Research for Social Change* and the special edition on nursing history published in 2004 in the *Canadian Bulletin of Medical History*. She is currently leading a team of researchers in examining issues of colonialism and nationalism in the history of nurses and their work.

**Cynthia Toman** is an associate professor with the School of Nursing and associate director of the Associated Medical Services Nursing History Research Unit at the University of Ottawa. In addition to publications on the history of Canadian nursing in academic journals, she is the author of *An Officer and a Lady: Canadian Military Nursing and the Second World War* (UBC Press, 2007) and co-editor of a special edition of the *Canadian Bulletin of Medical History* (2004) on nursing.

# Index

*Note:* "(f)" after a page reference indicates a figure; "CRCS" stands for Canadian Red Cross Society; "MSNM," for Margaret Scott Nursing Mission; "VON," for Victorian Order of Nurses

Bompas, William C., 44
Bonfield, 137, 142, 144, 146, 148, 150
Boschma, Geertje, 166
Bouchard, Jacqueline, 161-62, 162(f), 164
Bow, Malcolm R., 192n18
Bradbury, Bettina, 146
Bramadat, Ina, 108
Braybon, Gail, 9
British Columbia, public health programs in, 71
British Empire, 3, 10, 20-22
British nurses, 9, 22-24
Brown, Jennifer, 50
Buhler-Wilkinson, Karen, 70
Buies, Arthur, 115-16
Byrne Commission, 156-57
Byron Bay (NU), 66-67

Cairo, 8, 15, 16, 29
Cambridge Bay/Iqaluktuutiak (NU), 66-67
Cameron-Smith, Jean, 17
Canadian Army Medical Corps (CAMC), 8, 13, 20, 26, 27, 98-99
*Canadian Bulletin of Medical History*, 2
Canadian General Hospitals (CGHs): No. 4 (Toronto), 15; No. 5 (Vancouver), 15; No. 7 (Cairo), 16
Canadian Red Cross Society (CRCS), 91, 110; healthful living crusade, 92-93, 109, 110; Manitoba Division, 5-6, 91, 92, 93, 94, 95, 100, 101, 109; nurses (*see* outpost nurses; station nurses); Ontario Division, 97, 100, 112-13, 136, 142, 144, 150, 195n61
Canadian Stationary Hospitals (CSHs): No. 1, 14-15, 17, 29; No. 3, 15, 17, 36; No. 5, 16
Caroline (midwife), 48
Carter, Sarah, 50
Casey, F., 121
cautious caregivers, 5, 55, 61-65
*C.D. Howe* (ship), 62
Charleson, Eleanor, 14-15, 18-19, 38
childbirth, 4, 41, 43, 113, 126, 132, 133. *See also* midwifery; obstetrics
children: child welfare clinics, 87; child welfare nurses, 71; Inuit, 53-55, 60, 62. *See also* infant mortality
citizenship: Inuit and, 60; public health nursing and, 93
cleanliness, 58, 83
cleansers, 5, 54-55, 56, 64
Clint, Mabel, 8, 9, 12, 13, 14, 17, 19, 20-21, 22, 38
Collège Maillet (Saint-Basile, NB), 7, 153, 155, 158-59, 160-63, 164, 165

Collis, Elsie, 16
colonialism: military nurses and, 3, 9, 10, 12; northern health services and, 57
colonization, 6; British "home," 116; nurses and, 111, 113; Québec and, 115, 116
Committee for the Study of Nursing Education in the United States, 157
Connor, Ralph, 78
Conrad, Margaret, 27, 30
contact zones, 6, 40, 46, 52, 113, 126-34, 135
context-specific studies, 9
Cook, Tim, 28
Coombs, George, 78
Coombs, Mary, 78
Copeland, Donalda McKillop, 53-55, 54(f), 56, 58-61, 64, 68, 69
Copeland, Harold, 53, 54(f), 60-61
Copeland, Patsy, 53, 54(f)
Coral Harbour/Salliq (NU), 53, 58
Cormier, Adrien, 155
Cormier, Clément, 155-56, 156(f), 158-59, 160, 161, 164, 165, 166
Cornish, F.C., 48, 51
Cornish, Mrs. F.C., 50, 51
correspondence. *See* letters
Côte-Nord (QC), 113; conditions in, 129; location of nursing settlement stations in, 123(f); nursing service to, 122; working conditions in, 133
Courville, Serge, 116
Cousineau, Jacques, 193n25
Couturier, Jacques-Paul, 160
Cox-Smith, D., 104
CRCS. *See* Canadian Red Cross Society (CRCS)
Curly, Joe, 59

Dafoe, Alan, 136, 144
D'Antonio, Patricia, 2
Dardanelles campaign, 29. *See also* Gallipoli campaign
David (nursing station caretaker), 66
Davies, Celia, 2
Davies, Megan, 71
de Kiriline, Gleb, 139
de Kiriline, Louise Flach, 6, 137(f), 140(f), 148(f); car owned by, 147; church activity, 150-51; community contacts, 150-51; and Dionne quintuplets, 136, 144, 152; dogsled, 147-48, 151; early life, 139-41; and emergency nursing, 144; and French Canadians, 150; identities of, 137-38, 141-45, 146, 152; letters, 138-39, 144-45, 146, 151, 152; and nursing colleagues, 149-50; as

outpost nurse, 136-38, 142-45, 146-51;
and physicians, 143-44, 151; relationships with other women, 150; in Russia,
139-40, 145-46; and social class, 149-50;
social life, 146, 148-49; Swedish nursing
education and practice, 143
Dempsey, Nurse, 108
Department of Indian Affairs, 48-49
Depression, 103, 104, 111, 115, 117, 122,
125, 134
Deslandes (QC), 132
Deutsch, John, 154, 155
Deutsch Commission, 154, 155, 158, 159,
160, 162-63, 164
diagnosis by nurses, 62, 122
diaries, 4, 12, 21, 29, 30
Dionne quintuplets, 6, 136, 144, 152
disease(s): cautious caregivers and, 61;
cleansers and, 58; CRCS and, 92; in
histories, 41-42; and indigenous
communities, 41; military nurses and,
15, 17, 19
district nursing, 181-82n11. *See also*
visiting nurses/nursing
Dodd, Dianne, 65, 111
Douglas, A.J., 79, 88
Drees, Laurie Meijer, 113
Dubinsky, Karen, 149
Duder, Karen, 27

Earle, Rebecca, 138
East Braintree station (MB), 96, 97, 99,
100, 102, 189n50
École des sciences hospitalières (Université
de Moncton). *See under* Université de
Moncton
Edmundston (NB): Hôtel-Dieu Hospital,
164; Université Saint-Louis, 154, 158, 159
education in New Brunswick, 153; of
francophones, 159, 161, 165; reform of,
154-57; Roman Catholic Church and,
154-55, 164-66; secularization of, 3,
164-65. *See also* nursing education
Eenerook ("Tommy"), 58-60
Elliott, Jayne, 97, 98, 100, 101, 111, 112-13
emergency nursing, 93, 144
empire: Aboriginal women and, 44;
meanings of, 10; white women and, 20.
*See also* British Empire; imperialism
Eudist congregation, 154, 155, 164, 165
Evans, W. Sanford, 74
Ewart, John S., 78

femininity: of de Kiriline, 152; of Fowlds,
27, 33, 39; hospital training schools
and, 31; military nurses and, 3, 9, 16(f),

17-18, 21; outpost nurses and, 98;
shopping and, 35; uniforms and, 23,
26(f), 36
First World War: employment of nurses
in, 25-26; Mediterranean theatre, 8-9,
10, 13-14; and national identity, 11; and
Swedish emigration, 141; western front,
8, 27. *See also* military nurses
Fisher Branch Station (MB), 91, 92, 99,
100, 101, 104-5, 107, 189n50
Fitzpatrick, David, 138-39
Flach, Hellevid (Neergaard), 138, 139
Flach, Sixten, 139
Forbes, Mildred, 10, 16(f), 19, 20, 172n7
Fort McPherson/Teet'lit Zhen (NT), 55,
66, 67
Fowlds, Don, 29, 33
Fowlds, Eric, 33
Fowlds, Helen Lauder, 25-39, 26(f), 37(f);
autograph album recording impressions
of Lemnos, 14; on British nurses, 22-23,
24; career, 26; on Charleson, 18-19;
circulation of goods with family/relatives,
33-34; diaries of, 4, 18-20, 26, 27, 29-30,
33, 38; early life, 26; enlistment, 26; on
funerals of nurses, 17; as ideal type of
nurse, 33; identity within family, 34;
and leaks regarding working conditions,
19-20; letters, 4, 12-13, 25, 26, 27, 29-30,
33-34, 36-38, 39; in Mediterranean, 29;
and men, 36-37, 38; as modern "new"
woman, 25-26, 39; on Salonika, 21;
shopping, 34-35, 39; social life, 26, 33,
38, 39; on superiors, 33, 38-39; travel,
25; uniform of, 35
francophones of New Brunswick, 154;
education, 159, 161, 165; nursing
education, 6-7, 159, 161, 164, 165, 166
Fraser, Mrs. A.M., 77-78
French Canadians: birth rate, 114-15, 134;
colonization and, 6, 115; de Kiriline
and, 138, 150; infant mortality among,
114; protection and regeneration of
"race," 6, 111, 115, 134; settlement in
northern Québec, 111, 115, 116
Frenette, Yves, 117

Gagnon, Bishop, 160, 165
Gallipoli campaign, 8, 13-14. *See also*
Dardanelles campaign
Galt, Cecily, 14
Gant, M.R., 91, 101, 102, 103-4
Gardener, Marg, 61-62
Gaspésie (QC), 113; conditions in, 121,
132, 133; landscape in, 131-32; locations
of nursing stations in, 119(f)

## ENVIRONMENTAL BENEFITS STATEMENT

**UBC Press** saved the following resources by printing the pages of this book on chlorine free paper made with 100% post-consumer waste.

| TREES | WATER | ENERGY | SOLID WASTE | GREENHOUSE GASES |
|---|---|---|---|---|
| 7 | 2,538 | 5 | 326 | 611 |
| FULLY GROWN | GALLONS | MILLION BTUs | POUNDS | POUNDS |

Calculations based on research by Environmental Defense and the Paper Task Force.
Manufactured at Friesens Corporation